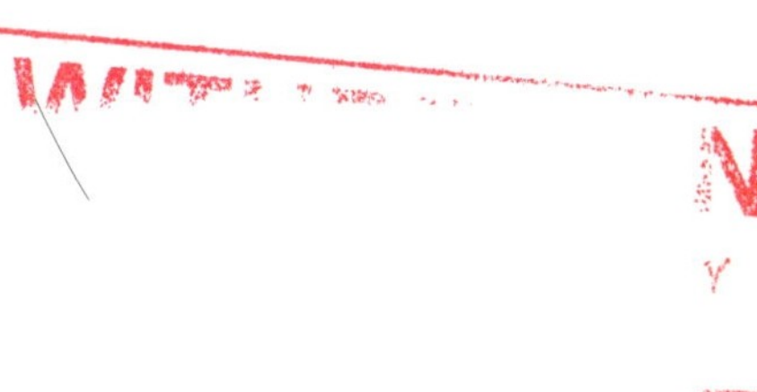

ADVANCES IN

Pharmacology and Chemotherapy

VOLUME 17

ADVISORY BOARD

ADVANCES IN

Pharmacology and Chemotherapy

EDITED BY

Silvio Garattini

Istituto di Ricerche Farmacologiche "Mario Negri" Milano, Italy

A. Goldin

National Cancer Institute Bethesda, Maryland

F. Hawking

Commonwealth Institute of Helminthology St. Albans, Herts., England

I. J. Kopin

National Institute of Mental Health Bethesda, Maryland

Consulting Editor

R. J. Schnitzer

Mount Sinai School of Medicine New York, New York

VOLUME 17—1980

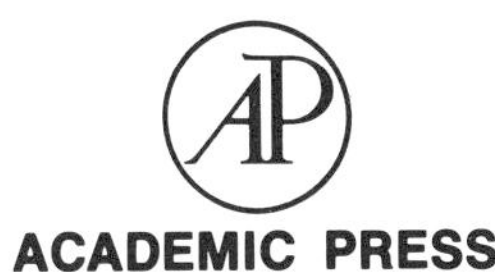

ACADEMIC PRESS

A Subsidiary of Harcourt Brace Jovanovich, Publishers

New York London Toronto Sydney San Francisco

ACADEMIC PRESS, INC.
111 Fifth Avenue, New York, New York 10003

United Kingdom Edition published by
ACADEMIC PRESS, INC. (LONDON) LTD.
24/28 Oval Road, London NW1 7DX

LIBRARY OF CONGRESS CATALOG CARD NUMBER: 61–18298

ISBN 0–12–032917–4

PRINTED IN THE UNITED STATES OF AMERICA

80 81 82 83 9 8 7 6 5 4 3 2 1

CONTENTS

Screening for and Evaluation of Anticoccidial Activity

John F. Ryley

Information Services of the International Cancer Research Data Bank (ICRDB) Program in Cancer Chemotherapy and Pharmacology

John H. Schneider

Dihydrofolate Reductase: Binding of Substrates and Inhibitors and Catalytic Mechanism

Jill E. Gready

Distribution and Classification of Airway Histamine Receptors: The Physiological Significance of Histamine H_2-Receptors

N. CHAND

In Vitro Methods to Predict for Patient Response to Chemotherapy

DANIEL D. VON HOFF AND LARRY WEISENTHAL

Macrophage Activation for Nonspecific Tumor Cytotoxicity

RICHARD M. SCHULTZ AND MICHAEL A. CHIRIGOS

Prenatal and Neonatal Toxicology and Pathology of Heavy Metals

LOUIS W. CHANG, PAUL R. WADE, JOEL G. POUNDS, AND KENNETH R. REUHL

Salicylates: Molecular Mechanism of Therapeutic Action

DAVID C. ATKINSON AND HARRY O. J. COLLIER

Physiological and Pharmacological Determinants of Sensitivity and Resistance to 5-Fluorouracil in Lower Animals and Man

BACH ARDALAN, DAVID COONEY, AND JOHN S. MACDONALD

CONTRIBUTORS TO THIS VOLUME

Numbers in parentheses indicate the pages on which the authors' contributions begin.

BACH ARDALAN (289), *Laboratory of Toxicology, Developmental Therapeutics Program, Division of Cancer Treatment, National Cancer Institute, Bethesda, Maryland 20205, and Department of Medical Oncology, City of Hope National Medical Center, Duarte, California 91010*

DAVID C. ATKINSON (233), *Pharmacology Section, Toxicology Department, Corporate Research Division, Miles Laboratories, Inc., Elkhart, Indiana 46515*

N. CHAND (103), *Department of Physiology, Downstate Medical Center, State University of New York, Brooklyn, New York 11203*

LOUIS W. CHANG (195), *Department of Pathology, University of Arkansas for Medical Sciences, Little Rock, Arkansas 72205*

MICHAEL A. CHIRIGOS (157), *Laboratory of Chemical Pharmacology, Developmental Therapeutics Program, Division of Cancer Treatment, National Institutes of Health, Bethesda, Maryland 20014*

HARRY O. J. COLLIER (233), *Research Department, Miles Laboratories, Ltd., Stoke Poges, Slough SL2 4LY, England*

DAVID COONEY (289), *Laboratory of Medicinal Chemistry and Biology, Developmental Therapeutics Program, Division of Cancer Treatment, National Cancer Institute, Bethesda, Maryland 20205*

JILL E. GREADY (37), *Physical Chemistry Laboratory, South Parks Road, Oxford OX1 3QZ, England*

JOHN S. MACDONALD (289), *Cancer Therapy Evaluation Program, Division of Cancer Treatment, National Cancer Institute, Bethesda, Maryland 20205*

JOEL G. POUNDS (195), *Department of Health and Human Services, Food and Drug Administration, National Center for Toxicological Research, Jefferson, Arkansas 72079*

KENNETH R. REUHL (195), *Division of Biological Sciences, National Research Council of Canada, Ottawa KIA OR6, Canada*

JOHN F. RYLEY (1), *Imperial Chemical Industries Ltd., Pharmaceuticals Division, Mereside, Alderley Park, Macclesfield, Cheshire SK10 4TG, England*

JOHN H. SCHNEIDER (25), *International Cancer Research Data Bank Program, National Cancer Institute, Bethesda, Maryland 20205*

RICHARD M. SCHULTZ (157), *Immunology and Connective Tissue Research, Lilly Research Laboratories, Eli Lilly and Company, Indianapolis, Indiana 46206*

DANIEL D. VON HOFF (133), *Department of Medicine, Division of Oncology, University of Texas Health Science Center at San Antonio, San Antonio, Texas 78284*

PAUL R. WADE (195), *Department of Pathology, University of Arkansas for Medical Sciences, Little Rock, Arkansas 72205*

LARRY WEISENTHAL (133), *Section of Hematology-Oncology, Veterans Administration Medical Center, Long Beach, California 90822, and Department of Medicine, University of California, Irvine, Irvine, California 92717*

ADVANCES IN PHARMACOLOGY AND CHEMOTHERAPY, VOL. 17

Screening for and Evaluation of Anticoccidial Activity

JOHN F. RYLEY

Imperial Chemical Industries Ltd.
Pharmaceuticals Division
Mereside, Alderley Park, Macclesfield
Cheshire, England

I. Introduction

Prophylactic chemotherapy of coccidiosis in chickens has been an essential factor in the amazing growth of the broiler industry witnessed over the last four decades. During this period a succession of drugs has fallen by the wayside due to developing drug resistance or the introduction of more active, less toxic, wider-spectrum compounds. For several years now the ionophore monensin has enjoyed the bulk of the market, but if past experience is anything to go by, there will always be the need for newer and better anticoccidial drugs. The search for novel activity in this field is not easy, as witnessed by the slender progress made over the past few years; it is the purpose of this article to review considerations pertinent to operating a large-scale anticoccidial research program.

ISBN 0-12-032917-4

A. Screening or Evaluation?

Considerable confusion seems to exist—particularly in the minds of those outside the pharmaceutical industry—as to what drug screening involves and how it differs from drug evaluation. In discussing screening techniques, it is vital to appreciate the purpose of the screening exercise and to be aware of the limitations of such systems. Although we might wish it otherwise, it is not yet possible to take a disease entity, sit down and design a drug, synthesize the compound, and hit the target at the first attempt. Seldom does one even land by chance directly on a drug. The most usual sequence of events is to discover activity in a compound, tested either quite empirically or following chemical synthesis with a particular hypothesis in mind, and then by a process of chemical manipulation and modification—very often along lines dictated by little more than trial and error—arrive at a compound with sufficient activity and a combination of other properties to warrant development of the compound as a commercial drug.

This somewhat empirical approach requires that large numbers of compounds be tested if there is to be any chance of success; we investigated perhaps 20,000 compounds for anticoccidial activity before discovering activity in the quinolones, and then synthesized around 300 other quinolones before developing methyl benzoquate for use in the field.

If such a program of drug hunting is to be carried out over a matter of years rather than centuries, then the initial testing procedures have to be very simple. This is screening. The purpose of screening is simply to provide a yes/no answer to the question: is there sufficient interaction between this compound and the disease entity to warrant more detailed investigation? The essentials of a screening procedure include such features as simplicity of operation, unambiguity of interpretation, and high throughput of compounds week after week. It matters little if a screen lets through moderate numbers of compounds which will be rejected at a later stage of evaluation; it is important however that the reverse does *not* occur, i.e., the screen rejects compounds of potential interest in the final disease situation (false negatives).

Once the possibility of therapeutic interest in a compound has been identified by the screen then a program of evaluation begins—which may often last no longer than one or two experiments—to confirm and then investigate the limitations of this activity. Early evaluation experiments may be no more than modifications of the initial screen, with however adequate replication of treatments, to investigate the degree of activity in a compound. If interest in a compound is maintained, then subsequent evaluation experiments will have to be specially designed to investigate the particular properties and limitations of the compound, comparing these with the behavior of established drugs under the same conditions and constraints. Although the therapeutic properties of the compound will have the most urgent practical significance, studies at this stage to determine the point of action in the life cycle, whether the compound is coccidicidal or coccidistatic, and something about the biochemical basis for its activity will be of interest—and may indeed be relevant to its method of use.

It is the purpose of this article to discuss various alternative procedures for screening for anticoccidial activity and to indicate modifications to these methods and other techniques useful in the early stages of the evaluation of promising compounds.

B. Screening for Anticoccidial Activity

In many parasitic disease situations an animal model has to be used in the laboratory. Thus in looking for antimalarial drugs one may use the model of *Plasmodium berghei* in the mouse. It is a big jump from this situation to *Plasmodium falciparum* in man. With poultry coccidiosis however we are in a position to screen and evaluate compounds right away against the actual parasites of interest in the actual host of interest, and the majority of anticoccidial screening has in fact been carried out in chickens.

There has been some dispute concerning the number of valid species of coccidia to be found in the domestic fowl, but probably six are of potential economic importance. A study of the various anticoccidial drugs introduced since the sulfonamides in the early 1940s indicates that some have activity restricted to one or a few species of coccidia, while most of the later discoveries are "wide-spectrum" in their activity. Because of this possibility of restricted activity, we feel it preferable to screen initially against two species if at all possible; one should be a representative of the "hemorrhagic" species *Eimeria necatrix* or *E. tenella,* while the other should be a representiative of the "intestinal" species *E. acervulina, E. brunetti, E. maxima,* or *E. mivati. E. tenella* presents far fewer technical problems than *E. necatrix,* particularly in connection with the large scale production of oocysts for inoculation, and is almost universally accepted for screening purposes. Of the intestinal species, *E. brunetti* we feel is the best practical proposition; severe disease can be produced by relatively low inocula and high yields of oocysts are readily obtainable at passage. Although *E. acervulina* also reproduces well, very high inocula have to be used to produce severe weight depression, while in our hands *E. maxima* produces relatively few oocysts and is not adequately pathogenic for screening purposes.

Given adequate animal facilities, technical effort, and availability of compounds, *in vivo* anticoccidial screening can be readily sustained with a high throughput. Careful consideration of the parameters to be followed can result in marked savings of technical effort. One of the main drawbacks of a screen in chickens is the amount of compound required for an initial test; our current requirements are 700 mg for each species. With the reproduction of the life cycle of *E. tenella* in chick embryos (Long, 1965) and the subsequent establishment of *E. tenella* in tissue culture (e.g., Doran, 1970) the possibility of alternative screens arose. To us the most interesting aspect of these alternatives was the possible saving of compound—and therefore access to more compounds, available only in small quantity—but other factors such as economy in animal facilities, technical input, and use of animals for experimental purposes may be pertinent.

II. Screening in Embryos or Tissue Culture

A. The Use of Chick Embryos for Screening

Following the introduction of the chick embryo system by Long (1965), we investigated the model as a potential screening tool (Ryley, 1968). Embryos inoculated on the ninth day of incubation with 10^5 sporozoites of *E. tenella* died 5 days later following massive hemorrhages. Anticoccidial drugs were injected into the allantoic cavity at the time of inoculation and minimum levels which prevented mortality due to coccidiosis were determined. Mortality before day 5 was ascribed to drug toxicity or nonspecific causes. Drugs were tested at a maximum level of 10 mg/embryo,[1] and active or toxic ones retested at doses of 5, 2.5, 1, 0.5 . . . etc. mg/embryo; 6 embryos were used for each drug level. Drugs showing activity in the embryo included methyl benzoquate, amprolium, buquinolate, diaveridine, clopidol, sulfaquinoxaline, and dinitolmide although relative activities did not always match relative activities in the chick. No activity however could be demonstrated for nicarbazin, furazolidone, nitrofurazone, glycarbylamide, trithiadol, and three experimental compounds which also showed some activity in the chick. We concluded that because of these false negatives, the embryo system was not satisfactory as a screening tool, but might have applications in studies on the nature of activity of specific drugs (Fig. 1).

Long (1970) reported "a more sensitive method" for assessing infections in embryos which involved counting focal lesions in the chorioallantoic membrane (CAM) and has subsequently used oocyst production, par-

[1] All drug weights or concentrations quoted refer to actual material used; in the case of salts, the concentration of active substance will be less.

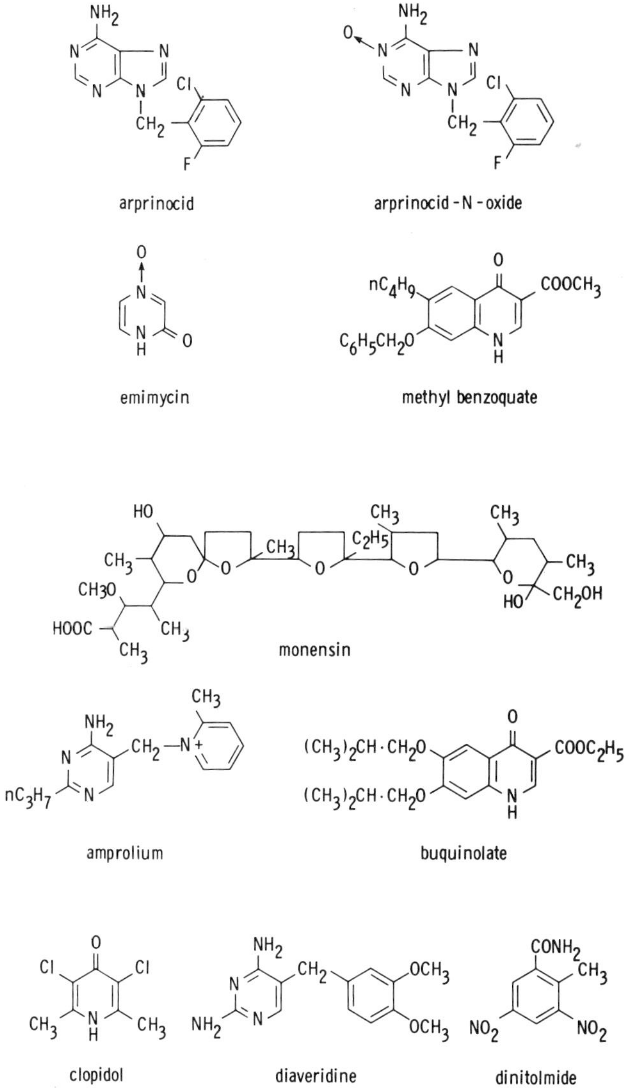

arprinocid

arprinocid-N-oxide

emimycin

methyl benzoquate

monensin

amprolium

buquinolate

clopidol

diaveridine

dinitolmide

FIG. 1. Structural formulas of compounds.

ticularly with embryo-adapted strains, as an alternative parameter. In a most interesting and useful study, Long and Millard (1973) examined 9 drugs with three different levels of coccidial challenge and determined minimum effective levels using mortality, CAM lesions, and oocyst pro-

furazolidone

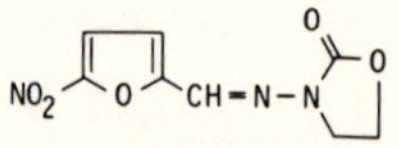

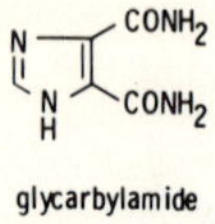

glycarbylamide

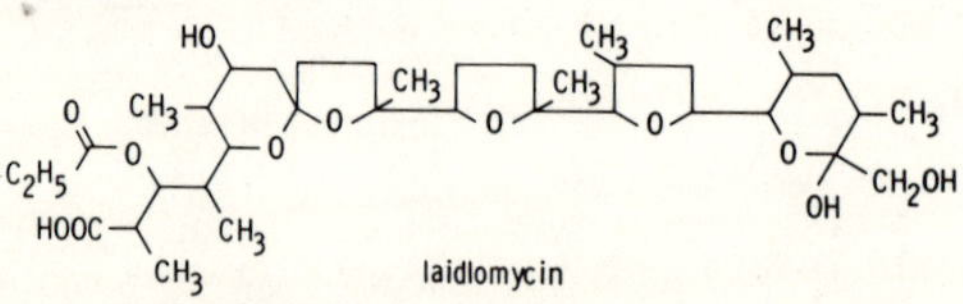

laidlomycin

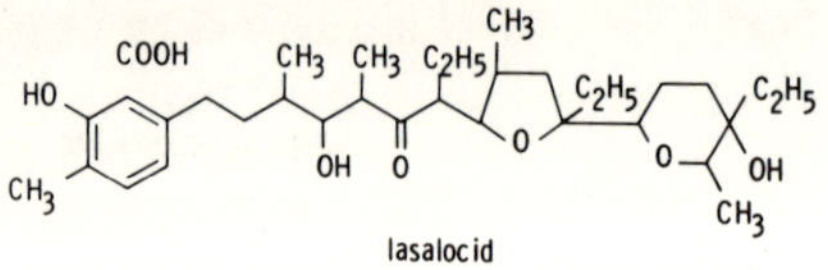

lasalocid

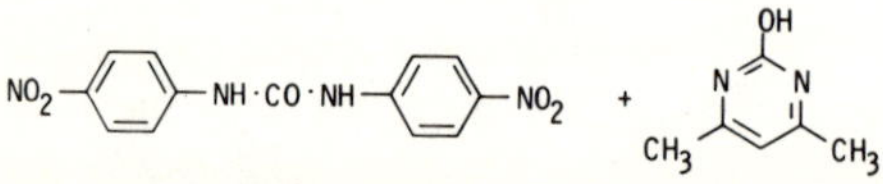

nicarbazin

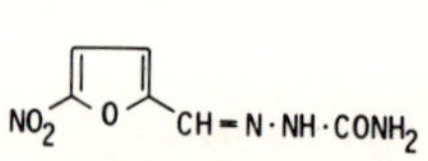

nitrofurazone

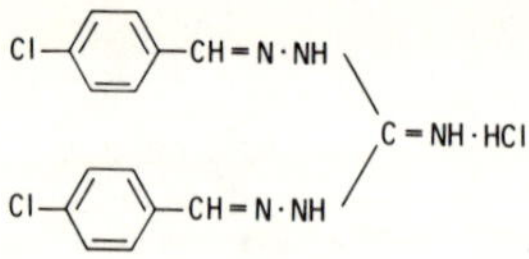

robenidine

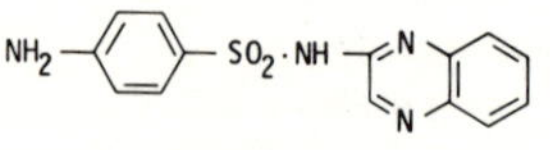

sulfaquinoxaline

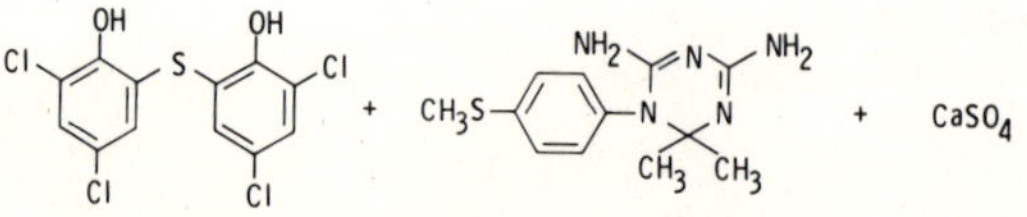

(bithionol 50%) (methiotriazamine 10%) (40%)

Trithiadol

FIG. 1 (*continued*).

duction as criteria for activity. Groups of 6–10 embryos were used, with initial drug levels of 1, 0.1, and 0.01 mg/embryo; drugs were administered the day before inoculation. Although they concluded that "inhibition of CAM focal lesions and oocyst production proved to be more sensitive parameters than mortality of infected embryos,'' the summary data presented in their Table 2 suggest rather the opposite (and more fortunate) conclusion. In 5/9 cases, *more* drug was required to give 95% protection from CAM lesions than from mortality while in only 1/9 cases was the reverse true. Oocyst production was a more sensitive measure of activity in 4/9 cases and a less sensitive one in 2/9 cases. The situation was little different when 50% protection was considered. These comparative data are extremely useful and important when considering the possible use of the embryo system for drug screening. Embryo mortality is easy to determine by simply candling the eggs; CAM focal lesion counting is an extremely messy and time-consuming procedure as is counting oocysts produced. There is absolutely no point in following these latter two parameters if they do no more than provide information more readily obtainable by observations on mortality alone. Certainly lesion counting or oocyst counting could not be used in a high throughput screen unless a great deal of technical effort was available just at the time of reading the test. More recent work using ionophores has cast further doubt on the validity of the embryo model; we found no activity for monensin, lasalocid, or laidlomycin at partially toxic levels (0.2, 0.05, 0.05 mg/embryo respectively), although activity for these compounds is readily demonstrable in the chick.

Work in embryos is labor intensive and requires aseptic techniques for much of the time. Group sizes are similar to those needed for a chick screen. We do not consider it realistic to screen in embryos with an initial level below 10 mg/embryo. Although this would result in some economy in compound for test, there seem to be no other advantages for an embryo screen, and in view of the high incidence of false negatives, we remain convinced that the system is not satisfactory as a screening tool. We are awarc of one institution in the UK, two in the U.S., and one in Czechoslovakia that have used an embryo screen for a limited period, but in all cases they have abandoned it.

B. Anticoccidial Screening in Tissue Culture

It is little more than a decade since the possibility of cultivating occidia in tissue culture was first mooted. A tremendous input of effort has led to the establishing of workable systems of cultivation with a limited number of species, both avian and mammalian, while exploitation of these systems has produced a series of studies on the *in vitro* activity of a variety of individual drugs and the setting up of anticoccidial screening programs in a number of pharmaceutical establishments. The whole situation, including a description of techniques and our analysis of the validity of the model, is reported in detail elsewhere (Ryley and Wilson, 1976a).

E. tenella can be readily cultivated in monolayers of chick kidney cells as far as second generation schizogony, and less readily as far as oocyst production. The sexual phase is more readily obtained with some strains than others, but cyclical maintenance *in vitro* has not yet been achieved. *E. necatrix* will develop readily as far as second generation schizogony, but in view of the fact that oocyst production in chickens to produce material for inoculation is none too reliable in our hands, we prefer *E. tenella* for screening purposes; *E. necatrix* however can be used *in vitro* for specific studies. *E. brunetti* can also be cultivated *in vitro* as far as second generation schizogony, but in our hands the system is too unreliable for a routine screen, and should be reserved for specific studies. Embryo-adapted *E. mivati* has also been reported to grow in culture, while Naciri-Bontemps (1976) claims to have grown *E. acervulina* in chicken kidney cells. We have no experience with these species, and for screening purposes therefore have been effectively limited to *E. tenella*.

The prime attraction for us of the tissue culture screen is the quantity of compound required; we normally use 10 mg, simply because the facilities for accurately weighing 1 mg or less are not readily available. When compared with the 700 mg requirement for our chick screen, the advantage is obvious; we have access to thousands of additional compounds available in too small a quantity to be screened *in vivo*. Chick kidney cultures are set up, and 2–3 days later they are inoculated with sporozoites of *E. tenella* and treated with drug. Sporozoites may be freshly prepared on each occasion, or can be produced in bulk and stored in liquid nitrogen. As cleaning of sporozoites on a glass bead column is desirable, preparation in bulk and storage is in the long run time saving. Four days after inoculation, the monolayers are fixed, stained, and examined with an inverted microscope for the presence or absence of clusters of second generation schizonts. The use of multiwell disposable plastic dishes makes it possible to work with large numbers of individual cultures—well over 1000 a week is not difficult. Because toxicity is extremely variable in a random selection of compounds, we initially screen at a series of 5 threefold dilutions. In view of the relatively low *in vitro* activity of a number of established anticoccidials, we start with a maximum level of 81 ppm (i.e., 81, 27, 9, 3, and 1 ppm in the first instance). If activity or toxicity is found at 1 ppm, then further threefold compound dilutions are tested to establish minimum levels of activity and toxicity.

From the technical point of view, the tissue culture screen has little advantage over a chick screen. Careful, aseptic working is required throughout. It is not possible to dispense with animal facilities, since these are necessary to produce material required for inoculation purposes and for further evaluation of compounds active in culture.

The biggest problem with the tissue culture screen is the interpretation of the results obtained and deciding whether a compound should be rejected or taken forward to testing in chickens. Absolute activities have ranged from 50 ppm for dinitolmide on some occasions to 0.0005 ppm for laidlomycin and for methyl benzoquate with some strains. Our analysis of some 11,550 compounds screened *in vitro* indicates that the absolute activity in culture gives no indication of the activity, if any, which might be expected in the chick. Emimycin, one of our most interesting leads, was active at only 3 ppm in culture, but active in the chick, while a number of compounds with perhaps one hundred times this *in vitro* activity were without interest in the chick. Not only can the absolute activity of a compound be misleading, so too can relative activities within types. Thus in the ionophore field, high relative activities *in vitro* and promising therapeutic ratios have on a number of occasions raised false hopes, dashed when sufficient material became available for test *in vivo*. With a situation like this we find it virtually impossible to say whether a compound active *in vitro* is worth testing *in vivo*, and particularly when resynthesis would be necessary for chick testing to say how worthwhile it is likely to be to expend the necessary effort. Over and above this however is the problem of false negatives. In our paper (Ryley and Wilson, 1976a) we drew attention to chemical series where no *in vitro* activity could be found in compounds which showed some activity in the chick; we have subsequently found further examples of this situation. Although the degree of *in vitro* activity in these cases—which would have been missed by relying on tissue culture alone as a prescreen—was limited, constituting a chemical lead rather than a usable drug, we have been even more disturbed to find that arprinocid, presently undergoing field development, shows no *in vitro* activity separable from toxicity in our hands. Comparative studies carried out with a number of compounds have indicated that *in vitro* potency can be influenced by the strain of coccidia and type of host cell used (Latter and Wilson, 1979). In the case of arprinocid, although the compound is inactive in kidney tissue culture, it is active if embryonic liver cells are used. It would appear that arprinocid is not anticoccidial in its own right, but needs to be metabolized, most probably to its N-oxide, for activity to occur. The N-oxide of arprinocid is active in chick kidney tissue cultures and is produced from arprinocid by microsomal preparations from chick liver; a metabolite active in chick kidney tissue cultures is produced from arprinocid by preincubation with embryonic liver cultures. Although the use of embryonic liver rather than chick kidney tissue cultures would solve the detection problem in the case of arprinocid, such a change would not get over all the problems of false negatives. Thus we feel we have with our tissue culture system an unacceptable situation with false negatives similar to that found with embryos. Of the two, the tissue culture system is to be preferred, since the technical and physical factors involved in high-throughput screening are less, and compound requirements are at least one order of magnitude smaller.

We continue to screen in tissue culture compounds which would not otherwise be tested at all, but believe that the most useful line of attack is to attempt modification to the *in vivo* screen to reduce compound requirements.

III. Screening in the Chicken

Starting from a description of our current *in vivo* screens, I wish to investigate the problem of sensitivity of methods for detection of drug activity, to comment briefly on some of the parameters which can be measured to evaluate activity, to consider other factors involved in screens, and to indicate lines along which the screen may be modified to reduce requirement for compound or for further evaluation of active compounds.

A. Chick Screen

At the time of writing, cock chicks of a laying strain (Warren Sex-Sal link F) 9–10 days of age are sorted in groups of eight so that the average weight of each group in the test is within a 10 gm weight range; there is little control of weight distribution within the individual groups. Chickens are housed in cages arranged 48 to a rack, with usually two racks per test. Water is supplied via automatic trigger cups, and 700 gm food is supplied from a trough within the cage, the trough being provided with a piece of $\frac{3}{4}$ in. gridweld mesh resting on the food to prevent undue wastage. The food is that proposed to the Coccidiosis Discussion Group (Ryley and Betts, 1973), formulated without antibiotics, growth promoters, or anticoccidials, and is deficient in vitamin K. Compounds for test are incorporated into the diet at a concentration of 1000 ppm (0.1%) for initial screening. Medicated food is supplied from the time of grouping on day -1. On day 0, 24 hours after the start of medication, birds are inoculated with the minimum number of oocysts as determined in a previous culture titration to give 100% mortality in untreated controls (*E. tenella*) or a marked weight depression (*E. brunetti*). All birds are weighed on day 3, and the average weight gain for each group over days -1 to 3 is calculated (calculations including the weights of any birds which died). Since coccidial infection does not influence weight gain appreciably until after this time, poor weight gain during this period gives as indication of compound toxicity. Fecal blood is scored visually on an arbitrary scale of 0–3 from day 4 onwards (*E. tenella*), or fecal consistency is scored on a scale of 0–3 (*E. brunetti*); birds which die are weighed and recorded, and all survivors are weighed on day 6 (*E. brunetti*) or day 7 (*E. tenella*). Average weight gains are calculated over the period days 3–6 or 7, again taking into account the weights of birds which have died (weight of survivors + weight of corpses − weight of birds on day 3 all divided by 8). Weight gains of treated birds during this second part of the test reflect the anticoccidial activity of the compound, complicated in some cases by toxicity revealed in the first part of the test. Control weight gains during the first part of the test are of the order of 25–50 gm per bird, and in the second part of the test 30–50 gm for noninfected controls, while infected controls usually show a loss in weight of 10–20 gm. The activity of a compound is assessed on the basis of control of weight gain, mortality, and fecal blood in the case of *E. tenella* or weight gain alone in the case of *E. brunetti*. Compounds showing activity are retested to confirm the result, and progressively lower incorporation rates are used to determined the minimum effective level.

B. Screen Sensitivity

The purpose of the screen is to detect activity. In the normal course of things, we are not looking initially for a drug, but for a chemical lead to a drug. Chemical modification of a molecule can lead to a tremendous increase in activity; with the quinolones, methyl benzoquate is around 500 times more active against *E. tenella* than our lead compound. It is important therefore that the screen should employ the most *sensitive* methods of picking up activity. There would seem to be almost as many varieties of screen as there are laboratories in the field, and screens vary both in the severity of challenge used and in the parameters followed to assess activity. In some cases there is an assumption that the lower the challenge, the more sensitive the test and the more realistic the system in relation to the field situation, while in other cases there is a belief that some parameters are more sensitive indicators of activity than others. Some laboratories use a single species, others (ourselves included) use two species in different birds, while at least two laboratories have at various times run a screen with a mixed infection of *E. tenella* and *E. acervulina*. In the latter case, low inocula are used, birds are examined for the presence of cecal lesions at postmortem on day 5, and feces obtained just before killing are examined for the presence of *E. acervulina* oocysts. We have examined 4 compounds at a range of concentrations using the two extremes of challenge; in one case a mixture of *E. tenella* and *E. acervulina* was used with inocula which failed to produce mortality, while in the other case our usual screen aimed at 100% control mortality was employed. The various treatments were each given to 2 replicates of 8 chicks, and the comparison was done twice; the combined results of the two experiments are given in Table I. In the screen with the low mixed inoculum, feces were collected on day 5 over the 2 hours preceding killing, shaken in a tube with saturated salt solution, and allowed to stand, and a surface sample was taken with a loop for microscopical examination. Oocysts were recorded as absent (0), plenty (+), or few (±). Birds were killed following collection of feces and cecal lesions were recorded as absent (0), present (1), or minimal (0.5); an average lesion score was calculated for each group (maximum 1.00).

TABLE I

COMPARISON OF TWO SCREENING METHODS IN CHICKENS[a]

	Inoculum					
	5000 *E. tenella* + 5000 *E. acervulina*		600,000 *E. tenella*			
				Average weight gain		
Treatment (ppm)	Lesion score	Oocysts	Percentage mortality	−1 to 3	3 to 7	Fecal score
Noninfected control	0.00	−	0.0	31.6	39.3	0
Infected control	0.98	+	96.9	26.8	−17.6	3
Arprinocid 250	0.00	−	0.0	2.4	13.1	0
Arprinocid 125	0.00	−	0.0	19.0	36.2	0
Arprinocid 62	0.04	−	6.3	25.7	21.0	1.5
Arprinocid 31	0.66	+	62.5	27.8	−9.5	3
Arprinocid 15	0.90	+	93.8	23.5	−12.1	3
Monensin 242	0.17	−	18.8	21.5	18.9	1
Monensin 121	0.45	±	46.9	30.0	−3.7	2.5
Monensin 60	0.76	+	84.4	29.2	−16.6	3
Monensin 30	0.86	+	100.0	28.4	−15.6	3
Methyl benzoquate 10	0.00	−	0.0	23.0	31.4	0
Methyl benzoquate 5	0.00	−	15.6	28.8	19.6	0
Methyl benzoquate 2.5	0.12	−	43.8	28.4	13.1	0.5
Methyl benzoquate 1.2	0.53	±	62.5	21.6	−4.6	1.5
Methyl benzoquate 0.6	0.72	±	93.8	27.4	−7.7	2.5
Emimycin 500	0.08	−	0.0	30.0	29.4	0
Emimycin 250	0.55	−	28.1	29.1	3.7	2.5
Emimycin 125	0.65	−	56.3	18.9	−4.7	3
Emimycin 62	0.90	−	78.1	16.4	−7.1	3
Emimycin 31	0.97	±	81.3	21.8	−13.9	3

[a] Each treatment was given to 4 replicates of 8 chicks.

It will be seen that the lowest level of arprinocid to show up markedly by the criterion of reduced mortality was 62 ppm, and this same level had an appreciable effect on weight gain control; appreciable fecal blood was produced. Although the challenge was considerably less where lesion scores were measured at day 5, 62 ppm arprinocid was still needed to give a marked reduction in score or suppression of oocyst production, i.e., this test is *not* more sensitive when looking for activity. Very similar conclusions can be reached in the cases of the other three drugs. It may at first sight seem that with emimycin, oocyst production in the case of the mixed infection was a more sensitive indication of activity; the effect is in fact due to a greater sensitivity of *E. acervulina* to the drug—which was of course the point of using the mixed infection.

Comparing the two basic methods of screening therefore, we see that using a low challenge with *E. tenella* does not enable activity in a compound to be detected at a lower level by the criterion of lesion scores than using a heavy challenge and following mortality and/or weight gain. It is however considerably easier to count dead bodies and weigh birds than it is to kill, cut up, and examine birds and examine feces microscopically, and for a given amount of available effort, the heavy challenge screen will allow a greater throughput of compounds. The only disadvantage by comparison is that rather more effort is required producing oocysts for inoculation purposes. A fourfold saving of oocysts for inoculation purposes can be made by using a diet deficient in vitamin K; the use of this deficient diet does not interfere in any way with the detection or evaluation of anticoccidial activity, but merely gives an apparent increase in pathogenicity of hemorrhagic species of coccidia (Ryley and Hardman, 1978).

The experiments of Table I involved 4 replicate groups of 8 chicks for each level of each drug. In a normal *screen* test, only one group would be used at one level, and from the point of view of economy of compound, it would be advantageous to use less than 8 chicks in this one group. If mortality is to be used in assessing a compound, it is essential that control mortality is very high—verging on 100%—in order to pick up significant changes due to drug activity. Table II indicates the spread of mortality on 4 occasions on which 48 groups of 8 chicks were given moderate inocula and fed unmedicated diet. The lower the challenge, the greater the spread of mortality among the 48 replicates. Were these groups medicated with compounds being screened it would be difficult to interpret results without repeated retesting.

We compared the same four compounds using two widely differing inocula of *E. brunetti* (Table III). Control mortality with *E. brunetti* in our routine screens is usually low, and variable from experiment to experiment, so that we seldom take it into account in interpreting the tests. As

TABLE II

MORTALITY SCATTER WITH MODERATE INOCULA OF *E. tenella*

Inoculum	Overall percentage mortality	Number of cages with *x* deaths								
		0	1	2	3	4	5	6	7	8
35,000	32.3	4	6	15	13	4	4	1	1	0
100,000	46.1	0	3	7	11	14	8	4	1	0
200,000	74.5	0	0	0	4	3	5	19	13	4
300,000	87.0	0	0	0	0	0	3	11	19	15

TABLE III

SCREEN TESTS WITH *E. brunetti*[a]

Treatment (ppm)	Inoculum: 200,000 Oocysts				2000 Oocysts	
	Percentage mortality	Average weight gain −1 to 3	Average weight gain 3 to 7	Fecal score	Average weight gain −1 to 3	Average weight gain 3 to 6
Noninfected control	0.0	34.0	40.0	0	35.1	31.9
Infected control	62.5	23.5	−24.6	3	26.8	−10.1
Arprinocid 250	0.0	5.1	16.8	0	8.0	13.3
Arprinocid 125	0.0	16.0	24.8	0	22.3	16.5
Arprinocid 62	0.0	28.5	31.9	0	23.5	30.8
Arprinocid 31	18.8	27.1	−10.9	2	30.9	29.9
Arprinocid 15	18.8	30.8	−11.8	2	23.6	−0.3
Monensin 242	0.0	21.1	19.1	0	19.5	18.5
Monensin 121	0.0	30.3	−1.4	2	27.3	23.3
Monensin 60	6.3	29.8	−8.8	2	34.9	15.5
Monensin 30	25.0	29.8	−23.6	3	27.6	10.5
Methyl benzoquate 5	0.0	26.8	27.5	0	23.8	32.9
Methyl benzoquate 2.5	0.0	32.3	12.8	0	30.4	32.9
Methyl benzoquate 1.25	12.5	34.3	−12.6	2	36.3	11.0
Methyl benzoquate 0.6	31.3	28.8	−22.3	2	31.0	−10.0
Methyl benzoquate 0.3	81.3	28.5	−29.6	3	28.3	−4.4
Emimycin 250	0.0	26.1	34.3	0	32.4	34.3
Emimycin 125	0.0	30.8	21.6	0	34.6	30.8
Emimycin 62	0.0	32.5	13.9	0	28.8	27.8
Emimycin 31	18.8	29.5	−8.5	1	33.0	22.0
Emimycin 15	25.0	32.5	−18.8	2	28.1	7.5

[a] Each treatment given to 2 replicates of 8 chicks.

with the *E. tenella* experiments of Table I, arprinocid at 250 and 125 ppm and monensin at 242 ppm showed some toxicity as indicated by reduced weight gains in the first part of the test. There was an appreciable control weight depression during the second half of the test with an inoculum as low as 2000 oocysts, and all four compounds showed an appreciable effect on this weight gain at one dilution or more lower than in the case of birds given 200,000 oocysts, i.e., when weight gain (but not mortality) is to be the parameter followed, the lowest inoculum consistent with producing a marked depression in the infected controls is advantageous to the sensitivity of the test.

C. Other Parameters

Oocyst production is often used in an attempt to quantitate the severity of an infection. This can be a very misleading procedure, since in some light infections where tissue damage is less during the asexual phase of reproduction, the subsequent oocyst production can be *higher* than with a heavy infection (Williams, 1973; Reid, 1975). In the experiments of Tables I and III oocyst counts were carried out on all groups which survived long enough to produce adequate feces; an additional series of chicks was used with an inoculum of 2000 oocysts of *E. tenella*. Comparison of the data of Table IV with that of Tables I and III will indicate that in no case was oocyst production a more sensitive criterion of activity in a particular species than mortality and/or weight gain; in most cases, higher concentrations of drug were required to suppress or appreciably reduce oocyst production. Oocyst counting is an extremely laborious and timeconsuming exercise; even the qualitative procedure used with *E. acervulina* took several hours. There is absolutely no point in a screen test wasting valuable effort to produce data less useful than that obtained more easily by following other parameters.

We were very intrigued by claims (U.K. Patent 1338520; International Minerals & Chemical Corporation, 1973) that benzyl-adenines—of which arprinocid is one—can suppress sporulation of oocysts. This could be a most useful feature in a drug which would limit build-up of infection in a flock, and might be looked for in a screen test if a simple method of observation could be developed. Arprinocid is recommended for use at 60 ppm, while weight gain depression is appreciable at 125 ppm due to toxicity. Surprised at the apparently low therapeutic ratio, we have investigated levels of 100, 75, and 45 ppm also in the experiments of Tables I, III, and IV and in a number of additional tests. In these tests we have not only counted oocysts, but also isolated oocysts and allowed them to sporulate in dichromate. In no case have we found evidence of markedly reduced sporulation in oocysts derived from birds treated with arprinocid.

TABLE IV

OOCYST PRODUCTION IN SCREENING EXPERIMENTS[a]

Treatment (ppm)	Inoculum						
		600,000 *E. tenella*[b]			200,000 *E. brunetti*[c]		
	5000 *E. acervulina*	Oocysts	Percentage sporulation	2000 *E. tenella*	Oocysts	Percentage sporulation	2000 *E. brunetti*
Infected controls	+	—	—	16.89	—	—	10.98
Arprinocid 250	–	0.00	—	0.00	0.00	—	0.00
Arprinocid 125	–	0.00	—	0.00	0.00	—	0.00
Arprinocid 62	–	8.49	83	1.17	0.00	—	0.00
Arprinocid 31	+	—	—	8.34	3.69	70	0.23
Arprinocid 15	+	—	—	13.40	2.88	72	14.26
Monensin 242	–	2.18	88	0.64	3.69	—	2.47
Monensin 121	±	9.80	87	6.87	8.94	—	4.62
Monensin 60	+	—	—	6.57	6.01	—	12.68
Monensin 30	+	—	—	16.76	—	—	15.97
Methyl benzoquate 10	–	2.07	91	0.00	—	—	0.00
Methyl benzoquate 5	–	15.00	93	0.00	0.38	—	0.42
Methyl benzoquate 2.5	–	8.50	93	0.05	1.42	—	6.05
Methyl benzoquate 1.2	±	18.69	92	0.58	3.96	—	13.50
Methyl benzoquate 0.6	±	—	—	2.24	3.65	—	12.31
Emimycin 500	–	4.25	90	0.00	—	—	—
Emimycin 250	–	21.72	92	0.43	0.00	—	0.15
Emimycin 125	–	10.05	89	6.58	0.83	—	0.24
Emimycin 62	–	—	—	16.47	3.09	82	3.43
Emimycin 31	±	—	—	15.62	4.29	—	11.96

[a] Oocyst counts expressed as millions per bird.

[b] From experiment of Table I.

[c] From experiment of Table III.

Subsequent papers by Ruff *et al*. (1978) and Tamas *et al*. (1978) show that the effect on oocyst sporulation is variable between strains and species. Oocysts which do sporulate are no less infective when inoculated into susceptible birds, and it seems doubtful that the use of arprinocid at 60 ppm would stop the cycling of coccidia in a flock. Inclusion at the screening stage of observations on the ability of oocysts to sporulate would add considerably to the work-input of the screen, would require more compound for a longer period of medication, and would require the use of lower inocula so that birds would survive to produce oocysts; it is probably more sensible to delay such observations until the evaluation stage with active compounds.

Other parameters which have been used in evaluating coccidial infections include hematocrit, serum albumin, serum carotenoids, and food conversion ratio. Although in the final evaluation of a new anticoccidial, food conversion is one of the most important criteria to follow, usefully accurate figures are difficult to obtain using single groups of just a few birds in cages, and is not, we feel, a useful parameter at the initial screening stage. Blood parameters are time consuming to measure and again give no useful information not more readily obtained by other means.

D. Economy in Compound for Test

In a large-scale screening operation, one of the greatest difficulties is obtaining sufficient compounds in sufficient quantity for screening. Anything which can be done to cut down the requirement for compound—provided it does not destroy the validity of the test—is useful. Younger birds eat less food over the period of the test than older birds, but require more heat (which can make working conditions unpleasant) and are more liable to suffer loss through nonspecific causes; we consider 9 days old at the start of the experiment optimal. Birds of a laying strain eat less food than broilers of the same age; although they also grow less, they are nevertheless suitable for screening purposes, where it is the interaction between drug and parasite which is of prime importance. Group numbers are important; although we have used groups of 8 for many years, it should be possible to reduce numbers considerably without losing all meaning to the test. The initial screening level of the compound is important. As we are looking for a lead rather than a ready made drug, we are more likely to find one if we screen at a high incorporation rate. We have used 1000 ppm as the initial rate, and have had few problems with toxicity, although others screen initially at 250 ppm or even lower. The necessary period of medication is interesting. The only compounds we know which need to be given before rather than from the time of inoculation to show optimal activity are the ionophores; obviously medication for 1 or 2 days prior to inoculation is going to use more compound. We have published point and type of action studies on 17 compounds, describing experiments in which medicated food was withdrawn at various times after inoculation. When mortality and weight gain at 7 days is considered, assessment of activity would be unchanged in $\frac{7}{17}$ cases if plain food had been given from 3 days onward, in a further $\frac{6}{17}$ cases from 4 days, and in only $\frac{3}{17}$ cases from 5 days. In a screen test, little would probably be lost therefore if medication was only given to say 4 days after inoculation, thus giving a worthwhile saving of compound.

IV. Cage Evaluation Experiments

Work in chickens so far considered has been aimed at screening, i.e., giving a yes/no answer to the question: is there sufficient interaction between this compound and the disease entity to warrant more detailed investigation? When the answer is "yes," we repeat the test, and investigate reduced incorporation rates until a minimum effective level has been determined. Before proceeding to floor pen trials, it is desirable to evaluate the compound further in single-species and mixed-species infections, comparing its behavior with that of commercially available anticoccidials. It is necessary to evaluate the compound against all the important species of coccidia, and to investigate possible strain variation by comparing the responses of a number of recent field isolates. It is important at this and subsequent stages to obtain adequate dose–response data, since although a recommended incorporation rate may have been chosen on biological and/or economic grounds, subsequent field experience may require a change in level (such as has happened with methyl benzoquate, robenidine, monensin, and lasalocid) and the relevant data should be available. We examine an experimental compound at a series of at least 5 doubling incorporation rates to obtain a realistic dose–response curve, while using the standard drugs at their recommended levels. Using groups of 8 chicks, we replicate each treatment 6 to 8 times, depending on the design of the experiment and the number of cages available. As with screening, the most important parameters to follow are mortality, weight gain, and fecal score. Although oocyst production is not an entirely satisfactory parameter for indicating the degree of coccidiosis control, it is desirable at this stage to prolong the experiment for several days and follow oocyst production, isolating oocysts for observations on ability to sporulate; oocyst production should be expressed in terms of oocysts per bird per day rather than oocysts/gram feces. The information provided will be useful when considering build-up of infection in a flock and ability to cycle in the presence of drug—leading to drug resistance. Extra birds may be included in the test for lesion scoring at intervals, although food conversion and lesion scores are probably best studied at the floor pen stage; hematocrits and serum albumin and carotenoids are probably not worthwhile determining at any stage.

V. Drug Resistance Studies

The ultimate fate of all anticoccidial drugs is drug resistance. The speed at which this has become a problem in the field has varied considerably from compound to compound. It is not at this stage possible to predict accurately from laboratory experiments just how soon it will become a problem in the field with a particular compound, but some sort of experimentation will need to be done (see Ryley and Betts, 1973; Ryley, 1980). Serial passage can be carried out in chickens using conditions of low drug pressure—repeated low incorporation rates with moderate coccidial challenge—or intensive drug pressure—massive coccidial challenges at each passage with steadily increasing drug incorporation rates. Alternatively drugs may be studied using the "microbroiler" technique of Ryley and Betts (1973), where a mixed population of coccidia is maintained in litter and exposed to drug pressure in a series of batches of chicks kept on the litter and supplied with medicated food.

The chick embryo system can be used for serial passage of coccidia in the presence of drug in order to produce resistant strains (Chapman, 1974, 1976). Experimentally this system may have advantages in cutting down possibilities of cross-contamination in the laboratory, but results obtained are even more difficult to extrapolate to a field situation than ones obtained in laboratory chickens. An embryo-adapted strain of *E. tenella* has been used in some of these resistance studies, being especially convenient because of enhanced oocyst yields at passage, but as this adapted strain is not generally available and adaptation cannot readily be achieved with one's own strains, the idea is not of practical significance. Cyclical passage of coccidia in cell culture has not yet been achieved, so this system is inapplicable in the context of developing drug resistance.

The embryo and cell culture systems can also be used—with the limited species of coccidia that will grow in them—to characterize drug-resistant strains and investigate problems of cross-resistance. Although it is preferable to carry out such studies in the chicken, inadequate facilities for large experiments with many replicates may make the *in vitro* techniques more appropriate. Again, in a situation where only small quantities of experimental compounds were available, we found the cell culture system very useful for cross-resistance studies in a group of ionophores.

VI. Point and Type of Action Studies

It is interesting to have information on the point in the life cycle at which a compound acts and whether this activity is coccidistatic or coccidicidal. Such information is useful when considering the likely effects of withdrawal or interruption of medication—intentional or otherwise—and the likely effect of drugs prophylaxis on the development of flock immunity. Of prime importance is what the drug actually does in the chicken with the recommended level of incorporation, and as most drugs are used prophylactically rather than therapeutically, the most interesting aspect is what happens to the parasite under conditions of continuous medication. Chickens are given food medicated with the recommended level of drug, challenged with coccidia, and killed at daily intervals for histology. By this means we have shown that in the presence of methyl benzoquate or clopidol, development of *E. tenella* is held up at the intracellular sporozoite stage (Ryley, 1967), while in the presence of robenidine, large multinucleate first generation schizonts accumulate, but are unable to proceed to merozoite differentiation (Ryley and Wilson, 1971). Similar studies have been reported with a number of other drugs (Ryley and Wilson, 1975, 1976b; Ryley *et al.*, 1974). In order to detect by histological means inhibited first generation parasites, it is necessary to use massive inocula of coccidia; in order to be relevant to the field situation, the recommended level of drugs should be used. Such methods give clear-cut results with drugs such as methyl benzoquate and robenidine, but in other cases, where parasite control is not complete, e.g., monensin, lasalocid, amprolium, the pattern of activity may be more difficult to interpret. The histological picture may indicate an overall reduction in parasite numbers, with abnormal parasites of all stages being present. Although not so relevant to the field situation, it may be interesting to delay the start of medication until 1–4 days after inoculation in order to study potential effects against later stages of the parasite. Such studies are more relevant in drugs being considered for therapeutic rather than prophylactic use.

Are such parasites alive or dead, i.e., is the drug coccidistatic or coccidicidal? Information on this point can be obtained by discontinuing medication after varying periods and observing birds for relapse as indicated by mortality, fecal blood, weight loss, lesions, or oocyst production. In this context however it is essential to take note of the degree of parasite control achieved during the period of medication; drugs which give only partial suppression or control will allow immunity to develop, and there will be no relapse on drug withdrawal (Ryley and Wilson, 1976b), i.e., a misleading conclusion may be reached.

There would seem to be little point in using embryos for such studies, since histology will still be necessary to observe inhibited parasites, and drug-withdrawal studies are not possible. On the other hand, cell cultures are useful in that observations can be made on whole parasites rather than fragments of parasites in sectioned material, and the possibility exists of making continuous observations on individual parasites in the presence of drug. Delayed medication and drug-removal studies are also possible in cell culture—although in the latter context the warning of Wilson (1976) concerning the difficulty in removing drugs from cultures should be heeded—but the results may not always accurately reflect the situation in the chick.

Embryo and cell culture systems are useful where attempts are to be made to antagonize the activity of drugs with various growth factors (Ryley, 1968; Ryley and Wilson, 1972a) or to study particular facets of drug activity where it is desirable to eliminate influences from the host. Thus we were puzzled by the fact that methyl benzoquate affected the course of infection with *E. tenella* in the chick only when present from the time of inoculation, whereas with *E. brunetti*, delayed medication was possible without foregoing control. Studies in embryos (Ryley, 1967) followed by intravenous dosing experiments in chickens indicated that the difference in response was due to the superficial location of all stages of *E. brunetti* in the intestinal mucosa contrasted with the deep-seated location of the second generation of schizogony of *E. tenella* coupled with the inability of the drug due to its poor solubility to penetrate deeply into the tissues. Again we were concerned that some drugs are wide-spectrum in activity, whereas others show good activity against only a limited number of species of coccidia. Are these differences due to real differences in susceptibility of the different species of coccidia, or are they a reflection of the distribution and metabolism of the various drugs in the chick? We were able to shed some light on this question by determining minimum effective levels of a number of drugs against *E. tenella, E. necatrix,* and *E. brunetti* in the chick and in cell culture (Ryley and Wilson, 1972b). In the case of some drugs (e.g., sulfonamides), differences in absolute activity between the species as measured under the same conditions in cell culture were reflected in similar differences in the chick, while in other cases (e.g., dinitolmide, methyl benzoquate), relative absolute activities as measured in cell culture were considerably modified by metabolism or distribution in the chick.

VII. Conclusions

The purpose of screening is to examine a large number of compounds to see whether in any case there is sufficient interaction between the compound and the parasite to warrant a more detailed investigation. It is preferable to carry out this screening *in vivo*, but if *in vitro* prescreens are to be used, they should not reject compounds having potential *in vivo* interest. In the context of coccidiosis, both the cell culture and chick embryo systems are unreliable in that they will reject some compounds active in the chick, and are far from quantitative in their predictive value. The cell culture system is probably the lesser of the two evils, imposing far less demands on quantity of compound necessary for investigation; the system is also useful in studies on the point and type of action of an anticoccidial drug. The most sensitive criteria for detecting activity in the chick are mortality, weight gain, and fecal score; it is preferable to screen against two species—*E. tenella* and *E. brunetti*—and to use sufficiently severe infections to allow the parameters chosen to be used effectively. Cage evaluation experiments can be based on the primary screening system, modified to give adequate replication of treatments and observations on oocyst production. They should be comparative in nature, using as many commercially available anticoccidials and species of coccidia as possible, and should generate dose–response data for the compound under investigation. Studies on the development of drug resistance, the type of activity of the compound under investigation, and the point in the life cycle at which it acts should be carried out in chickens, but particular facets of these studies may be confirmed or more conveniently carried out in cell culture or embryos.

References

Chapman, H. D. (1974). *Parasitology* **69,** 283–290.
Chapman, H. D. (1976). *Parasitology* **73,** 275–282.
Doran, D. J. (1970). *Proc. Helminthol. Soc. Wash.* **37,** 84–92.
Latter, V. S., and Wilson, R. G. (1979). *Parasitology* **79,** 169–175.
Long, P. L. (1965). *Nature (London)* **208,** 509–510.
Long, P. L. (1970). *Z. Parasitenk.* **33,** 329–338.
Long, P. L., and Millard, B. J. (1973). *Avian Pathol.* **2,** 111–125.
Naciri-Bontemps, M. (1976). *Ann. Rech. Vét.* **7,** 223–230.
Reid, W. M. (1975). *Avian Dis.* **19,** 802–811.
Ruff, M. D., Anderson, W. I., and Reid, W. M. (1978). *J. Parasitol.* **64,** 306–311.
Ryley, J. F. (1967). *J. Parasitol.* **53,** 1151–1160.
Ryley, J. F. (1968). *Parasitology* **58,** 215–220.
Ryley, J. F. (1980). *Adv. Vet. Sci. Comp. Med.* **24,** 99–120.
Ryley, J. F., and Betts, M. J. (1973). *Adv. Pharmacol. Chemother.* **11,** 221–293.
Ryley, J. F., and Hardman, L. (1978). *Parasitology* **76,** 11–20.
Ryley, J. F., and Wilson, R. G. (1971). *Z. Parasitenk.* **37,** 85–93.
Ryley, J. F., and Wilson, R. G. (1972a). *Z. Parasitenk.* **40,** 31–34.
Ryley, J. F., and Wilson. R. G. (1972b). *J. Parasitol.* **58,** 664–668.
Ryley, J. F., and Wilson, R. G. (1975). *Parasitology* **70,** 203–222.
Ryley, J. F., and Wilson, R. G. (1976a). *Parasitology* **73,** 137–148.

Ryley, J. F., and Wilson, R. G. (1976b). Parasitology **73,** 287–309.
Ryley, J. F., Wilson, R. G., and Betts, M. J. (1974). *Parasitology* **68,** 69–79.
Tamas, T., Olson, G., Smith, D. A., and Miller, B. M. (1978). *Poultry Sci.* **57,** 381–385.
Williams, R. B. (1973). *Parasitology* **67,** 279–288.
Wilson, R. G. (1976). *Parasitology* **73,** 283–286.

ADVANCES IN PHARMACOLOGY AND CHEMOTHERAPY, VOL. 17

Information Services of the International Cancer Research Data Bank (ICRDB) Program in Cancer Chemotherapy and Pharmacology

JOHN H. SCHNEIDER

International Cancer Research Data Bank Program
National Cancer Institute
Bethesda, Maryland

I. Introduction

Modern information services are becoming an increasingly vital link in the research process. They provide a systematic mechanism for widespread and rapid dissemination of new research results to scientists and clinicians who are in the position to use the research results.

Classic methods of communication depend on person-to-person contacts, occasional browsing through or regularly covering a few journals, or attending a few scientific meetings each year. These methods are no longer adequate to cope with the flood of information being generated by scientists from some 100 countries around the world. The results of their efforts are published in thousands of journals and presented at hundreds of scientific meetings each year. No individual can begin to cover all the sources that have useful information.

ISBN 0-12-032917-4

Instead, scientists must now rely on services that systematically cover the significant sources of information on a given topic and convert it to a form that is easily available to scientists on a selective, targeted basis. Use of such services is essential, if the results of research are to be effectively disseminated.

The International Cancer Research Data Bank (ICRDB) Program of the National Cancer Institute (NCI) serves the purposes just outlined. This Program was developed in response to a Congressional mandate stating that NCI shall:

> Collect, analyze, store, and disseminate all data useful in the prevention, diagnosis and treatment of cancer . . . and disseminate, insofar as feasible, the results of cancer research undertaken in any country for the use of any person involved in cancer research in any country.

In order to accomplish this objective, the International Cancer Research Data Bank (ICRDB) Program has developed three on-line computer data bases containing cancer information. These can be searched to supply requested information to scientists throughout the world in a matter of minutes, or for more complicated searches or service to remote areas, in a matter of several days.

In addition, the ICRDB Program has developed publications that are automatically sent to researchers to keep them aware of research in progress by other scientists who are working in the same field of research. Other publications automatically provide scientists with monthly abstracts of published papers related to their current research.

This article describes these services in some detail and mentions other aspects of the ICRDB Program and its present and past activities, stressing technical information services for scientists working in fields of cancer chemotherapy and pharmacology.

II. Collection of Data

Three major types of cancer-related information collected by the ICRDB Program are described in the following sections.

A. Abstracts of Published Literature

About 3000 different scientific journals are screened on a regular basis to identify all articles dealing with cancer. The subject areas covered are listed in Table I.

For most of these areas, all articles dealing with the topic indicated are selected. The only significant exceptions are anecdotal papers dealing

TABLE I

MAJOR SUBJECT AREAS COVERED BY THE ICRDB PROGRAM

Anticancer agents
Screening and isolation of natural and synthetic agents
Characterization, synthesis, and physical properties
Experimental pharmacology and toxicology
Clinical trials of anticancer agents:
Phase I, II, and III trials
Related clinical pharmacology and toxicology
Supportive care of patients
Rehabilitation following cancer therapy
Carcinogens
Chemical carcinogens
Carcinogens in diet, water, air
Other environmental carcinogens
X-Ray and ultraviolet radiation
Nuclear radiation and other radiation
Occupational carcinogens
Oncogenic viruses and their mechanism of action
Pharmacology and toxicology of carcinogens
Metabolism and mechanism of action of carcinogens
Effects of carcinogens on nucleic acids and proteins
Cancer epidemiology
Cancer biology
Cancer immunology
Cancer virology
Cancer biochemistry
Cancer cytology and histology
Genetic, familial, and other host factors in cancer
Other biology of cancer

with single case histories and articles dealing exclusively with the chemistry of anticancer agents or carcinogens. Such chemistry articles are abstracted in detail by Chemical Abstracts Service (CAS). Most chemists would look for chemistry information in a CAS publication.

Because of the broad scope of cancer, nearly 45,000 articles dealing with the topics listed in Table I are selected each year. When publisher permission has been granted, the author abstract is used. If this is not possible, abstracters with biomedical backgrounds prepare abstracts of all selected articles. The fact that *abstracts* are prepared for all articles is significant because many information services provide only titles and citations, thereby requiring the user to locate the article in order to find any information about the results. In contrast, the use of abstracts will, in most cases, be sufficient to determine whether the article is sufficiently valuable to justify reading the original article. In many cases, the abstract alone will provide enough information to avoid the time and effort needed to locate the article.

Once the abstracts are prepared, they are entered on magnetic tape in a standardized format that is needed for input into a computer system. Speed of processing receives particular emphasis. All issues of journals must be screened within 5 days after receipt. Magnetic tapes containing the abstracts must be prepared within 30 days for English language articles and within 45 days for articles in other languages.

Abstracts of about 12,000 cancer-related papers presented at meetings are also collected each year. These abstracts are particularly useful because they often describe very recent results which will not be available as a formal publication for many months, or in some cases a year or more. I am not aware of any other information service that provides this type of timely, useful data.

Cancer-related abstracts are also prepared summarizing books, chapters in books, theses, reports by government agencies, and other monographs. Thus, published literature dealing with cancer is covered in a very thorough and comprehensive fashion by the ICRDB Program through its data collection activities.

B. Descriptions of Current Cancer Research Projects

If scientists are aware of other researchers who are working on the same problem, the possibility of collaboration is greatly facilitated, and unnecessary duplication of effort can be avoided. For this reason, the ICRDB Program collects descriptions of current cancer research projects from countries around the world and disseminates them to scientists in a highly targeted fashion.

In the United States, most government agencies as well as other organizations that support research (such as the American Cancer Society) send copies of current research project descriptions to the Smithsonian Science Information Exchange (SSIE). These descriptions include most of the pharmacology and toxicology research projects in the United States.

In order to use and expand on this large collection effort, the ICRDB Program has established a Current Cancer Research Project Analysis Center (CCRESPAC) at SSIE. CCRESPAC staff are in contact with data coordinators in some 60 different countries who act as focal points for collecting descriptions of cancer research projects from scientists in those countries. The staff of the International Union Against Cancer (UICC) located in Geneva, Switzerland, contact and work with the data coordinators in each country. Through their combined efforts, many countries have established procedures by which preparation of a project description for the ICRDB Program is required at the time a request for funding of a cancer-related research project is submitted to a granting agency.

C. Outlines of Clinical Cancer Protocols

The third type of data collected by the ICRDB Program consists of detailed outlines of protocols of clinical trials for different types of cancer. Since most of these trials are supported by the U.S. government, many of the protocols are easily available within the National Cancer Institute. Others are collected throughout Europe and other countries by the European Organization for Research on the Treatment of Cancer (EORTC).

III. ICRDB Data Bases for Cancer Researchers

Information collected by the ICRDB Program is stored in computer files called "data bases." There are three cancer data bases:

1. CANCERLIT which contains abstracts of about 200,000 cancer-related articles, meeting abstracts, and other publications;
2. CANCERPROJ which contains descriptions of some 20,000 current cancer research projects; and
3. CLINPROT which has detailed outlines of nearly 2000 experimental clinical protocols currently being tested for treatment of a wide variety of human cancers.

These three cancer data bases are collectively referred to as the CANCERLINE System. This name reflects the fact that the data base contains cancer information which can be searched "on-line" by using typewriter-like terminals that are directly connected through telephone lines (i.e., "on-line") to a distant central computer.

In the case of the CANCERLINE system, the data bases are resident in a computer at the National Library of Medicine in Bethesda, Maryland, where they are part of a large Medical Literature Analysis and Retrieval (MEDLARS) System. This system is linked by an extensive communication network to terminals in some 800 locations in the United States and numerous locations in 12 other countries.

Use of the cancer data bases in Europe will be greatly expanded as a result of a new European telecommunications system called EURONET. When fully implemented, EURONET will make it possible for scientists in almost any laboratory throughout Europe to have easy access to the cancer data bases which reside on computers in several European countries.

For developing countries which lack the telecommunications system for searching data bases, the ICRDB Program supports a project called Cancer Information Services for Developing Countries (CISDC). Under this project, staff at the British Library search the ICRDB data bases in response to requests from scientists who are working in developing countries. A limited number of copies of complete articles are also provided as part of the CISDC project. As a result, scientists in every country throughout the world have relatively easy access to the cancer data bases.

IV. Searching of Cancer Data Bases and Indexing of Biomedical Information

Searching of cancer data bases in response to requests from individual scientists is usually performed by trained "search analysts" or "search specialists," who work at each location that is authorized to use the MEDLARS System. After discussing the type of information that is needed with a scientist, the search specialist formulates a "search strategy" or "search profile" consisting of various technical words and terms that will be used, in combination, to retrieve the requested information from the computer system. These terms are then typed into the computer on the typewriter-like terminal, and sample title or abstracts are immediately printed at the terminal or displayed on a TV screen. Based on examination of this initial trial retrieval, the terms are often changed slightly to make the search broader and more inclusive or more narrow.

All the CANCERLINE data bases can be searched by use of "free-text" search strategy which means that the name of any drug, carcinogen, or any other word or combination of words that appears in the title or text of an abstract can be used to retrieve information. In addition a "controlled vocabulary" consisting of a fixed set of index terms or subject categories can also be used if each item of the information has been indexed using this vocabulary.

One advantage in using a controlled vocabulary which is limited to a fixed set of terms is that many search specialists lack the in-depth knowledge of biomedical terminology that would permit them to formulate a thorough search strategy using free-text searching. Instead, they feel more confident in using a fixed set of indexing terms, such as the 14,200 Medical Subject Headings (MeSH) terms that are used to index data in the MEDLARS System of the National Library of Medicine. When MeSH terms or the controlled vocabularies are used, searchers are relying on the ability of the indexers to identify correctly all the subject headings that would be most useful for retrieving an abstract.

Another method for indexing involves the use of detailed hierarchical classifications which permit each item of information to be indexed under multiple categories in the classification. These categories are arranged in a very logical fashion so that all related information is grouped together in neighboring categories, regardless of individual words or terms used in the title or text of the abstract to describe the information.

The advantages of using such a hierarchical classification have been described in detail previously (Schneider, 1971). A five-level hierarchy has been developed jointly by the ICRDB Program and the SSIE to index all research project descriptions. This classification provides a very powerful tool for retrieving all projects that deal with a narrow subject area such as the pharmacology, toxicology, metabolism, characterization, or mechanism of action of a specific agent. They also make it very easy to narrow a search or to broaden a search by going to a higher or lower level of the classification.

One of the most useful searching methods for retrieving information from a data base is called Automatic Selective Dissemination of Information (Automatic SDI). When this method is used, the search profile or search strategy which has been developed jointly by a scientist and a search specialist is permanently stored in the computer. Each month this profile is automatically activated to search through all the new data entered during the past month, and a printout of all the new information is automatically sent to the scientist who placed the original request. In this way, the scientist automatically receives a monthly list of abstracts dealing directly with fields of most interest to him. The cost of this service is very low since no on-line communication time is required. Instead, only minimum time is required for the computer to execute off-line a previously stored search.

The advantages of this type of SDI system are much greater than is generally realized. A pilot SDI system which was tested several years ago (Schneider, 1971) showed that scientists are unaware of a high percentage of information that is directly relevant to their research and that they rate as being "useful."

In this pilot SDI system, abstracts of articles from 12 journals dealing exclusively with cancer were matched against the research subject areas of 104 principal investigators of research grants for a 1-year period. This was accomplished by using a detailed hierarchical decimal classification covering all areas of cancer research to index both the scientific content of the articles and the research subject areas.

During the trial, abstracts of more than 5000 articles that matched the scientist's research areas were sent to the researchers. Of these, 1305 articles were rated as being "very useful." (The same articles were also almost always rated as being "directly related" to current research.) On an evaluation sheet, scientists checked that they did not known about the research described in 76% of these "very useful" articles before they were published. They had not seen 61% of these "very useful" articles before they received an abstract through this test SDI system. At the second level (out of four possible levels of usefulness), the scientists did not know about the research presented in 88% of the papers rated as being of "definite but limited use" before the research was published. They had not previously seen 72% of these "definitely useful" articles. (The same articles were almost always rated as being of "direct but limited relation" to current research projects.)

This trial clearly demonstrated that the type of SDI systems just described bring the attention of researchers to many useful articles that are directly related to their research and of which they would otherwise be unaware. Clearly, the information contained in these articles will help to increase the efficiency and productivity of research.

V. Publications Used to Disseminate Cancer-Related Information Automatically

The following sections describe major publications used to disseminate widely information collected by the ICRDB Program.

A. CANCERGRAMS

The SDI service just described provides data specifically tailored to the information needs and interests of individual scientists. In order to disseminate information automatically on a much broader scale, the ICRDB Program has identified about 65 major topic areas within the overall area of cancer research. Each month all the abstracts being added to the CANCERLIT data base that deal with each of these 65 areas are identified.

Scientists at three Cancer Information Dissemination and Analysis Centers (CIDACs) review the newly added abstracts, select those that are most significant for each area, and arrange them into the most logical categories. These selected and organized abstracts for each of the 65 subject areas are published in a series of 65 different publications called CANCERGRAMS. Each month more than 20,000 of these current awareness bulletins, each containing about 70–100 abstracts, are mailed to approximately 10,000 principal investigators of cancer research projects.

Selected CANCERGRAMS that deal with agents and topics of greatest interest to pharmacologists and toxicologists are listed in Table II.

TABLE II

CANCERGRAMS of Greatest Interest to Pharmacologists and Toxicologists[a]

Antitumor and antiviral agents—experimental therapeutics, toxicology, pharmacology
Antitumor and antiviral agents—mechanism of action
Short-term test systems for carcinogenicity and mutagenicity
Environmental and occupational carcinogenesis
Dietary aspects of carcinogenesis
Chemical carcinogenesis—azo dyes, aryl amines, and related compounds
Chemical carcinogenesis—nitroso compounds
Chemical carcinogenesis—polycyclic aromatic hydrocarbons, and related compounds
Chemical carcinogenesis—miscellaneous agents
Mechanisms of carcinogenesis—activation and metabolism of carcinogens
Mechanisms of carcinogenesis—macromolecular alterations and repair
Mechanisms of carcinogenesis—oncogenic transformation
Modification of carcinogenesis

[a] Many other CANCERGRAMS deal with the use of anticancer agents to treat specific types of cancer and with carcinogenesis of specific organ systems.

B. Special Listings

A similar series of publications is derived from information in the CANCERPROJ data base. These publications, which are designed to disseminate information about some 50 different areas of cancer research, are called *Special Listings of Current Cancer Research*.

These *Special Listings* are published annually, and are automatically sent to each of the scientists working on the 200–500 projects described in each *Special Listing*. The knowledge of similar research programs that are currently underway in some 60 different countries around the world is expected to promote collaboration between investigators and to avoid unnecessary duplication of research activities. Examples of *Special Listings* likely to be of most interest to pharmacologists and toxicologists are listed in Table III.

C. Compilation of Clinical Protocol Summaries

Of special interest to pharmacologists is an annual publication containing about 2000 outlines of protocols currently used in clinical trials for the therapy of many types of human cancer. Information for this *Compilation* is taken from the CLINPROT data base. Future editions of the *Compilation* will include outlines of tumor immunotherapy protocols which, in the past, have been published as a separate volume.

TABLE III

SPECIAL LISTINGS OF GREATEST INTEREST TO PHARMACOLOGISTS AND TOXICOLOGISTS

Preclinical studies of pharmacokinetics, effectiveness, and mechanisms of action of anticancer drugs
Isolation, synthesis, and screening of anticancer agents
Occupational and environmental carcinogenesis
Carcinogenic substances in food and drugs, and related epidemiology
Azo dyes, aryl amines, aliphatics, and various other organic and inorganic chemicals
Polycyclic aromatic hydrocarbons
Nitroso compounds
Effects of chemical carcinogens on nucleic acids, proteins, and chromosomes
Modification of chemical carcinogenesis in model systems
Antiviral agents and procedures

D. ONCOLOGY OVERVIEWS

Each year about 30 of these OVERVIEWS will be published. Each OVERVIEW deals with a specific topic currently of high interest to cancer researchers and contains 100–600 abstracts of relevant literature published in recent years. Examples of past OVERVIEW titles dealing with pharmacology and toxicology of chemical agents are: "Carcinogenicity of Vinyl Chloride and Related Compounds," "Aflatoxin and other Mycotoxin Carcinogenesis," "Artificial Sweeteners and Other Sugar Substitutes," "Carcinogenic Contaminants of Water Supplies," "The Role of Asbestos in Human Cancer," and "The Role of Metals in Carcinogenesis."

E. DIRECTORY OF CANCER RESEARCH INFORMATION RESOURCES

A *Directory of Cancer Research Information Resources* listing publications and other information services in all fields of cancer is also available. Much of the information in this *Directory* would be of use to scientists working in areas of pharmacology and toxicology.

VI. Scientist-to-Scientist Communication Projects

The ICRDB Program also provides support for projects that promote direct international collaboration between cancer scientists. One project called the International Cancer Research Technology Transfer (ICRETT) Program provides funds that permit individual scientists to work for a brief period of time with scientists in another country in order to collaborate on a project of mutual interest.

TABLE IV

EXAMPLES OF SCIENTIST-TO-SCIENTIST COMMUNICATION PROJECTS SUPPORTED BY THE ICRDB-PROGRAM

Type of project	Description of the project
ICRETT[a]	Studies on hydrocarbon metabolism in cell culture
ICRETT	Cytostatic and antitumor properties of ribonuclease dimers
ICRETT	Effect on cytosine derivatives on enzymatic methylation of DNA
ICRETT	Determination of polyamines in urine
ICREW[b]	Prognostic parameters of drug response obtained with the aid of cell separation techniques
ICREW	New approaches to the study of environmental hepatocarcinogenesis

[a] International Cancer Research Technology Transfer Program.
[b] International Cancer Research Workshop Program.

Another type of support is provided by the International Cancer Research Workshop (ICREW) Program. Under this program, catalytic funds are provided to support in part the costs of workshops dealing with specific cancer research areas. Examples of ICRETT and ICREW projects that have been supported by the ICRDB Program in fields of pharmacology and toxicology are listed in Table IV.

This paper has outlined some of the major publications and other technical information services of the ICRDB Program that are of most interest to pharmacologists and toxicologists. Readers are urged to request searches of the data bases described in this paper and to contact the International Cancer Research Data Bank Program for information on how to obtain copies of the various publications listed in this paper. It is hoped that many of the services provided by the ICRDB Program will be of considerable value to researchers working in areas of pharmacology and toxicology.

REFERENCE

Schneider, J. H. (1971). *Science* **173,** 300–308.

ADVANCES IN PHARMACOLOGY AND CHEMOTHERAPY, VOL. 17

Dihydrofolate Reductase: Binding of Substrates and Inhibitors and Catalytic Mechanism

JILL E. GREADY

Physical Chemistry Laboratory, Oxford, England

I. Introduction

Dihydrofolate reductase (DHFR) (tetrahydrofolate NADP$^+$ oxidoreductase, EC 1.5.1.3) catalyzes the NADPH-dependent reduction of 7,8-dihydrofolate (DHF) to 5,6,7,8-tetrahydrofolate (THF) (see Fig. 1):

$$\text{DHF} + \text{NADPH} + \text{H}^+ \underset{\text{DHFR}}{\rightleftharpoons} \text{THF} + \text{NADP}^+ \qquad (1)$$

THF is a coenzyme in a number of 1-carbon transfer reactions (Rader and

ISBN 0-12-032917-4

Huennekens, 1973) but from the pharmacological viewpoint its most important function is in the reaction whereby deoxyuridylate (dUMP) is converted to thymidylate (dTMP) by thymidylate synthetase (EC 2.1.1.45):

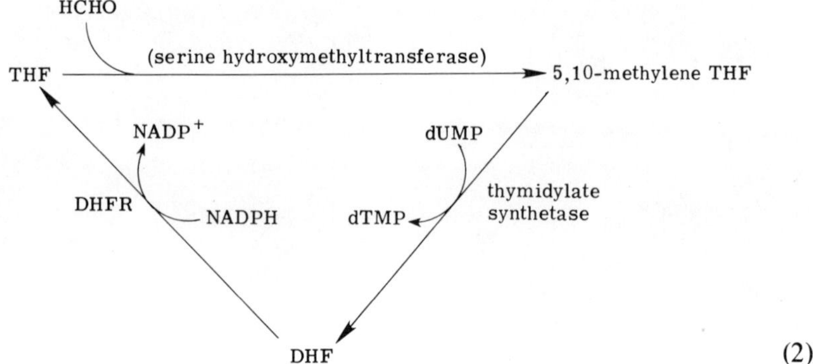

(2)

The reaction producing thymidylate is unique among those involving the THF coenzymes because here THF is used not only as a source of a 1-carbon fragment but also as a reductant and hence is used in substrate rather than coenzyme amounts: THF must be regenerated via the DHFR-catalyzed reaction in order to maintain the cellular pool of THF derivatives. Inhibition, then, of DHFR leads to a deficiency of thymidylate and thus to disruption of nucleic acid synthesis: this mechanism for interfering with DNA synthesis is thought to provide the biochemical basis for the antifolate class of drugs that have found clinical applications in the treatment of neoplastic and microbial diseases (Blakley, 1969). In bacteria, the so-called "thymine-less death" occurs when DNA synthesis is blocked but synthesis of RNA and protein continues: the thymine starvation not only halts cell proliferation but also leads to irreversible cell damage including degradation of DNA (Danenberg, 1977). Some secondary metabolic effects of DHRF blockage will be noted in Section VI.

Aminopterin (Fig. 1) was first synthesized more than 30 years ago (Seeger *et al.*, 1947) as possible antimetabolite of folic acid and shortly afterward was found to be beneficial in treating some cases of leukemia (Farber *et al.*, 1948). Its exact mode of action was not discovered until it was found upon the identification and purification of DHFR to be a powerful inhibitor of this enzyme (Futterman, 1957; Osborn *et al.*, 1958; Zakrzewski and Nichol, 1958).

No comprehensive review of the literature on DHFR has appeared since the work of Blakley (1969). Some extended discussions (Hitchings and Burchall, 1965; Baker, 1967; Roberts, 1977) have been published and,

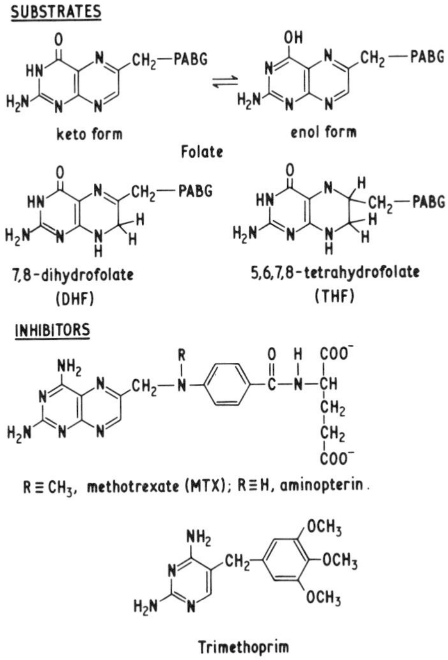

FIG. 1. Substrates and inhibitors of DHFR. The predominant tautomer of the substrates is the keto form.

in addition, there are several collections of papers in symposium volumes (Iwai *et al.*, 1970; Bertino, 1971; Pfleiderer, 1976; Kisliuk and Brown, 1979). As seen from the contents, the present treatment will be primarily from the biochemical and physicochemical viewpoints and will cover theories of substrate and inhibitor interaction with the enzyme together with related cellular aspects of folate biochemistry. The detailed discussion will be restricted to the class of inhibitors closely related structurally to the substrates (e.g., aminopterin). However, a great many classes of nonclassical inhibitors have been discovered in the course of the search for pharmacologic agents for use in cancer and antimicrobial chemotherapy; these are expected to bind to the enzyme somewhat differently than do the substrates and analog inhibitors (Baker, 1967). Indeed, following the rationale developed by Baker (1967), much of the synthetic effort has had the deliberate aim of exploring possible additional inhibitor binding sites adjacent to the active site in order to thereby introduce species-specific chemotherapeutic properties into the drug molecule. Recently attempts have been made, using correlation analysis, to systematize some of the synthetic and biochemical data of Baker and others with the view to relating chemical structure and electronic properties of inhibitor molecules with biological activity (Hansch and Silipo, 1974; Silipo and Hansch, 1975, 1976; Fukunaga *et al.*, 1976; Yoshimoto and Hansch, 1976; Hansch *et al.*, 1975, 1977; Blaney *et al.*, 1979; Dietrich *et al.*, 1979a,b). Another theoretical approach has sought to map the shape and size of the DHFR receptor site by correlating empirical results from a number of inhibitor studies (Simon *et al.*, 1977).

The search for species-specific drugs has had considerable success for antimicrobial agents: for instance, the usefulness of trimethoprim (Fig. 1) as an antibacterial agent arises from a 30,000-fold greater affinity for bacterial than for mammalian DHFR (Roberts, 1977). Other results of inhibitor specificity are reviewed by Burchall and Hitchings (1965) and Burchall (1971, 1973). On the other hand, this approach had little success in antineoplastic chemotherapy: future developments in more effective and selective antifolate agents will involve exploitation of cellular differences such as drug transport and metabolism (Section V) rather than enzyme differences.

In recognition of the pharmacological importance of DHFR, biochemical studies have proceeded with the dual aims of understanding the inhibitor binding mechanism and elucidating the substrate binding and reaction mechanisms. Improved methods of enzyme isolation and purification developed during the 1970s (e.g., Dann *et al.*, 1976) have made possible the detailed studies of the enzyme and its substrate and inhibitor complexes described here. However, because the enzyme is normally present in cells in only small amounts, problems in large-scale production and purification have meant that the bulk of the studies have been on bacterial rather than mammalian DHFRs.

One other important biological feature relates to the biosynthetic pathways for the production of DHF. Most microorganisms synthesize DHF directly from a simple pteridine precursor by coupling 7,8-dihydropteroate and glutamate whereas mammals require folic acid as a vitamin and produce THF via a two-step reduction catalyzed by DHFR (Wood, 1976):

$$\text{Folate} + 2\text{NADPH} + 2\text{H}^+ \xrightarrow{\text{DHFR}} \text{THF} + \text{NADP}^+ \quad (3)$$

It is not known why some bacteria have retained/attained the ability to absorb and reduce folate when they are capable of *de novo* synthesis of DHF. Although the differences (not well-characterized) between folate-reducing and folate-nonreducing DHFRs themselves do not seem to offer great potential for the development of more selective drugs, the differences in transport properties between folate-absorbing and folate-nonabsorbing cells are now being investigated as a new avenue for achieving selective activity (Section V).

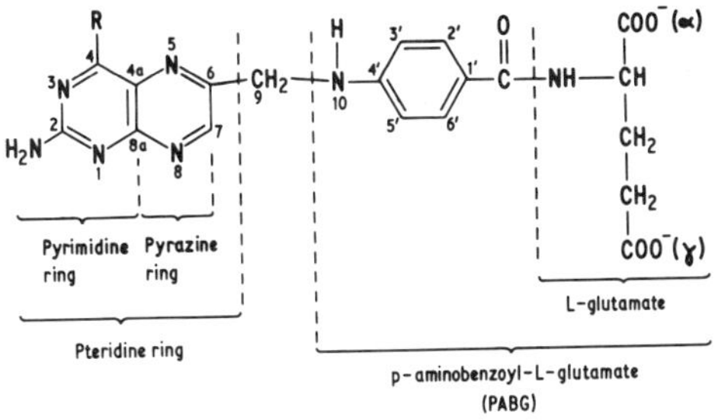

FIG. 2. Structure and numbering of the folate analog molecule.

Aminopterin [and methotrexate (MTX)] is an essentially stoichiometric inhibitor of all DHFRs although, as can be seen from Fig. 1, it differs only slightly in structure from the natural substrates. Despite the intense study documented here the origin of the difference in binding to the enzyme—specifically binding of the pteridine moiety (Fig. 2)—between the substrates and classical inhibitors has still not been fully defined. The present degree of characterization of the enzyme structure should encourage more efforts in the future in rational synthesis of new drugs.

The discussion begins with a review of critical aspects of enzyme structure as revealed by a comparison of the known amino acid sequences of a number of DHFRs and X-ray crystallographic studies on enzyme-inhibitor complexes. A major emphasis in this article will be in relating the biochemical and physicochemical evidence to these essential features of the enzyme and to the physicochemical properties of the substrate and inhibitor molecules themselves.

II. Critical Aspects of the Enzyme Structure

A. AMINO ACID SEQUENCES

As a consequence of the development of the improved methods of purification previously mentioned, complete and partial amino acid sequences are now available for DHFRs from a number of sources, predominantly bacterial. Complete bacterial sequences have been obtained for an MTX-resistant strain of *Escherichia coli* (MB1428) [Bennett *et al.*, 1978; note this reference supersedes an earlier sequence published by Bennett (1974a)], a trimethoprim-resistant strain of *E. coli* (RT500) (Stone *et al.*, 1977), an MTX-resistant strain of *Lactobacillus casei* (Bitar *et al.*, 1977; Freisheim *et al.*, 1978), and an MTX-resistant strain of *Streptococcus faecium* (Gleisner *et al.*, 1974; Peterson *et al.*, 1975a). A partial sequence of 51 N-terminal residues (Batley and Morris, 1977) and 29 elastase peptides (Morris *et al.*, 1974) has also been reported for an MTX-resistant strain of

L. casei: differences between these (London) studies and those of the American group (above) are noted by Freisheim *et al.* (1978) and are further discussed by Matthews (1979). Also, there is some evidence from the residue composition studies (Freisheim *et al.*, 1978; Dann *et al.*, 1976) that the enzyme from the American and London strains of *L. casei* may not be identical. At this point it should be noted that the X-ray studies on the DHFR–MTX–NADPH complex were carried out using enzyme from a *L. casei* strain isolated at yet another laboratory (Pastore *et al.*, 1974b). Also very recently work has been reported on the isolation and properties—including the sequence of the first 42 N-terminal residues—of two other strains (MB3746 and MB3747) of trimethoprim-resistant *E. coli* (Poe *et al.*, 1979).

The only complete mammalian enzyme sequence reported to date is that from an MTX-resistant line of mouse lymphoma L1210 cells [Stone *et al.*, 1979; note corrections to an earlier sequence by Stone and Phillips (1977)]. Partial sequences have been reported for beef liver enzyme (Bauman and Wilson, 1975; Peterson *et al.*, 1975b) and for mouse sarcoma 180 enzyme (Rodkey and Bennett, 1976): these have been compared with that of L1210 enzyme by Stone *et al.* (1979). In addition, some residue composition data have been reported for pig liver enzyme (Poe *et al.*, 1976) and beef liver enzyme (Kaufman and Kemerer, 1976).

Some general conclusions based on the published sequences can be made: these refer not only to specific conserved areas of structure essential for an understanding of the enzymes' binding and catalytic functions but also to the degree of homology between enzyme from different sources—particularly bacterial and mammalian—which may be useful in understanding drug-binding specificity. A comparison of complete sequences from four different sources is given in Fig. 3: the sequences are aligned following Stone *et al.* (1979). Some proliferation has arisen in the literature in the numbering of the sequences. The initial numbering from the *E. coli* MB1428 sequence (Bennett, 1974a) is no longer advisable due to insertions and a deletion in the revised sequence (Bennett *et al.*, 1978). The numbering of the *L. casei* enzyme (Freisheim *et al.*, 1978) is used in the discussion of the *L. casei* DHFR–MTX–NADPH X-ray structure (Matthews *et al.*, 1978): this numbering is given in italics in Fig. 3 for future reference to the X-ray results for both the *E. coli* and *L. casei* structures.

One outstanding feature of Fig. 3 is the presence of two highly conserved regions: the first at the NH_2-terminal end extends from residue 1 to 78, the second from residue 109 to 146. Early suggestions linked these to two domains binding substrate—and presumably inhibitor—and dinucleotide, respectively (Gleisner *et al.*, 1974). However, it is now known from

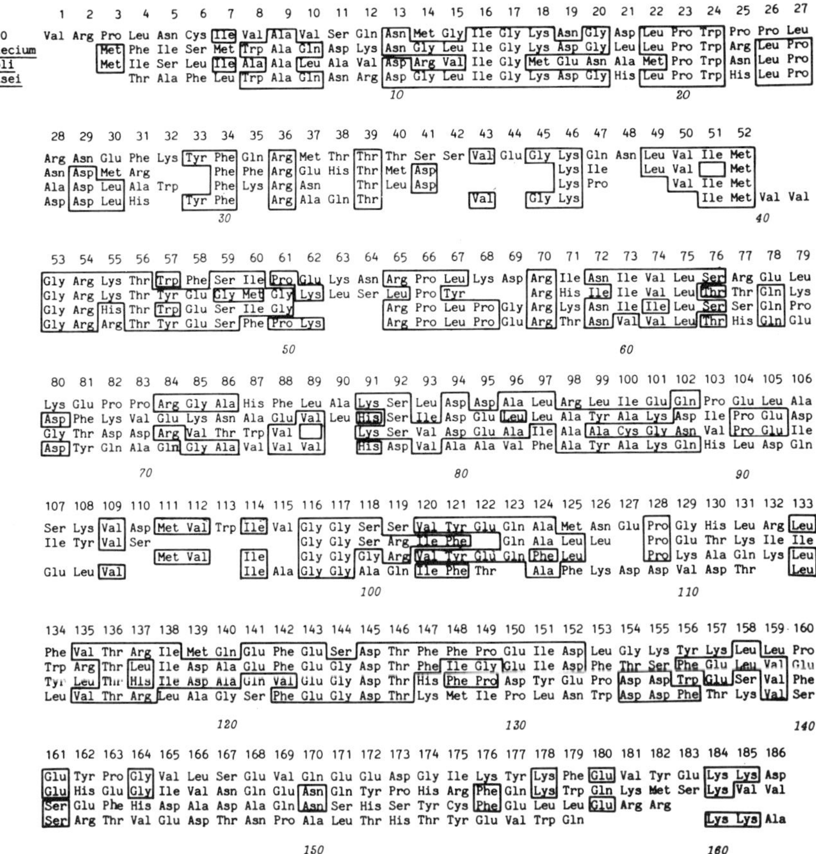

FIG. 3. Comparison of amino acid sequences of the DHFRs from mouse L1210 cells (186 residues; MW 21, 458), *S. faecium* (167 residues; MW ~ 20,800), *E. coli* RT500 [159 residues; MW for MB1428 (see text) 17,958], and *L. casei* (162 residues; MW 18,322). Complete numbering above the sequences refers to the L1210 enzyme while the incomplete numbering (in italics) is that for the *L. casei* sequence. Boxed areas indicate regions where two or more sequences are identical.

the X-ray studies (Section II,B,1) that there is considerable overlap in inhibitor and coenzyme binding to these two regions. Also early attempts (Bennett, 1974a) to find homologies between the DHFR sequence and the sequences of larger dehydrogenases, that might be ascribed to dinucleotide binding sites of common origin, subsequently proved negative (Bennett, 1974b; Peterson *et al.*, 1975a).

Comparison of the three bacterial sequences by Freisheim *et al.* (1978)

showed that the *L. casei* enzyme sequence had 29 and 34% identities, respectively, with the *E. coli* and *S. faecium* enzymes. Comparison of the first 67 highly conserved residues indicated that *L. casei* and *S. faecium*, both folate-requiring organisms, had a 54% identity in this region with a mean base change per codon of 0.55 whereas the analogous figures for *L. casei/E. coli* and *E. coli/S. faecium* were 0.82 and 0.88, respectively. Comparison with the L1210 enzyme, which is slightly larger than any of the bacterial enzymes, still shows approximately 30% identity with each of them (Stone *et al.*, 1979). Also, with the exception of the COOH-terminal 30 or so amino acids, the residues which are common to the mammalian and bacterial enzymes are distributed throughout the lengths of the molecules, suggesting that all the enzymes have similar overall structures (see Section II,B for comments on *E. coli* and *L. casei* backbone structures). As there are indications in the literature of larger monomeric DHFRs (MW up to 40,000: Roberts, 1977) it would be interesting to know in which regions the sequences of these differ from those of the smaller enzymes.

The above comparisons do not yield a ready explanation as to why trimethoprim has a 30,000-fold greater affinity for bacterial DHFRs than for mammalian enzymes (Roberts, 1977). The mode of binding of trimethoprim is not understood (Section III,B): however, the recent studies on trimethoprim-resistant strains of *E. coli* (Poe *et al.*, 1979) may pinpoint the mechanism for development of drug resistance at the molecular level. Preliminary results for the first 42 NH_2-terminal residues of trimethoprim-resistant *E. coli* MB3746 and 3747 strains show identical sequences with *E. coli* RT500 except for MB3747 having Ile instead of Met at position 22 (Fig. 3).

The sequence of the *E. coli* MB1428 enzyme is not given in Fig. 3. When presenting the revised sequence Bennett *et al.* (1978) report that it differs at only three positions from the RT500 sequence of Stone *et al.* (1977)—at positions 141 (Glu for Gln), 165 (Asn for Asp), and 177 (Lys for Glu)—and that these changes can all be related by single base changes in the DNA coding. However inspection of the published data reveals another change at position 92 (Asn for Ser).

A particularly noteworthy feature of the revised sequence for the L1210 enzyme (Stone *et al.*, 1979) is that the amide assignments for residues 29 and 30 (Asn and Glu) have been reversed from those reported earlier (Stone *et al.*, 1977). Stone *et al.* (1979) state that the change followed reinvestigation prompted by results for the bovine liver enzyme. As is apparent from Fig. 3 the altered assignments deprive residue 29 of fully conserved status as an aspartate residue: as this residue has been strongly implicated in both binding and reaction processes (Sections III,B and

III,F) its essential role will need to be reassessed. Some speculative comments on this point are noted in Section III,B,1.

B. X-Ray Crystallographic Studies

X-Ray crystal structure results, at 2.5 Å resolution, are available for the binary complex of MTX-resistant *E. coli*–DHFR and MTX (Matthews *et al.*, 1977) and for the ternary complex of MTX-resistant *L. casei*–DHFR, MTX, and NADPH (Matthews *et al.*, 1978). These studies have defined the overall shape of the enzyme molecule, identified regions of secondary structure and binding areas for inhibitor and cofactor, and helped to explain the existence of some of the highly conserved residues. There are indications (Sections III,B and III,D) of differences between the protein conformational structures in the enzyme–MTX and enzyme–substrate complexes: hence, direct analogy from the X-ray results to a description of enzyme–substrate binding is not possible although Matthews *et al.*(1978) provide arguments for a close correspondence (Section II,B,1). X-Ray crystallographic studies on the native *L. casei* enzyme are also in progress (Roberts, 1977).

The discussion will be in two parts: general features, and the implications of specific residue interactions. Section references to further chemical or biochemical information will be indicated.

1. *General Aspects*

The polypeptide backbone is folded into an eight-stranded β-sheet beginning at the NH_2-terminus and ending with a single antiparallel strand at the COOH-end. The course of the backbone of the *L. casei* enzyme is structurally quite similar to that of the *E. coli* enzyme despite a sequence homology of only about 29%. About 30% of the backbone is involved in the β-sheet structure, the remaining secondary structure consisting of several helices and interconnecting loops. A primary sequence alignment for the *L. casei* and *E. coli* enzymes was obtained by assuming that deletions and insertions would occur so as to minimize disruptions of important secondary and tertiary features: this alignment differs slightly from that proposed by Bitar *et al.* (1977).

The extent of the similarity in backbone geometries between the *E. coli* –MTX binary complex and the *L. casei* ternary complex might superficially appear to disagree with the CD and NMR spectroscopic results on DHFRs from several sources (Sections III,D,2 and III,D,4) which indicate that the enzyme–MTX complex undergoes some additional conformational changes on binding NADPH. There is no real conflict, however: it is not possible to ascribe these changes to backbone rather than simple side chain orientations. Also, it should be noted that backbone differences observed in the X-ray structures cannot be unambiguously assigned to the effects of NADPH binding rather than to species differences. It seems clear, however, that no major reorganization of secondary structure occurs when NADPH binds, in contrast, for instance, to NAD^+ binding to lactate dehydrogenase where backbone movements of up to 11 Å are observed (Holbrook *et al.,* 1975).

The overall connectivity and structure of DHFR was compared by Matthews *et al.* (1977) with that of a number of NADH-dependent dehydrogenases using topological maps. It was found that the spatial arrangement but not the connectivity was nearly the same for the two enzyme classes: this led to the conclusion that a similar preferred mononucleotide binding structure had been arrived at by convergent evolution. The X-ray results for coenzyme binding necessitated some revision of this view as it was found that NADPH binds in a position shifted one β-strand from the location expected on the basis of the above structural comparisons (Matthews *et al.,* 1978).

At the level of residue binding contacts some similarities are preserved although they are not directly analogous: a conserved glycine (Gly-117 in Fig. 3) at geometrically equivalent postitions is close to the adenosine ribose of bound NAD^+ in the dehydrogenases but in van der Waals contact with the pyrophosphate group in the *L. casei* complex—this difference resulting from the relative translation of the coenzyme across one β-strand in the *L. casei* enzyme. Also an aspartate residue which H-bonds with the 2′-hydroxyl of the adenosine ribose in NAD^+ in the dehydrogenases is replaced by a conserved arginine (Arg-54 in Fig. 3) at the corresponding geometrical location in DHFR. It was expected (Matthews *et al.,* 1977) that this arginine would interact with the 2′-phosphate of NADPH: this prediction was borne out by the results for the *L. casei* complex despite the one β-strand shift, because the arginine side chain when fully extended is about 5 Å longer than an aspartate side chain (Matthews *et al.,* 1978). But despite these similarities there is still a major difference between DHFR and the other nucleotide dehydrogenases, namely, that there is no separate binding domain for NADPH in DHFR. Instead the substrate and coenzyme binding functions are carried out by overlapping portions of the primary sequence.

Methotrexate is bound in a cavity which is 15 Å deep and cuts across one whole face of the enzyme. It is bound in an open conformation with its pteridine ring nearly perpendicular to the aromatic ring of the *p*-aminobenzoyl group: the overall conformation is similar in both the binary and ternary complexes (Matthews *et al.,* 1978). The pyrimidine end of the pteridine ring is buried in a primarily hydrophobic pocket. Most of the face of the pyrazine ring is completely exposed to solvent in the binary complex but covered by NADPH in the ternary complex in a manner that would allow reduction of DHF at N(5) — N(6) as required in an active enzyme–substrate complex (Section III,F). One side of the cavity provides a binding site for the nicotinamide ring of NADPH while the remainder of the coenzyme molecule fits in a shallow groove. More than half the MTX and coenzyme interactions are with the first 50 residues (of *L. casei* and *E. coli* enzymes), many of which are strongly conserved as indicated in Fig. 3. A summary of specific interactions is given in the next section.

Matthews *et al.* (1978) advanced a number of reasons to support a close correspondence between the binding in the enzymically active DHFR–DHF–NADPH complex and the DHFR–MTX–NADPH complex. Thus, the orientation of the pteridine ring to the plane of the nicotinamide ring (about 45°) with the C(6) of MTX at a distance of about 4.5 Å above C(4) of nicotinamide was consistent with the then available experimental evidence (Section III,F) indicating hydride transfer from NADPH to C(6) of DHF. Also the transferable hydride ion at C(4) of nicotinamide directed toward the pyrazine is on the A side in accord with the experimental results for the stereospecificity of hydride transfer (Section III,F). Furthermore, the above authors noted that the observed binding interactions in the inhibitor ternary complex appear to account well for strictly conserved residues among a number of DHFRs, although the details of this argument require some minor modifications in the light of more recently available sequences presented in Fig. 3.

However, as spectroscopic evidence (Section III,D) suggested that MTX, folate, and DHF are each bound slightly differently, Matthews *et al.* (1978) also investigated another possibility—that originally proposed some time ago by Baker (1967)—that of completely different orientations of the pteridine ring of substrates and inhibitors within the binding site. They reported that model building experiments confirm the possibility of a complete turning over of the pteridine moiety with respect to the rest of the MTX molecule while still maintaining a reasonable fit within the binding pocket (Section III,B,3). The model experiments indicate that this flip could be achieved while still maintaining the close approach of C(4) of the nicotinamide ring to C(6) of the pteridine ring. Very recent results (Charlton *et al.*, 1979) have now shown that this inverted pteridine orientation for the substrates, folate and DHF, is indeed the case. These results are discussed more fully in Sections III,A,6 and III,F.

The question of the source of the proton which is transferred ultimately to N(5) of DHF during reduction is considered in detail in Section III,F. On the basis of the X-ray results Matthews *et al.* (1978) suggest Asp-29 and Thr-136 as two possible sources on the enzyme. Although reference to Fig. 3 shows that Thr-136 is totally conserved, the most recent results indicate that Asp-29 is not and hence proposed roles in catalysis and inhibitor binding need to be reevaluated.

2. *Specific Binding Interactions*

While the X-ray studies have provided evidence for specific binding interactions, they cannot provide information about the stabilizing influence of individual interactions in the total binding scheme which is of the utmost importance chemically and, hence, pharmacologically. Experimental results for the binding energetics, including cooperative binding of inhibitor and substrate fragments and the relative importance of the various binding areas, are given in Section III,B,4.

Some information about interactions between specific enzyme residues and MTX in both the binary and ternary complexes is summarized in Table I, in a manner similar to that of Matthews *et al.* (1978). The numbering is that for *L. casei* DHFR (Fig. 3). In view of the evidence for interactions of structurally equivalent residues presented in Table I, the sequence alignment in Fig. 3 is questionable in some instances—possibly even for Leu-*54*. It is noteworthy that the numbers of interactions are identical except for Leu-*19* in the *L. casei* case. Although 9 out of the 13 side chain interactions are with residues conserved between the two species, only 4 (possibly 5 with Leu-*54*) are with totally conserved residues while one other residue is conserved among bacterial DHFRs (Fig. 3). It is suggested (Matthews *et al.*, 1978) that the proximity of the Leu-*19* side chain to the pyrazine ring in the ternary complex is the result of a conformational change on NADPH binding: the analogous residue in the binary complex, Met-*19,* is over 7 Å away from any part of the pteridine ring. Also, the extra interaction provided by the side chain contact of Leu-*19* (or presumably Met-*19* in *E. coli*) with MTX may partially explain the enhanced binding of MTX to DHFR in the presence of NADPH (Section III,C) (Matthews *et al.*, 1978). It is likely, however, that small changes in conserved interactions, or interaction between the inhibitor and coenzyme, are responsible for most of the cooperative effect.

Residues involved in the two hydrophobic pockets binding the pteridine and benzene rings are indicated in Table I. Discussion of the importance of the Asp-*26* interaction and of H-bonding on the pyrimidine ring is deferred to Section III,B. Note that the fact that aminopterin (Fig. 1) is an almost equally potent inhibitor compared with MTX suggests that the Leu-*54* interaction with the N(10)-methyl group is not of vital importance.

The glutamate portion of MTX is bound at the enzyme surface with the Arg-*57* side chain H-bonded to the α-carboxyl group. The glutamate side chain moiety is held in different conformations in the two complexes and

TABLE I

INTERACTIONS BETWEEN DHFR AND MTX FOR THE *E. coli* BINARY AND *L. casei* TERNARY COMPLEXES[a]

MTX constituent	*E. coli*	*L. casei*	Type of interaction, comments
Pteridine ring	Ile-*4*	Leu-*4*	Hydrophobic
	Carbonyl of Ile-*4*	Carbonyl of Leu-*4*	H-bond to 4-NH_2; Section IIIB,2
	Peptide *5–6*	Peptide *5–6*	Hydrophobic or pi–pi; approaches N(1), C(2), 2-NH_2, and N(3)
	Ala-*6*[b]	Ala-*6*[b]	Hydrophobic
		Leu-*19*	Hydrophobic, pyrazine ring; see text
	Asp-*26*[c]	Asp-*26*[c]	Charge interaction and H-bonds; approaches N(1), 2-NH_2, and N(8); Section III,B,1
	Leu-*27*	Leu-*27*	Hydrophobic
	Phe-*30*[b]	Phe-*30*[b]	Hydrophobic
	Ile-*96*	Carbonyl of Ala-*97*	van der Waals/hydrophobic
	Thr-*116*[b]	Thr-*116*[b]	H-bond to 2-NH_2; Section III,F
		(nicotinamide-ring of NADPH)	(hydrophobic)
N(10) methyl	Ser-*48*	Ser-*48*	Hydrophobic; see text
p-Aminobenzoyl	Leu-*28*	Leu-*28*	Hydrophobic
	Ile-*49*	Phe-*49*	Hydrophobic; see Mathews *et al.* (1978)
	Leu-*54*	Leu-*54*	Hydrophobic, may be fully conserved; see Fig. 3
Glutamate	Lys-*31* or water	His-*28*	Charge interaction; see text
	Arg-*57*[b]	Arg-*57*[b]	Charge interaction and α-carboxyl H-bond

[a] Residue numbering is that for *L. casei* (Fig. 3). Structurally equivalent residues are on same line.

[b] Residues conserved in 4 DHFRs.

[c] Residues conserved among the 3 bacterial DHFRs.

also interactions differ in the two asymmetric units of the binary complex. There are indications in the literature (Section IV,B) that the glutamate side chain binding is relatively nonspecific and not essential for the enzymic process.

For the purpose of understanding the pharmacological action of inhibitors of DHFR the specific details of NADPH binding (Matthews *et al.*, 1979) are pertinent to a limited extent because of the enhancement of inhibitor binding in the ternary complex (Section III,B,4) which, in turn, implies that coenzyme binding will be involved in the enzyme blocking under physiological conditions. In the ternary complex, NADPH assumes an open conformation in contrast to the free solution case where a folded conformation with parallel stacking of the bases is thought to predominate (Matthews *et al.*, 1978). The adenine and nicotinamide bases [$C(6_a)$ — $C(2_n)$] are oriented almost perpendicularly and separated by 17 Å in the ternary complex. An unusual feature of the NADPH conformation when bound to DHFR is a deviation of almost 60° in the torsion angle about the C(5′) — O(5′) bond in the adenosine component, $\sigma_a = 122°$, from a value of approximately 180° found for 5′-nucleotides in mono- and dinucleotide crystal structures and in solution. This deviation in torisonal angle had previously in fact been quantitatively identified by some ^{31}P NMR results (Feeney *et al.*, 1975). Matthews *et al.* (1978) note the possibility of using this sort of structural information in designing new inhibitors containing parts of both substrate and cofactor and cite one example—lactate dehydrogenase—where this has already been achieved (Everse *et al.*, 1972). Further details of coenzyme binding are given in Sections III,C and D.

III. Physicochemical Aspects

A. Properties of Folates and Inhibitor Analogs

1. *General*

Blakley (1969) reviewed in detail the then current literature on the physicochemical properties of folates and pterins (pterin ≡ 2-amino-4-oxopteridine: see Fig. 2) and their 2,4-diaminoanalogs: only the most pertinent recent additions to the subject are discussed here. It is appropriate, however, to reiterate some major features of the earlier work in preparation for the discussion on the proposed mechanisms for binding to DHFR and the enzymic reduction, and, also, to restate some only partially resolved problems of pteridine chemistry that appear to be neglected in current discussions of these processes (e.g., Matthews *et al.*, 1977, 1978). The most notable feature of the folate literature is that there are two different approaches: that pursued by organic chemists studying the properties and reactions of pterins in the context of general pteridine and heterocyclic chemistry (Pfleiderer, Visconti, von Philipsborn, Albert, and co-workers) and that of biochemists and pharmacologists who are specifically interested in those pterin analogs involved in biological reactions.

Some general conclusions from pteridine chemistry (e.g., Albert, 1967) provide simple rationalizations for many of the observed biological properties and reactions of folates. The polarized — C = N — bonds of the pteridine ring system reduce the aromatic stabilization, although electron-releasing groups such as OH and NH_2 increase the stability. Conversely these substituents render the reduced derivatives less stable. In the pterin ring system the pyrazine ring is more susceptible to nucleophilic attack than the pyrimidine ring. Once aromaticity of the pyrazine ring is destroyed by one reduction step, the second reduction proceeds more readily (Section III,A,7): the observation that enzymic reduction of DHF proceeds more rapidly than that of folate may thus have a partly straightforward chemical foundation, although wide variation in the rate of enzymic reduction of folate relative to that of DHF, depending on the enzyme source, implies some contribution from the enzyme. These general considerations also indicate why protonation of the pyrazine ring should be preferred in the reduced folates and their 2,4-diamino counterparts although it is now established that protonation of the fully oxidized compounds occurs intially in the pyrimidine ring (Section III,A,2). Reduction of the pyrazine ring would also be expected to lead to a loss in planarity of the pteridine ring system: this prediction has been recently confirmed by X-ray crystallographic (Section III,A,6) and NMR results (Section III,A,5).

Two other aspects of pteridine chemistry are relevant to the purpose of this article—tautomerism and covalent hydration. Blakley (1969) noted that, although in general α-hydroxy heteroaromatics would be expected to exist in equilibrium between enolic and cyclic amide forms, the evidence for 4-hydroxy pteridines favors the cyclic amide structure (shown in Fig. 1). However, the possibility that an appreciable amount of the enol form is present at equilibrium was not discounted. More recent work (Elguero *et al.*, 1976) does not appear to have changed these conclusions. Theories that implicate binding of the enol form to DHFR are discussed in Section III,B,2. Covalent hydration in pteridines has attracted considerable attention (Albert, 1976, 1967; Ewers *et al.*, 1976): here a molecule of water is added reversibly across a — C = N — bond, multiple (nucleophilic) additions also being observed. Blakley (1969) noted that pterin and its 6-alkyl derivatives do not undergo detectable hydration at neutral pH and more recent studies also have not implicated hydration in folates or the 2,4-diamino analogs. However, the accumulated studies indicate that the phenomenon is a sensitive indicator of electron distribution in the ring system not only as a function of substituents but also under varying conditions of solvent, ionization state, etc. and may be able to provide some insight into the reactivity of the ring when bound to the enzyme by specific interactions. The site and extent of hydration also depend on the relative aromatic stabilization of the hydrated species and thus information in addition to that which can be obtained from ground state quantum mechanical calculations (Section III,A,8) of the electronic distribution is available.

One physical property of the present compounds which displays marked differences between folate and its reduced derivatives, and between folate and its 2,4-diamino analogs, is its relative insolubility in water. Blakley (1969) noted this unexpected characteristic and ascribed it to possible H-bonding or π-stacking intermolecular interactions. The results of ^{1}H NMR experiments using pH- and temperature-dependent techniques have suggested that this is due to the formation of dimers—but not higher aggregates—at increased concentrations (Pastore, 1971; Poe, 1973; Poe and Hoogsteen, 1978). MTX has a much lower degree of association than folate although parallel studies on N^{10}-methylfolate suggested this was partly due to the N(10) methyl group (Pastore, 1971). The studies of Poe and Hoogsteen (1978) showed a negligible degree of concentration-dependent association for THF. Poe (1973) proposed a head-to-tail coplanar ring stacking model for the dimers: on this model steric effects due to nonplanar substituents in the pyrazine ring in DHF and, also, a nonplanar pteridine ring in THF would account for reduced association compared with folate but the difference between folate and aminopterin is most likely due to different potentials for hydrophobic bonding in the two ring systems.

2. *Acid–Base Behavior*

Despite a great deal of early interest in possible differences between protonation sites in folates and their 4-amino 4-deoxy derivatives—as differential protonation had been implicated in theories of substrate and inhibitor binding (Baker, 1976)—it is only fairly recently that comprehensive results correlating measured pK_as with specific protonation sites have been available. Poe (1977) has redetermined the acidic dissociation constants for folic acid, DHF, N^{10}-methylfolic acid and MTX and summarized earlier results for THF and pterin. While earlier studies relied mainly on comparisons with model compounds and UV spectral changes, the more recent use of NMR methods has clarified some of the protonation site assignments.

For the purpose of this article the most pertinent pK' results [see Poe (1977) for experimental conditions] are as follows. For folic acid: N(1), pK' 2.35; N(10), pK' 0.20; N(5), p$K' < -1.5$; amide N(3), pK' 8.38. For DHF: N(5), pK' 3.84; N(1), pK' 1.38; N(10), pK' 0.28; amide N(3), pK' 9.54. For THF: N(5), pK' 4.82; N(1), pK' 1.24; N(10), pK' -1.25; amide N(3), pK' 10.5. For MTX: N(1), pK' 5.71; N(10), pK' 0.50; N(5), p$K' < -1.5$. The most noteworthy features are the shift in initial protonation from the pyrimidine to the pyrazine ring upon reduction of folate as predicted on general gounds in the previous section [note, also, indications that dihydroaminopterin is initially protonated on N(5) (Erickson and Matthews, 1972; Section III,B,1, and earlier work by Kisliuk and Levine (1964)] and the increased basicity of N(1) in the 2,4-diamino analogs compared with folate. The dissociations of the γ-carboxyl and α-carboxyl groups of MTX and THF are close to those of benzoylglutamate (p*K*s of 4.99 and 3.49, respectively) while solubility problems preclude their determination for DHF and folate (Poe, 1977).

3. *UV Absorption Spectra*

In the present context the major interest in the UV spectra of the folates and analogs has been in assigning the protonation sites of the free species and, more recently, in attempting to detect changes in the ionization state of substrates and inhibitors when bound to the enzyme. The interpretation of these latter studies (discussed in Sections III,B,1 and III,D,1) has been complicated by three factors: (1) some ionizations are not accompanied by significant UV spectral changes; (2) theoretical assignments of the pteridine spectra are not available with the result that changes produced solely by the enzyme environment are not understood; and (3) protonation in the bound state differing in site from that in free solution would be difficult to detect, particularly in view of factor 2. Spectral data for a large number of pteridines have been tabulated by Blakley (1969): the spectra show little fine structure. In accord with results for dissociation constants for the pterin and benzoylglutamate moieties showing similar constants in corresponding positions compared with folate (Poe, 1977), the UV absorption has been observed to be similarly additive suggesting little interaction between the two ring systems (although note complications at acid pH) (Huennekens, 1968). These results refer, of course, to molecules in their preferred solution conformation—presumably open (Section III,A,8): the X-ray results for the inhibitor complexes indicate a different orientation of the two ring systems but there is no suggestion of a close interaction.

4. *Resonance Raman Spectra*

Very recently Saperstein *et al.* (1978) obtained the resonance Raman spectra of MTX, aminopterin, folate, and N^{10}-methylfolate in the visible and UV regions, in basic and neutral aqueous solution. The spectrum for MTX in acidic solution—used for the enzyme complex spectral difference experiment discussed in Section III,D,3—was also reported. Tentative assignments for some features include a stretch in the phenyl ring (1615–1600 cm^{-1}), a pteridine ring stretch region (1410–1330 cm^{-1}) showing differences for the 2,4-diamino and 2-amino-4-oxo compounds, and a region at 1215–1180 cm^{-1} sensitive to the substitution at N(10). Assignment of other features was precluded by the lack of data for suitable model compounds.

5. *NMR Spectra*

The use of NMR in determining the ionization/protonation sites of the folates and analogs has been previously mentioned. Apart from general studies of the electronic and conformational structure which will be listed below, one important application of the technique has been the determination of the conformation of the tetrahydropyrazine ring of THF. The ^{1}H NMR results of Poe and Hoogsteen (1978) suggested that THF is a roughly equal mixture of two half-chair conformations, one with the C(6) proton axial and the other with the C(6) proton equitorial. The authors note that this lack of conformational preference is surprising considering the bulky C(6) substituent—6-methyltetrahydropterin, for instance, strongly prefers its 6-methyl group to be equitorial—but, also, point out the possible biological advantage of this conformational flexibility in increasing the versatility for binding to the different enzymes utilizing the cofactor and its derivatives. On the other hand the ^{1}H NMR studies of tetrahydropteroic acid and THF in 1 *N* NaOD solution of Furrer *et al.* (1978) showed that the tetrahydropyrazine ring exists in a half-chair configuration with a pseudoequitorial position of the C(6) side chain. The same conformation of the tetrahydropyrazine ring was obtained more recently for 5,10-methenyl-THF (Khalifa *et al.,* 1979). Further study of this conformational flexibility—particularly with respect to experimental conditions such as pH—is indicated.

A large number of NMR studies on pterin derivatives have been published recently: the sole use of ^{1}H NMR for this purpose suffers the disadvantage that pteridines possess only a relatively few nonexchangeable hydrogens. In consequence ^{13}C and ^{15}N NMR techniques have also been employed. The most relevant ^{1}H NMR studies are: pterins and their mono- and dications (Dieffenbacher *et al.,* 1966; Dieffenbacher and von Philipsborn, 1969); 5-formyl-6,7-dimethyl-H_4-pterin and 5,6,7,-trimethyl-H_4-pterin (Bieri and Visconti, 1974); 6-methyl-H_4-pterin and 5,6-dimethyl-H_4-pterin (Weber and Visconti, 1975); 6,7-dimethyl-H_4-pterin and 5,6,7-trimethyl-H_4-pterin (Weber and Visconti, 1976); 2,4-diamino pteridines and their 5,6,7,8-tetrahydro derivatives (Konrad and Pfleiderer, 1970); folates and MTX (Pastore, 1971; Poe, 1973); and THF analogs (Weber, 1976). ^{13}C NMR studies are available for pterin (Müller and von Philipsborn, 1973; Ewers *et al.*, 1974); folate, MTX, and other pteridines (Ewers *et al.*, 1973); DHF and THF (Frick *et al.*, 1974; Frick, 1976); H_4-pterin derivatives (Schirks *et al.*, 1976); and covalent hydration in pteridines (Ewers *et al.*, 1976). Schwotzer *et al.* (1978) have recently published ^{15}N NMR results for pterin and folic acid derivatives.

6. *X-Ray Structure Studies*

X-Ray crystallographic studies of folic acid or its reduced derivatives and of MTX have not been done: in the case of folic acid this is due to lack of success in obtaining crystals suitable for analysis (Camerman *et al.*, 1978). However, as the most needed structural information is that of the pteridine ring and in view of the negligible interaction between the two ring systems, X-ray structural studies on the pterin analogs should suffice. The most pertinent aspects are the degree of planarity of the ring system and, particularly, the configuration of the pyrazine portion and those of its substituents in various stages of reduction. More accurate information on bond length asymmetries for the atoms constituting the ring would be useful particularly to improve the input coordinates for quantum mechanical calculations (Section III,A,8).

Several crystal structures for dihydropterin and tetrahydropterin derivatives have been published recently. The structure for 6-methyl-7,8-dihydropterin monochloride-monohydrate (Bieri, 1977) showed a planar ring system protonated on N(5). The structure for 5-formyl-6,7-dimethyl-5,6,-7,8-tetrahydropterin (Bieri and Visconti, 1977a) indicated a distinctly flattened configuration: the two methyl substituents were in a cis-configuration, with the C(6) group axial and the C(7) group equitorial. The study of 5,6,7-trimethyl-5,6,7,8-tetrahydropterin-dihydrochloride-monohydrate (Bieri and Visconti, 1977b) showed a molecule, protonated at N(1) and N(5), in which C(6) deviates markedly from the mean plane of the other five atoms in the pyrazine ring: the C(6) methyl group is again axial. [The latter two compounds have also been studied by ^{13}C NMR (Bieri and Visconti, 1974)]. The crystal structure of xanthopterin (6-oxo-pterin)-hydrochloride (Bieri *et al.*, 1976) displayed an angle of about 2° between the planes of the pyrimidine and pyrazine rings. Also, finally, the structure of pteridine itself has been recently redetermined (Shirrell and Williams, 1975).

One final point concerns the configuration at C(6) of the naturally produced diastereoisomer of THF. The absolute stereochemistry at C(6) of the biologically active diastereoisomer of folinic acid has recently been defined as being (S) by X-ray studies on 5,10-methenyl THF (Fontecilla-Camps *et al.*, 1979). In very recent experiments, Charlton *et al.* (1979) enzymically reduced DHF to THF and converted THF to folinic acid: the active diastereoisomer of folinic acid was formed thereby defining the absolute stereochemistry at C(6) of the naturally produced THF as being (S). In an associated experiment (Charlton *et al.*, 1979) in which folate was enzymically reduced using (4*R*)[4-$^2H_1$]NADPH, the stereochemistry of the reduction at C(7) was determined by use of NMR methods on the resultant deuterated THF: the deuterium label had replaced the proton on C(7) which is cis to that on C(6), i.e., the *7-pro-S* hydrogen.

7. *Reduction Potentials*

Studies of the redox reactions of pterins in free solution show that the reaction pathway is determined by experimental conditions: Scrimgeour (1976) has summarized the available studies. It is generally agreed that polarographic reduction of 6-alkyl-pterins (and folate) initially produces the 5,8-dihydro derivative, but that it rapidly isomerizes to the 7,8-dihydro compound (Scrimgeour, 1976; Lund, 1976; Kretzschmar and Jaenicke, 1971). Scrimgeour (1976) states that reduction of the pterins to the 7,8-dihydro derivatives and then to the 5,6,7,8-tetrahydro derivatives is thermodynamically irreversible. The oxidation of the tetrahydroderivatives is thought to proceed to the 7,8-dihydro derivatives via the quinonoid-dihydro compound (Scrimgeour, 1976). Both oxidation and reduction are believed to be acid catalyzed. The 5,6-dihydro compounds have not been observed and the 5,8-dihydro compounds have not been isolated or clearly characterized physicochemically (Whiteley, 1971). The reduction potential of the pterin/5,8-dihydropterin couple at pH 7 has been estimated as −0.51 V (Kretzschmar and Jaenicke, 1971), that for 7,8-DHF/THF at pH 7.4 has been calculated as −0.18 V (Rothman *et al.*, 1973), and that for quinonoid-dihydropterin/tetrahydropterin was determined to be +0.15 V at pH 7 (Archer *et al.*, 1972).

To a certain extent these results do not provide a basis for understanding the enzyme-catalyzed reductions. First, the enzyme-catalyzed reduction of DHF to THF is known to be reversible in the presence of the $NADP^+$/NADPH couple. Second, the available evidence (Section III,F) does not support initial reduction of folate to 5,8-dihydrofolate in the biological process. Another point is that the results of polarographic and other studies indicate that reduction of the 7,8-dihydro compounds occurs via the protonated form as in other azomethine compounds (Lund, 1976): this is rationalized in terms of initial protonation of N(5) resulting in a displacement of electronic charge toward N(5) which facilitates nucleophilic addition of a hydride ion to the adjacent carbon [C(6)]. This is the basis of the proton-hydride mechanism for the DHFR-catalyzed reaction proposed by Huennekens and Scrimgeour (1964) which is reexamined in Section III,F,1.

8. *Quantum Mechanical Calculations*

Experimental difficulties in characterizing the sites of protonation of the folates and analogs stimulated attempts to determine this information theoretically by the use of molecular quantum mechanics (Perault and Pullman, 1960, 1961; Collin and Pullman, 1964; Neely, 1967, 1971; Kapoor, 1973; Gund *et al.*, 1977). Mixed success was achieved in predicting the protonation sites: this is due not only to necessary mathematical approximations inherent in the different computational procedures but also to basic limitations on predicting such solvent-dependent properties from calculations on isolated molecules.

More recently quantum chemical methods have been used in interpreting the NMR spectra of pterins (Bieri, 1976) and in studying conformations (Gund *et al.*, 1977). In the latter study the CNDO/II method was used to partially search the conformational freedom of the three major rotational angles in 7,8-dihydropteroylamide (i.e., glutamate residue omitted)—about the C(6) — C(9), C(9) — N(10), and N(10) — C(4′) bonds (see Fig. 2). Not surprisingly it was found that the extended form of the molecule was preferred although the preference was not very strong and more folded forms would not be expected to involve much strain. In fact the X-ray results for the enzyme–inhibitor complexes indicate that the pteridine and glutamyl moieties of MTX are not maximally separated from each other: this involves a nonparallel arrangement of the two ring systems.

B. Substrate and Inhibitor Binding Mechanisms

The primary emphasis of the models for inhibitor binding to DHFR has been in attempting to explain the large differences in tightness of binding between the 4-amino derivatives and the 4-keto substituted pteridine ring of the substrates: by illustration, Blakley (1969) notes that aminopterin binds 10,000–50,000 times (6–8 kcal/mole) more tightly to DHFRs than does folate. This feature has not yet been clearly explained. By contrast, considerably less attention has been accorded to the binding mechanisms for the *p*-aminobenzoyl and glutamate portions, although it should be noted a great deal of synthetic effort has gone into developing new potential inhibitors which would bind to and exploit species-specific differences in the "hydrophobic" site, thought to bind the *p*-aminobenzoyl group of folate analogs (Hitchings and Burchall, 1965; Baker, 1967): particularly as a result of the X-ray crystallographic results (Section II,B,2), these binding interactions are quite well characterized spatially and their relative contribution to the total binding of folate analogs has recently been determined (Roberts, 1977; Birdsall *et al.*, 1978; Section III,B,4).

Studies with folate and nonfolate analogs have shown that the primary requirement for a DHFR inhibitor is a 2,4-diaminopyrimidine ring (Hitchings and Birchall, 1965; Roberts, 1977): almost all the studies on nonfolate analog inhibitors designed to explore the species-specific possibilities of the hydrophobic binding site(s) have incorporated a 2,4-diaminopyrimidine ring—or a minor variation with the carbon atoms at positions equivalent to 4a or 8a in Fig. 2 replaced by nitrogen—into the inhibitor structure. However, while it is tempting to conclude that the conservation of strong binding properties to DHFR by a number of classes of inhibitors containing the 2,4-diaminopyrimidine ring implies similar binding of this moiety to the enzyme, the evidence accumulated by Baker (1967) suggested this was probably not the case. Also recent UV and NMR studies (Hood and Roberts, 1978; Cayley *et al.*, 1979) suggest that the 2,4-diaminopyrimidine ring of trimethoprim (Fig. 1) is not bound analogously to the pteridine ring of MTX.

The major portion of this section will review the numerous proposed mechanisms for the binding of the pteridine ring of substrate and inhibitors. The earlier alternatives will also be discussed: some of these such as the inverted-pteridine ring theory have been reaired recently (Matthews *et al.*, 1978), while others—for example, bound folate in the enol form (Zakrzewski, 1963)—have fallen into disfavor without any totally conclusive evidence being advanced against them (however, note Hood and Roberts, 1978). In order to assist the structure of the discussion the origin of the difference between 2-amino-4-keto-pteridine (pterin) and 2,4-diaminopteridine ring binding can be considered within the following categories.

1. Due to differences in the properties of the isolated substrate and inhibitor molecules that are reflected straightforwardly in the strengths or types of interactions on binding, otherwise similarly, to the active site—for example, potential for forming H-bonds.
2. Due to differences in the properties of the isolated molecules that are manifested in a complex manner when bound in a similar orientation in the active site—for example, protonated/deprotonated behavior or keto-enol tautomerism.
3. Due to a combination of simply—and complexly—expressed properties of the two classes of compounds that results in significantly different modes of binding to the active site region—for example, inverted pteridine ring.

It is also important to note here that although the experimental information on binding constants provides free energy differences for the interaction of substrates or inhibitors with the enzyme, the rationalizations of binding behavior in terms of numbers and strengths of different types of enzyme–substrate interactions are descriptions of enthalpy differences. The importance of entropy difference terms was recognized early (Zakrzewski, 1963) but had received little attention until very recently: Subramanian and Kaufman (1978) have reported calorimetric results for chicken liver DHFR and other experiments on *L. casei* DHFR are in progress (Roberts, 1978). The results of Subramanian and Kaufman (1978) indicate that at 25° the binding of NADPH and $NADP^+$ is characterized by small negative enthalpies and large positive entropies whereas the binding of folate, DHF, and MTX is accompanied by large negative enthalpies and small negative entropies: the substrate/inhibitor results differ qualitatively from those of Zakrzewski (1963). By studying the effects of varying the buffer on the observed heats of binding, Subramanian and Kaufman (1978) showed that the enthalpy of the MTX–enzyme interaction demonstrates a *net* proton transfer associated with binding: the authors advance reasons to support the thesis that MTX abstracts a proton from the buffer solution and binds in the cationic state, although the experiments cannot directly distinguish this effect from abstraction of a buffer proton by an enzyme group, followed by proton transfer to (bound) MTX. It is suggested that the large entropy contribution involved in coenzyme binding is due to a conformational change, rather than desolvation of hydrophobic interaction effects.

1. *Protonation/Ionic-Bond Model*

The earliest attempts to explain the difference in binding between substrates and inhibitors containing a 2,4-diaminopyrimidine ring noted the marked increase in basicity which accompanies the replacement of the 4-keto group by a 4-amino group (Section III,A,2) and proposed that a higher degree of protonation of the 2,4-diamino compounds (when bound) might lead to tighter binding as the result of an extra coulombic interaction (Baker, 1959). This proposal prompted most of the activity aimed at discovering preferred protonation sites reviewed in Section III,A. In order to rationalize the apparent differences in the modes of binding of pyrimidyl and pteridinyl inhibitors, Baker and Shapiro (1966) extended the idea by postulating a delocalization of positive charge within the protonated heterocycle in the bound inhibitor. This would retain the coulombic interaction with an acidic function of the enzyme while still allowing the heterocycle to adopt one of a number of possible orientations or rotational conformers in the active site thus enabling the inhibitor side chains to maximize their binding with the enzyme hydrophobic sites, H-bonding sites, or glutamate binding site.

Baker (1967) also used the protonation idea in presenting a model for the binding of both substrates and inhibitors that would explain the pH binding (and reaction) profiles in terms of both a weakly acidic group on the enzyme and on the ionization state of the inhibitor or substate. Thus if Py and $\overset{+}{\text{HPy}}$ denote nonprotonated and protonated forms of a pyrimidine ring then two types of enzyme complex could be formed:

$$\begin{array}{ccc} \text{E—R—H} & \underset{\text{H}^+}{\overset{\text{OH}^-}{\rightleftharpoons}} & \text{E—R}^- \\ \updownarrow \text{Py} & & \updownarrow \overset{+}{\text{HPy}} \\ \text{E—R—H---Py} & & \text{E—R}'\text{---}\overset{+}{\text{HPy}} \\ \text{(I)} & & \text{(II)} \end{array}$$

The difference between (I) and (II) depends on the degree of association of the proton with either the enzyme of Py group—i.e., on their relative acidity or basicity in the bound complex. This will determine whether the interaction resembles more closely a salt link (ionic bond) or a hydrogen bond. Using this model Baker (1967) was able to rationalize the effect of pH or the inhibition of DHFR by a variety of 2,4-diaminopyrimidine and -pteridine compounds.

In recent years a great deal of evidence supporting or contradicting the above models has become available. Also, unfortunately, the scope of recent discussion has been limited to explaining differences between substrate and aminopterin analog binding, with the wider issues of binding of pyrimidyl-type inhibitors and pH behavior not being considered in the development of modified theories. Another set of information which has not been digested by current theories is that for the 4-thio compounds: McCormack (1976) reported that the 4-thio analog of MTX was surprisingly not a potent inhibitor of either L1210 cell, *Trypanosoma cruzi*, or *L. casei* DHFRs while similarly low activity has also been found for the 4-thio derivatives in the quinazoline series (Hynes *et al.*, 1974). The protonation or tautomeric behavior of these compounds has not been discussed. Early results on the 4-thio derivatives of the pyrimidine compounds found that inhibitory activity against *L. casei* was in the order N > S > O: this result was rationalized in terms of H-bonding potential (Section III,B,2) assuming a predominant thiol tautomer (Hitchings and Burchall, 1965).

The evidence for the protonation model is summarized below.

1. UV and Raman spectral experiments (Section III,D) support the thesis that MTX (and aminopterin and N^{10}-formylaminopterin) binds to bacteriophage T4, *E. coli*, porcine liver, L1210 lymphoma, chicken liver, and

L. casei DHFRs (Erickson and Mathews, 1972; Neef and Huennekens, 1975; Poe *et al.*, 1974a, 1976; Gupta *et al.*, 1977; Hood and Roberts, 1978; Subramanian and Kaufman, 1978; Saperstein *et al.*, 1978) in a protonated form closely resembling that of the free inhibitor in acidic solution. The corresponding results for binding of folate, DHF, and dihydroaminopterin (Erickson and Mathews, 1972; Poe *et al.*, 1974a; Gupta *et al.*, 1977; Hood and Roberts, 1978) are less clear-cut due to complexities in the UV difference spectra. Briefly though, they do not support the idea that folate, DHF, and dihydroaminopterin are bound significantly as protonated forms resembling those of the free molecules in acidic solution: it is not possible to say whether these molecules are bound with a proton attached at a site other than the most basic one in solution. Note, again, that the calorimetric experiments (Subramanian and Kaufman, 1978) indicate *net* proton transfer only for MTX. This point is particularly important for the folates because of the suggestions of prior protonation in the reaction mechanism (Section III,F) and because folate and DHF differ significantly in protonation behavior (Section III,A,2), the former being initially protonated on N(1) in solution and the latter on N(5). For the case of dihydroaminopterin the above qualification is also pertinent: if it is assumed that dihydroaminopterin would be protonated in the bound form on N(5) —as it appears to be in free solution (Section III,A,2)—then if it were bound in a similar manner to MTX, the N(5) protonated form would be unsuited for forming the salt-link implicated in MTX binding. However, if the bound species were protonated on N(1)—quite likely in view of point 2 below—pyrimidine ring interactions with the enzyme similar to those formed by MTX would be possible and the almost stoichiometric inhibition of DHFR by dihydroaminopterin (Zakrzewski *et al.*, 1962; Kisliuk and Levine, 1964; Erickson and Mathews, 1972) could be readily explained. Finally, UV experiments (Hood and Roberts, 1978) indicate that the 2,4-diaminopyrimidine ring of trimethoprim is protonated when bound to *L. casei* DHFR.

2. An interesting result of the UV spectral studies of Hood and Roberts (1978) is that the pK_a of MTX is raised from 5.35 to 8.55 ($\pm$ 0.1) on binding to *L. casei* DHFR. Thus the protonated form of MTX binds 1600 ($\pm$ 300) times more tightly to the enzyme than the neutral form. However, at pH 7.5 where MTX is bound 2000 times more tightly than folate the difference in charge state still accounts for only one-third of the difference in binding energy between the two compounds (4.5 kcal/mole). A similar analysis for trimethoprim shows that it too shows an increase in pK_a on binding, but only from 7.22 to 7.90 ($\pm$ 0.1): this provides further evidence for the previously mentioned conclusion that the 2,4-diaminopyrimidine ring does not bind analogously to the corresponding ring of MTX, although more recent evidence (Roberts, 1979) suggests that the difference

in pK shift between MTX and trimethoprim binding reflects a difference in the mode of binding of the unprotonated, not the more relevant protonated forms. Hood and Roberts (1978) have argued that two-thirds of the difference in binding energy between folate and MTX is due to different enzyme conformational states in the two binary complexes.

3. In addition to the UV results, the fact that MTX binds more weakly to DHFR at higher ionic strength while the dissociation constant for folate is independent of ionic strength has been mentioned (Poe *et al.*, 1974a) in support of the idea that the bond between the protonated heterocyclic ring and the enzyme is more of the nature of a salt link or ionic bond (depicted schematically as II) rather than a less polar H-bond (species I). [This effect should be distinguished from the complex effect of ionic strength on substrate activity (Blakley, 1969; Poet *et al.*, 1976) which has found no specific explanation.] Although the glutamate side chains of folate and its analogs are expected to be ionized throughout the range of physiological pH values (Section III,A,2) they have not been implicated in any strong salt link to the enzyme. The X-ray results (Section II,B,2) indicated they were located near the surface of the enzyme in a hydrophilic environment and hence a strong charge interaction with the enzyme is unlikely. The X-ray and NMR results for *L. casei* (Matthews *et al.*, 1978; Matthews, 1979; Birdsall *et al.*, 1977a) indicating a charge–charge interaction between the γ-COO^- group and His-31(nonconserved; see Fig. 3) should, however, be noted again. But earlier chemical evidence (replacement of glutamate by neutral or positively charged residues (Section IV,B)) also mitigates against a strong salt link with the glutamate group.

4. Reference to the summary of specific MTX–DHFR interactions shown in Table I indicates a close association between Asp-29 (L1210 DHFR numbering; Fig. 3) and N(1) of the pteridine ring. Matthews *et al.* (1977) report that N(1) of MTX in the binary complex is approximately equidistant (2.7 Å) from both Oδ1 and Oδ2 of Asp-29 which in turn are about 3.3 Å from the 2-amino group and N(8) respectively. The X-ray results for the binary complex indicate that this region of the hydrophobic pocket was inaccessible to water while in the ternary complex the hydrophobic crevice is completely blocked off from solvent by the nicotinamide ring (Matthews *et al.*, 1978). These results suggest that the pK_a of the aspartate side chain would be considerably higher than that of a solvent-exposed group ($\sim$ 3.9) in the ternary and probably also the binary complexes. It is not known whether the hydrophobic pocket in the free enzyme is inaccessible to solvent or what the ionization state of Asp-29 is for the free enzyme. The suggestion that the Asp-29 proton is involved in the reduction mechanism is discussed in Section III,F,1. The general conclusion that the Asp–COO^- . . . H–N(1) interaction corresponds to the

observed salt link (Matthews *et al.*, 1978). However, a direct proton transfer within the binding site would appear to contradict the calorimetric experiments (Subramanian and Kaufman, 1978) indicating a net proton transfer unless a proton were to be added somewhere else during MTX–enzyme complex formation.

However, the major weakness with this explanation is that DHFRs from two animal sources have now been found not to have an aspartate residue at the equivalent position in the sequence according to the sequence alignment shown in Fig. 3. Although an alternative proton source for the reaction (the so far fully conserved Thr-136; Section III,F) may be available if necessary, the explanation for a salt-link with inhibitors for the animal DHFRs does not seem straightforward.

Some speculative comments on this problem are advanced below. It is possible, of course, that the amide assignments for residues 29 and 30 in the mammalian DHFRs are still wrong, although, as noted in Section II,A, this aspect has already been accorded particular attention. However, the difficulties alluded to above depend not only on the assignment itself but also on whether the alignment given in Fig. 3 is correct, i.e., whether residue 29 in the L1210 enzyme is indeed structually equivalent to the aspartate residues of the bacterial enzymes—the structural equivalence of the aspartate residues of *E. coli* and *L. casei* DHFRs was demonstrated by the X-ray results. If one started looking for an indication that this was not so, then inspection of the surrounding residues in the mammalian and bacterial enzymes may provide one. Thus it can be noted that residues 25 and 26 are proline in the L1210 enzyme [and also in the bovine liver enzyme (Peterson *et al.*, 1975b) while residue 25 is also proline in the mouse sarcoma enzyme (Rodkey and Bennett 1976] but that proline at position 27 is conserved for the three bacterial DHFRs. Note also Leu-26 is conserved among the bacterial DHFRs. As it is well known that the occurrence of proline residues places constraints on the configuration the backbone may adopt in its immediate vicinity, these differences in the array of prolines in what is thought to be a critical region for pteridine ring binding are surprising. [Note the implication of the fully conserved Pro-23 and Trp-24 residues in coenzyme binding (Section III,E,2).] An additional observation from Fig. 3 is that Leu-30 which is conserved between the *E. coli* and *L. casei* enzymes and has been implicated in hydrophobic interactions with the pteridine ring on the basis of the X-ray results (Table I) is replaced by a glutamate residue in the L1210 and bovine liver sequences (according to the alignment in Fig. 3). Note also the chemical modification study results for Met-30 in *S. faecium* (Section III,E,6).

This discussion leads obviously to the speculation whether the peptide bond of the glutamate residue in the mammalian enzymes occupies the corresponding position to Asp-29 in the bacterial enzymes or whether the extra methylene group in the side chain of glutamate (pK_a in solution ~ 4.3) compared with aspartate could allow almost equivalent positioning of the carboxyl functions. Such structural organization would allow conservation of a salt-link to inhibitors for both mammalian and bacterial enzymes to be explained, while inevitable differences between the detailed geometry of the hydrophobic pocket may provide a reason for the as yet unexplained fact that the 2,4-diaminopyrimidine type inhibitor trimethoprim binds to bacterial enzymes 30,000 times stronger than to mammalian enzymes (Roberts, 1977). However, while this rationalization may partially account for inhititor binding properties it involves fundamental difficulties in understanding the evolution of the DHFRs, namely, why nonconserved acidic residues should be present in a hydrophobic bonding pocket if they are not involved in essential bindng of the substrate or in the reaction mechanism.

2. *Differing H-Bond Potential Model*

Other early attempts at explaining the differences in binding of the 4-amino and 4-keto molecules noted their different potentials for forming H-bonds with the substituted pteridine ring (Zakrzewski, 1963; Blakley, 1969). Thus the 2,4-diamino ring is capable of forming four H-bonds with an enzyme—N(1) and N(3) as donors and two hydrogen atoms of the 2- and 4-amino groups as acceptors—while the 2-amino-4-keto ring could also form four H-bonds, but now N(1) and the 4-oxo group would be donors while hydrogens on N(3) and the 2-amino group would be acceptors. If the substrates were to be bound to the enzyme in the enol form instead of as the keto tautomer (Fig. 1) then the same disposition of H-bond donor and acceptor sites as for the 2,4-diamino ring would be possible (Zakrzewski, 1963). However, the overall free energy for binding the enol form would be less than for the inhibitors because of the energetically unfavorable tautomerism required before productive binding to the enzyme could occur (Zakrzewski, 1963).

The empirical evidence presented to implicate such differences in the observed binding tendencies was not judged definitive (Blakley, 1969). On the basis of the X-ray results, Matthews *et al.* (1977, 1978) offered some comments which, again, do not permit a confident assessment. Thus, although for the *E. coli* DHFR–MTX complex it was found that the carbonyl oxygen of an isoleucine residue (see Table I) can donate an H-bond to the 4-amino group it was noted that the backbone amide of a glycine residue (Gly-*98*, Fig. 3) was only 3.2 Å from the 4-amino group and was so positioned that it could donate an H-bond to the 4-keto group of a similarly bound folate molecule. However, for the *L. casei* ternary complex a small conformational change compared with the *E. coli* structure in the region of Gly-*98* meant that there was no H-bond donor close to the 4-substituent of MTX which might interact with an oxo group on the folate molecule (Matthews *et al.*, 1978). But note in passing that Gly-*98* and Gly-*99* are fully conserved residues (Fig. 3). [Also, note implication of Gly-*99* in coenzyme binding (Section II,B,1).] No specific H-bond was found to N(3) in either DHFR–MTX complex although N(3) together with N(1), C(2), and the 2-amino group was involved in an interaction with a peptide bond suggested to be of a hydrophobic or pi–pi nature (Table I).

While the enol binding hypothesis may be thought improbable on evolutionary grounds (Roberts, 1977) there is no definite evidence to suggest it is wrong, although the absence of the expected changes in the UV spectrum between the keto and enol forms on substrate binding (Section III,D,1) may be proposed against it. Unfortunately, planned X-ray structure studies on the enzyme–substrate complexes are unlikely to resolve this question because of the inherent imprecision in locating hydrogen atoms.

3. *Inverted Pteridine Ring Model*

In line with Baker's (1967) general suggestion that different classes of inhibitors containing the 2,4-diaminopyrimidine ring might adopt varying orientations within the ring-binding site, the particular possibility that the pteridine ring of the 2,4-diaminofolate analogs might be bound in an inverted orientation compared with the pteridine ring of the substrates is evident. This question was investigated by model building experiments in conjuction with the X-ray studies (Matthews *et al.*, 1978): it was found that rotation of the C(6) — C(9) bond by 180° and a 30° rotation about the C(9) — N(10) bond of the bound MTX pteridine ring would allow N(1) and N(8) to exchange positions approximately with C(4) and N(5), respectively, while a reasonable fit within the substrate binding crevice was still maintained.

As the direction of hydride transfer to C(6) from NADPH is now known from the X-ray studies, it would be possible to discriminate directly the orientation of the substrate molecule in the binding site if the absolute configuration about C(6) of the naturally produced THF were known. As noted in Section III,A,6, Charlton *et al.* (1979) have now determined the absolute configuration of naturally produced THF: their results indicate that the inverted pteridine model is correct.

4. *Inhibitor Fragment Binding*

Results accumulated from the many empirical studies have provided some general indications as to the relative importance of the binding of particular sections of the folate analog molecule: the contribution of the 2,4-diaminopyrimidine ring has already been discussed and the results for glutamate and C(9) — N(10) bridge region binding are dealt with in Section IV,A and B, while the pyrazine ring is thought probably to contribute little (Baker, 1967). Roberts and co-workers have investigated the binding of two fragments of MTX, *p*-aminobenzoylglutamate (PABG; Fig. 2) and 2,4-diaminopyrimidine (DAP) to *L. casei* DHFR; preliminary results, including those from NMR experiements, were reviewed by Roberts (1977) while comprehensive studies in which the equilibrium constants were determined by fluorimetric methods are reported by Birdsall *et al.* (1978). Birdsall *et al.* (1978) found that DAP and PABG bind cooperatively to the enzyme, PABG binds 54-fold more tightly to the enzyme–DAP complex than to the enzyme alone, and the reciprocal nature of the effect was confirmed. Evidence was presented which suggests that the cooperativity is due to conformational change rather than a direct interaction between bound ligands, and also for the fragments occupying the subsites which bind the complete MTX molecule. In the latter regard it is suggested by Matthews (1979) that a second binding site for PABG found by Birdsall *et al.* (1977a) to be noncompetitive with MTX is a nonspecific hydrophobic pocket normally used to bind the adenine portion of NADPH.

As an indication of the binding energies involved it is found (Birdsall *et al.*, 1978) that under conditions where the binding constant of MTX is approximately $2 \times 10^9\ M^{-1}$ ($\Delta G - 12.0$ kcal/mole), the binding constant of DAP is 1.28 (±0.08) $\times\ 10^3\ M^{-1}$ ($\Delta G - 4.22$ kcal/mole), that of PABG is 0.83 (±0.07) $\times\ 10^3\ M^{-1}$ ($\Delta G - 3.97$ kcal/mole), and the cooperativity (54-fold) is approximately -2.35 kcal/mole.

The effect on binding and cooperativity of *N*-alkyl substitution of PABG or 5- and/or 6-substitution of DAP was also studied by Birdsall *et al.* (1978). Parallel experiments on fragment binding to enzyme–NADPH complexes indicate a cooperative effect for binding both fragments (4.5-fold for PABG; 8.7-fold for DAP) but with little effect on the cooperativity of binding of the fragments themselves.

C. Coenzyme Binding

Only a few general aspects of coenzyme binding with some relevance to the pharmacology will be mentioned here: full details of specific interactions determined from the X-ray study are given elsewhere (Matthews *et al.*, 1979).

Most kinetic experiments on the binding of coenzyme to preformed enzyme–inhibitor complexes and of inhibitor to enzyme–coenzyme complexes indicate that the binding mechanism to form the ternary complexes is not ordered (Blakley, 1969; McCullough *et al.*, 1971; Birdsall *et al.*, 1978). However, some other work notably on types of *S. faecium* DHFR indicated a sequential mechanism with NADPH binding first (Blakley *et al.*, 1971; Cocco *et al.*, 1977; Williams *et al.*, 1979). Some insight into this difference may be gained from two other experimental findings—cooperative binding and interconvertible forms of DHFR. The equilibrium constant results of Birdsall *et al.* (1978) for *L. casei* DHFR and those of Williams *et al.* (1979) for *S. faecium* DHFR implied cooperative binding of folate analogs and coenzyme in forming the ternary complexes. Very recently the London group have measured the cooperativity between coenzyme and inhibitors accurately—it can be large (up to 200 times) and depends strongly on the structure of both coenzyme and inhibitor (Roberts, 1979). The calorimetric studies of Subramanian and Kaufman (1978) on chicken liver DHFR suggested that ordered binding was not enthalpically required but that enhanced binding in the ternary complexes must have an entropic origin. Using stopped-flow fluorescence techniques to study the kinetics of coenzyme binding to *L. casei* DHFR, Dunn *et al.* (1978) found that the enzyme existed in at least two interconvertible forms whose relative proportions are pH dependent: NADPH binds rapidly and exclusively to one of the forms. Another study by Pattishall *et al.* (1976) indicated *E. coli* DHFR existed as two species showing large differences in their affinities for the inhibitors trimethoprim and pyrimethamine. The two species could be interconverted via formation of a common ternary complex formed after binding trimethoprim (or DHF) but not pyrimethamine: thus only the formation of the trimethoprim–NADPH–enzyme complex involves strong cooperative effects. The significance of the study of Poe *et al.* (1974b) showing two binding sites for NADPH on *E. coli* MB1428 DHFR is not known, although note the suggestion of Huennekens *et al.* (1971). Multiple NADPH binding sites for *E. coli* RT500 and *L. casei* DHFRs have not been detected (Roberts, 1979). In general, spectral studies (UV, CD, and NMR; Section III,D) and calorimetric work (Subramanian and Kaufman, 1978) indicate an enzyme conformational change on binding NADPH: as noted in Section II,B this is not consistent with the X-ray studies although some conformational rearrangement of a loop important in binding the nicotinamide mononucleotide portion of NADPH was observed on coenzyme binding (Matthews, 1979; but also note difference between *E. coli* and *L. casei* coenzyme complexes, Section III,D,3). Improved resolution of the NMR signals of specific residues in the binary and ternary complexes (e.g., Roberts, 1977; Blakley *et al.*, 1978) suggests a loss of conformational freedom on formation of the complexes.

There is strong evidence from ^{31}P NMR studies (Feeney *et al.*, 1975; Birdsall *et al.*, 1977b) and calorimetric studies (Subramanian and Kaufman, 1978) than the 2′-phosphate group of NADPH and $NADP^+$ binds to DHFR as the dianion. Neef and Heunnekens (1975) studied binary complexes of L1210 DHFR with NADPH, $NADP^+$, DHF, and MTX, and ternary complexes formed by admixing NADPH and MTX, $NADP^+$ and THF, and acid-modified NADPH and DHF with enzyme: all the complexes migrated as stable well-defined bands by electrophoresis and were also stable to extensive dialysis. There have been a number of studies on binding NADPH analogs or fragments including those of Williams *et al.* (1977), Birdsall *et al.* (1977b), and Subramanian and Kaufman (1978).

In summary the above studies strongly suggest that folate analog inhibitor ternary complexes rather than binary complexes will be the biologically important form. The extent to which ternary complexes of other classes of DHFR inhibitors are pharmacologically relevant has not been routinely studied. For further studies on *in vivo* DHFR-reduced inhibitors (Section IV,A) specific details of NADPH binding from the X-ray study should prove useful in avoiding substituent groups likely to interfere sterically with coenzyme binding, and also possibly for indicating new substituent sites for which catalytic function is maintained.

D. Spectral Studies of Enzyme Complexes

A bibliography of UV, Raman, CD, and NMR results and a brief description of some pertinent points are given below.

1. *UV Spectra*

Most interest in this technique has focused on its use in determining the ionization state of the pteridine ring of bound substrates and inhibitors by comparison of the spectral difference curves obtained from the free molecules and enzyme curves, with those for the binary complexes, at different pH values. In this respect similar difference spectra for MTX binding to T_4 bacteriophage (Erickson and Mathews, 1972), *E. coli* (Poe *et al.*, 1974a), L1210 lymphoma (Neef and Huennekens, 1975; Gupta *et al.*, 1977), porcine liver (Poe *et al.*, 1976), *L. casei* (Hood and Roberts, 1978), and chicken liver (Subramanian and Kaufman, 1978) DHFRs, indicating MTX bound in a form similar to that of the free molecule at acid pH, were observed (Section III,B,1). By contrast the difference spectra generated by folate binding to T_4 phage, *E. coli,* and *L. casei* DHFRs are markedly different (Hood and Roberts, 1978): although folate is a substrate for all these enzymes, its activity relative to DHF does vary greatly from one enzyme to another. The DHF binding spectra for *E. coli* and L1210 DHFRs were reported to be very similar while the folate binding spectra were slightly different (Gupta *et al.,* 1977).

The difference spectra for binding NADPH and $NADP^+$ to *E. coli* (Poe *et al.*, 1974b) and L1210 (Gupta *et al.*, 1977) DHFRs were virtually identical. The NADPH difference spectrum for binding to the porcine liver enzyme differs considerably from those for *E. coli* and L1210 DHFRs (Poe *et al.*, 1976). However, in all three cases part of the spectral change on coenzyme binding was attributed to perturbation of one (or more) enzyme tryptophan residues (see Section III,E,2). Difference spectra for NADPH binding to L1210 (Neef and Huennekens, 1975) and *L. casei* (Gundersen *et al.*, 1972) DHFRs have also been reported. In contrast virtually no spectral difference was found for NADPH binding to T_4 phage (Erickson and Mathews, 1972). Furthermore, although in this study no spectral changes were observed on addition of NADPH to binary complexes of folate, DHF, or aminopterin, a change was detected for the H_2-aminopterin case. Neef and Huennekens (1975) report UV spectra for enzyme–MTX–NADPH, enzyme–DHF–acid-modified NADPH, and enzyme–THF–$NADP^+$ ternary complexes.

Hood and Roberts (1978) have presented a detailed analysis of the pH dependence of *L. casei* folate and MTX binding spectra and discussed their relevance to the binding difference problem. The MTX difference spectrum is characterized by three main features: (1) a pH-dependent change which was ascribed to the altered ionization state of MTX when bound, (2) a pH-independent peak which was suggested to be due to a perturbation of the pteridine ring on binding, and (3) a feature attributed to perturbation of an enzyme tryptophan residue on binding (also observed for the trimethoprim case). As a result of the increase in the pK_a of bound MTX from 5.35 to 8.55 $\pm$ 0.1, it was calculated that more than 90% of MTX is bound in the protonated form at pH 7.0. However, the results suggest that only about one-third of the binding free energy difference between folate and MTX is accounted for by the presence for binding protonated MTX rather than the unprotonated form (Section III,B,1). By contrast the folate difference spectrum was independent of pH over the range 5.3 to 8.5: its features were not readily interpretable. The observed pH independence at lower pHs allowed the authors to set an upper limit of 4.3 to the pK_a for protonation of bound folate, while at the higher pH values it implied that the amide dissociation (solution pK_a 8.38; Section III,A,2) was unaffected by binding of the enzyme. In view of the picture of a hydrophobic pteridine binding site developed from the X-ray results (Sections II,B,1 and III,B,1) it is somewhat surprising that the enzyme shows no preference for the neutral over the negatively charged form. In summary of the folate results it is suggested that folate is bound in the normal keto form and at pH 7.0 is more than 90% in the neutral ionization state (Hood and Roberts, 1978).

2. *Raman Spectrum*

The visible and UV resonance Raman spectrum of the *E. coli* DHFR–MTX binary complex was obtained at pH 7.0 by Saperstein *et al.* (1978): it was found to be similar in band positions and intensities to that of MTX in 0.01 *M* HCl. Consideration of the assignments of the MTX Raman spectral features noted in Section III,A,4 suggests that the spectral changes due to protonation on binding to DHFR (in the region 1410–1330 cm^{-1}) are directed toward the pteridine ring.

3. *CD Spectra*

CD spectra of the enzyme and its binary and ternary complexes with substrates, inhibitors, and coenzymes have been reported for DHFRs from *S. faecium* (Freisheim and D'Souza, 1971; D'Souza and Freisheim 1972), *E. coli* (MB1428) (Greenfield *et al.*, 1972; Greenfield, 1975), L1210 cells (Gupta *et al.*, 1977), and two strains of *L. casei* (Reddy *et al.*, 1978; Hood *et al.*, 1979). These spectra have been compared by Hood *et al.* (1979) who conclude that although ligand binding to DHFRs shows a number of constant features there is marked species-to-species variation in many of the observed spectral changes: the major points are summarized below. In addition a CD study on DHFR from soybean seedlings has been reported by Reddy and Rao (1977).

The CD spectrum of the MTX-resistant *L. casei* DHFR (Hood *et al.*, 1979) in the peptide region (~ 220 nm) closely resembled that for the *E. coli* enzyme for which an approximate secondary structure content of 10% α-helix and 50–60% β-sheet was calculated (Greenfield *et al.*, 1972). However, the X-ray structure for the *E. coli* DHFR–MTX binary complex indicated 18% α-helix and 30% β-sheet (Matthews *et al.*, 1977) with a similar backbone pattern being observed for the *L. casei* ternary complex (Matthews *et al.*, 1978). The L1210 DHFR backbone CD pattern is distinctly different from that of the above two DHFRs and was suggested to imply approximately 15% α-helix and only 15–25% β-sheet (Gupta *et al.*, 1977). A full spectrum for *S. faecium* was not reported in the far UV region (D'Souza and Freisheim, 1972). For soybean seedling DHFR a helical content of about 5% was calculated by Reddy and Rao (1977). In the 250–350 nm region the CD spectra for *E. coli* (Greenfield *et al.*, 1972) and *L. casei* (Reddy *et al.*, 1978; Hood *et al.*, 1979) are comparable in amplitude while those from *S. faecium* and L1210 cells show 4- to 8-fold greater intensity: the spectra vary considerably in wavelength, however, reflecting species differences in content, distribution, and environment of tyrosine and tryptophan residues.

For *L. casei,* binding of $NADP^+$ leads to relatively small changes centered on the 285–290 nm region: these were correlated with perturbations of aromatic residues produced specifically by the nicotinamide ring (Hood *et al.*, 1979). For *S. faecium* there was very little change in the peptide region suggesting no conformational change was occurring on $NADP^+$ binding (D'Souza and Freisheim, 1972).

However the spectra for NADPH binding are quite different from those for $NADP^+$ binding: except for *E. coli* (Greenfield, 1975) and soybean seedling (Reddy and Rao, 1977), all DHFRs show enhancement of the negative band at 340 nm (due to the dihydronicotinamide ring). A substantial increase in the band at approximately 270 nm seen in both *L. casei* studies and for the L1210 case [but not for *E. coli* (Greenfield *et al.*, 1972), soybean seedling (Reddy and Rao, 1977), or *S. faecium* (Freisheim and D'Souza, 1971)] is attributed to interaction with a specific tryptophan residue (Hood *et al.*, 1979), based on arguments from the chemical modification studies (Section III,E,2) and the NMR studies which indicated different binding for NADPH and $NADP^+$ (Kimber *et al.*, 1977). Only slight changes in the peptide region were noted for NADPH binding to L1210 and *L. casei* (Hood *et al.*, 1979) DHFRs. The clear difference between NADPH binding to *E. coli* and *L. casei* indicated in the CD spectra is pointed out by Hood *et al.* (1979); this result may be significant in interpreting the X-ray results.

For folate and DHF binding the most consistent feature for the five DHFRs is a positive bond at 290–295 nm that, however, varies substantially in amplitude from one source to another; however, the band is not present for folate binding to soybean seedling DHFR (Reddy and Rao, 1977). Binding of MTX results in a marked increase in the negative CD band at 220 nm for the *L. casei,* L1210 and *E. coli* cases [but not for *S. faecium* (D'Souza and Freisheim, 1972)] which could reflect a reorganization of secondary structure but may also be due to a transition of MTX itself (Hood *et al.*, 1979). In a number of respects the spectrum for MTX bound to *S. faecium* DHFR differs from those of the other DHFRs indicating a unique binding environment (Hood *et al.*, 1979).

Addition of $NADP^+$ to the MTX–binary complexes of *E. coli* (Greenfield, 1975) and *L. casei* (Hood *et al.*, 1979) DHFRs has little effect on the CD spectra: note, however, that the NMR spectra (Way *et al.*, 1975; Feeney *et al.*, 1977a,b) do show an interdependence of MTX and $NADP^+$ binding. By contrast, addition of NADPH to the MTX–binary complexes shows marked effects on the CD spectra: these are similar for the *E. coli* (Greenfield, 1975), L1210 and (one) *L. casei* (Hood *et al.*, 1979) cases although surprisingly the other *L. casei* spectrum (Reddy *et al.*, 1978) is totally different. For the first three studies there is little change below 310 nm but the long wavelength transitions of bound MTX are substantially perturbed clearly indicating an electronic interaction between the pteridine and dihydronicotinamide chromophores (Hood *et al.*, 1979).

The CD spectra for the ternary complexes of trimethoprim and NADPH with *E. coli* (Greenfield, 1975) and *L. casei* (Hood *et al.*, 1979) DHFRs indicated a substantial difference from NADPH binding: furthermore, this difference was species specific. For the ternary complex between the antimalarial agent pyrimethamine, NADPH, and the *E. coli* enzyme (Greenfield, 1975) the CD results indicated no effect on the binding affinity of NADPH from prior pyrimethamine binding.

4. *NMR Spectra*

NMR spectra for DHFRs from *L. casei, S. faecium,* and *E. coli* have been reported: only the scope of this work and a few details are mentioned here.

a. L. casei. The bulk of the NMR work has been performed on DHFRs from strains of this organism, by two independent groups (Pastore *et al.*, 1974a, 1976; and the London group: Way *et al.*, 1975; Feeney *et al.*, 1975, 1977a,b; Birdsall *et al.*, 1977a,b; Roberts *et al.*, 1974, 1977; Kimber *et al.*, 1977, 1978). Pastore *et al.* (1974a) reported general features of ^{1}H NMR spectra for substrates, MTX, and coenzyme binding. The effect on the ^{13}C NMR spectra of binding of folate enriched by ^{13}C in the benzoyl carboxylic group to DHFR and to the DHFR–NADP^{+} complex was also studied (Pastore *et al.*, 1976). The London group have been able to resolve individual resonances for approximately 20 amino acids and to study the effect on these residues of binding of inhibitors, substrates, and coenzymes. The C(2)–H peaks of the imidazole rings of the six histidines were studied by ^{1}H NMR (Roberts *et al.*, 1974; Birdsall *et al.*, 1977a). The five [or possibly four (Matthews, 1979)] tryptophan residues and the five tyrosine residues have been studied by ^{19}F NMR on DHFR containing 3-fluoro Tyr and 6-fluoro Trp (Kimber *et al.*, 1977, 1978; Roberts *et al.*, 1977) while the Tyr residues have also been studied by ^{1}H NMR on selectively deuterated DHFR (Feeney *et al.*, 1977a). The ^{31}P resonances from NADPH, NADP^{+}, and the coenzyme fragment adenosine-2′-phosphate (Feeney *et al.*, 1975, 1977b; Birdsall *et al.*, 1977b) and the ^{13}C signals from coenzyme enriched in the 3-carboxamido carbon of the nicotinamide ring (Way *et al.*, 1975; Feeney *et al.*, 1977b), in a number of binary and ternary complexes, have been reported. The general ^{1}H NMR spectra are discussed in earlier papers of the series (Roberts *et al.*, 1974; Way *et al.*, 1975). Part of the London work has been reviewed by Roberts (1977) and very recently Matthews (1979) has given a comprehensive analysis of the results in relation to the *L. casei* complex X-ray structure (Matthews *et al.*, 1978, 1979). In general, the *L. casei* results show varying enzyme residue shifts for binding of folate compared with DHF, of both substrates compared with MTX, and of their ternary complexes.

Some features of coenzyme binding are of particular interest. The study of Feeney *et al.* (1975) indicated that the 2′-phosphate group of NADPH (and $NADP^+$) binds to DHFR in the dianionic form and that its pK_a must be reduced by at least 3 units compared with the solution value: in the X-ray structure of *L. casei* specific interactions with the 2′-phosphate group from the side chains of His-*64*, Thr-*63*, and Arg-*43* were found (Matthews, 1979). Stabilization of the dianion by an electric field associated with a nearby helix dipole has been proposed (Hol *et al.*, 1978). It is suggested that the dianion interactions may account for the 100-fold difference in K_m for NADPH and NADH seen for DHFR (Feeney *et al.*, 1975). Feeney *et al.* (1975) also found that one nucleotide of NADPH changes conformation about the C(5′) — O(5′) bond by at least 50° upon binding to the enzyme: this result is in agreement with the X-ray findings (Section II,B,2). The results for coenzyme binding indicate that any differences between NADPH and $NADP^+$ binding must be strongly localized at the binding site for the nicotinamide ring (Feeney *et al.*, 1977b).

b. S. faecium. ^{13}C NMR studies of the arginine, methionine, and tryptophan residues using [*methyl*-^{13}C]Met (Blakley *et al.*, 1978; London and Avitable, 1979), [*guanido*-^{13}C]Arg (Cocco *et al.*, 1977, 1978), and [γ-^{13}C]Trp (London *et al.*, 1979) DHFRs have been reported. Between four and six peaks can be resolved for the enzyme's eight Arg residues: on the basis of folate, MTX, and NADPH binding studies it was suggested (Cocco *et al.*, 1978) that Arg-36 and Arg-70 were involved in interactions with the α- and γ-carboxyl groups of folate or MTX, while Arg-54 was implicated in coenzyme binding (see also Section III,E,1). Two of the four tryptophan residues were found to generate unusual resonances: this was suggested to indicate slow exchange of residues between alternative stable conformations, specifically in the region around these Trp residues as no similar evidence was found from the [^{13}C]Met or [^{13}C]Arg studies (London *et al.*, 1979). Sharpening of these resonances on binding 3′, 5′-dichloro-MTX was interpreted as a locking of the enzyme region into one conformation.

c. E. coli. The ^{1}H NMR spectra of the MB 1428 enzyme—including a discussion of the five histidine residues—for folate and MTX binding were reported by Poe *et al.* (1975). Recently ^{1}H NMR spectra for the two similar trimethoprim-resistant strains, MB 3746 and MB 3747, were compared with that of the MB 1428 enzyme (Poe *et al.*, 1979).

E. Specific Amino Acid Residue Studies

Studies on chemical modification of arginine, tryptophan, lysine, cysteine, histidine, and methionine residues on a number of DHFRs have been reported.

1. *Arginine*

Vehar and Freisheim (1976) reported that treatment of MTX-resistant *L. casei* DHFR with phenylglyoxal results in complete loss of enzyme activity which is concomitant with modification of five out of a total of eight arginine residues. In the presence of NADPH two of the five Arg residues are protected from chemical modification with complete retention of enzyme activity. Reference to Fig. 3 indicates two fully conserved Arg residues—Arg-54 and Arg-70. As noted in Section II,B, Arg-54 has been implicated in binding to the 2′-phosphate group of NADPH, while Arg-70 is bound to the α-carboxyl group of the glutamate moiety.

2. *Tryptophan*

Enzyme modification studies of selective oxidation of tryptophan residues with *N*-bromosuccinimide (NBS) have been reported on DHFRs from chicken liver (Freisheim and Huennekens, 1969), *S. faecium* (Warwick *et al.,* 1972), *E. coli* (Williams, 1975) and *L. casei* (Liu and Dunlap, 1974; Freisheim *et al.,* 1977). Note from Fig. 3 that only Trp-24 is fully conserved although the four DHFRs have between three and five Trp residues.

For the chicken liver enzyme, complete loss of activity was correlated with the oxidation of one Trp residue while for the *S. faecium* case it corresponded to oxidation of 2 Trps. Both studies indicated that prior incubation of the enzyme with either NADPH or DHF protected the enzyme from NBS deactivation. However, as Williams (1975) found that both substrates and coenzyme react with NBS the observed protection may be due partly to competition between the enzyme and small molecules for NBS. Initial treatment of the *E. coli* enzyme (Williams, 1975) with NBS resulted in a 40% decrease in activity concomitant with modification of one histidine and possibly one methionine residue before Trp oxidation. However, this 40% NBS-deactivated enzyme possessed full binding capacity for MTX and NADPH with unaltered K_m values for DHF and NADPH: it was suggested that the initial modification affects the proton transfer step (Section III,F). Further treatment with NBS gradually reduced the activity to zero while the capacity to bind MTX and NADPH was also reduced.

The studies of NBS oxidation of an MTX-resistant *L. casei* DHFR (Liu and Dunlap, 1974; Freisheim *et al.*, 1977) indicated selective oxidation of only one Trp residue: the oxidation correlated with the extent of enzyme inactivation and loss of ability to bind NADPH. Treatment of the NADPH–enzyme complex with NBS indicated protection of both bound NADPH and enzyme from oxidation; the presence of folates did not protect the enzyme from NBS inactivation. The sensitive Trp residue was identified as Trp-24 by Freisheim *et al.* (1977): in the enzyme–inhibitor ternary complex the side chain of this residue was found to be in van der Waals contact with the carboxamide portion of the coenzyme (Matthews, 1979). Roberts and co-workers have recently shown that NBS oxidation of Trp-21 decreases folate binding by only a factor of 2, but decreases that of NADPH by a factor of 200 (Roberts, 1979).

3. *Lysine*

Vehar *et al.* (1976) reported that MTX-resistant *L. casei* is virtually completely and irreversibly inactivated by relatively low concentrations of dansylchloride, which can be correlated with modification of a single lysine residue: only one out of nine Lys residues is affected. Incubation with inhibitor or coenzyme protected against inactivation: it was suggested that the dimethylaminonaphthyl moiety was interacting with a Lys in a hydrophobic region at or near the active side, the ϵ-amino group of the residue possibly having an abnormally low pK_a. This lysine residue was later identified as Lys-18 (Freisheim *et al.*, 1979).

4. *Cysteine*

Williams and Bennett (1977) found that treatment of *E. coli* DHFR with 5,5′-dithiobis(2-nitrobenzoate) (DTNB) resulted in modification of the two cysteine residues, one very rapidly: modification did not affect activity, or inhibitor or coenzyme binding. However, the presence of both NADPH and MTX greatly reduced the rate of modification of the slowly reacting Cys in the binary complexes. Phenylmercuric acetate and $CuCl_2$ react preferentially with the slowly reacting Cys and cause enzyme inactivation: prior substrate or coenzyme administration prevents inactivation. The rapidly reacting Cys was identified as Cys-175 while the slowly reacting one is Cys-100. The earlier studies of Warwick and Freisheim (1975) with *S. faecium* DHFR found that DTNB modification of the single Cys residue completely inactivates the enzyme: pretreatment with NADPH or DHF protects against deactivation. The *S. faecium* strain for which the amino acid sequence is reported (Fig. 3) does not have a Cys residue: there are, indeed, no fully conserved Cys residues for the four DHFRs in Fig. 3.

5. *Histidine*

Greenfield (1974) studied the effect of histidine modification of *E. coli* DHFR using ethoxy formic anhydride. Of five His residues, two react quickly with a loss of 50–60% of activity: DHF, MTX, or folate protect one of these from modification but the activity is not protected at pH 7.2. Binding of NADPH to the stronger of the two *E. coli* binding sites (Poe *et al.*, 1974b) protects one of the two rapidly reacting His residues and also prevents loss of activity at pH 7.2. Binding of both MTX and NADPH protects both His residues. Note that there are no fully conserved His residues in DHFR (Fig. 3).

6. *Methionine*

Gleisner and Blakley (1975a,b) studied the effect of carboxymethylation of methionine residues of MTX-resistant DHFR by iodoacetate. The first study correlated loss of 90% activity with modification of the equivalent of two out of seven Met residues while the latter study established that in fact four residues were being modified to different extents. Tryptic digestion studies (Gleisner and Blakley, 1975b) determined the four affected residues at Met-30, Met-40, Met-60, and Met-182 (Fig. 3). Aminopterin, and to a lesser extent folate and DHF, and also NADPH could protect the enzyme from the inactivation: the inhibitor effect was ascribed to protection from carboxymethylation of Mets 30 and 60 which were presumed to be in the region of the substrate/inhibitor binding site. Modification of Met-30 was thought to be responsible for loss of activity. Modification of the fully conserved methionine residue, Met-52, was not mentioned as a source of the loss of activity.

F. Enzyme Reduction Mechanism

For pharmacological purposes, examination of the reduction mechanism for DHFR is relevant because of recent interest in a new class of antifolate agents—those designed to act as substrates for DHFR but as inhibitors of later steps in folate utilization, notably the action of thymidylate synthetase (Section VI). *In vivo* reduction is necessary in many cases because of instability to oxidation of the reduced derivatives. The results of the empirical studies on the effect of alterations to the C(9) — N(10) bridge region of folates reviewed in Section IV,A suggest that the heteroatom must be separated by at least one carbon unit from the pteridine ring if substrate activity is to be maintained: the underlying reason may be a straightforward chemical one—i.e., thermodynamic stability of the ring toward reduction (redox potentials for the bridge analogs are not available)—or may derive from unknown constraints imposed by the enzyme-catalyzed reaction mechanism. Disruption of essential binding interactions does not appear to be a primary consideration for the activity of these bridge analogs.

The treatment here will briefly review the historical ideas and evidence in the light of more recent information and also suggest alternative mechanisms. Many details of the mechanism have not yet been elucidated. In particular the difference between the enzyme-catalyzed folate reduction and that of DHF is not well understood: in consequence the difference between DHFRs which can catalyze the reduction of both folate and DHF and those which can only assist DHF reduction is not known. Note, however, that both enzyme types can bind folate although nonfolate-requiring organisms cannot actively transport is. This difference may have a major structural basis but is more likely to be due to subtle energetic causes—note that the published X-ray studies have been on both folate-utilizing (*L. casei*) and nonfolate-utilizing (*E. coli*) organisms. Also, it has not been definitely established whether or not MTX is reduced on the enzyme—and if not why not (Section II,B,1). The complex pH-dependent activity of DHFRs from different sources (Blakley, 1969) has also not been explained: earlier theories (Baker, 1967) sought to rationalize this behavior in terms of substrate binding alone. Low-temperature trapping experiments are currently being undertaken to characterize the mechanistic steps (Fink, 1979).

Historical and Recent Ideas

The reduction mechanism generally proposed in the literature is the so-called proton-hydride mechanism originally due to Huennekens and Scrimgeour (1964). According to this theory the enzyme-catalyzed reduction of folate or DHF is to be considered a two-step process; initial protonation of the nitrogen [i.e., N(5) or N(8) of the C = N bond], followed by nucleophilic attack on the adjacent carbon atom [i.e., C(6) or C(7)] by the hydride ion from NADPH. This rationale was derived by analogy with the general reduction properties of folates in solution (Section III,A,7) and is also consistent with mechanisms proposed for other dehydrogenases. (Dalziel, 1975). In the latter context Baker and Ho (1964) suggested that the proton was donated by an enzyme histidine residue: the recent amino acid sequence studies (Section II,A) have not revealed a totally conserved histidine residue and the X-ray studies failed to show a histidine residue anywhere near the pteridine binding pocket in either *L. casei* or *E. coli* DHFR (Matthews *et al.*, 1978).

Matthews *et al.* (1978) note that the only potential proton donors in the neighborhood of the pteridine ring (in the enzyme-inhibitor complexes) are Asp-29 and Thr-136 (Fig. 3): although the current sequence results still indicate Thr-136 as totally conserved, Asp-29 is now known to be Asn-29 in L1210 and some other mammalian DHFRs. In discussing the possibility of Asp-29 acting as a proton donor Matthews *et al.* (1978) suggest that the highly hydrophobic environment in the ternary complex of the crevice in which the side chain resides would raise its pK_a so that it would be unionized. Now, with the finding that the pteridine ring of the substrates is bound upside-down compared with that of MTX (Charlton *et al.*, 1979) but assuming a similar disposition of enzyme groups in the binding pocket to that indicated by the X-ray results, it is apparent that Asp-29 could now be close to N(5). On the other hand, for folate reduction it is probable that preprotonation of N(8) would be required in the first reduction step (see below), and hence it is difficult to visualize proton transfer from the Asp-29 group. As the Oγ of Thr-136 is H-bonded to the 2-amino group of the pteridine ring in the inhibitor complexes, this difficulty would also apply to its possible role as a direct proton donor. Other possible mechanisms for the source of the proton added during the reductions, or for pyrazine ring rearrangements such as were described for solution reductions (Section III,A,7) will be discussed below. However, as alternative proposals must account for experimental evidence for sites of hydride transfer during the enzymic process, these results will be summarized first.

It was generally assumed (Blakley, 1969) that hydride is transferred from NADPH to C(7), and subsequently to C(6), during the enzymic reduction of folate to THF, and to C(6) during the reduction of 7,8-DHF to THF. From the results of tritium or deuterium labeling experiments, evidence has been presented for tritium transfer to C(6) during enzymic DHF reduction (Lorenson *et al.*, 1967; Pastore and Williamson, 1968; Poe and Hoogsteen, 1974) although another tritium study (Zakrzewski, 1966) suggested that label was transferred only to C(7) during both folate and DHF reduction. Because of the greater activity of DHFRs toward DHF reduction compared with that of folate it has not been possible to positively identify the intermediate product in folate reduction. Thus it is not possible to discriminate directly between initial 5,6- or 7,8-reduction. On the basis of model studies of nucleophilic addition to folate by bisulfite (HSO_3^-) in which the monoadducts can be identified, Scrimgeour (1976) suggested initial 7,8-addition as the most likely. The results of Charlton *et al.* (1979) (Section III,A,6) demonstrate that during enzymic reduction of DHF, attack by NADPH must occur at the *re*-face of the ring. Furthermore, during enzymic reduction of folate, hydride is transferred from the *4-pro-R* position of NADPH to the *si*-face of C(7), so that the hydrogen transfer to both C(6) and C(7) involves the same face of NADPH and the same face of folic acid. Thus, orientation of the oxidized and reduced pteridine rings of the substrates when bound to the enzyme does not differ fundamentally, although the orientation is inverted compared with that of

MTX. As previously noted, the model building experiments of Matthews *et al.* (1978) performed to explore the inverted-ring hypothesis indicated that a close approach between C(4) of the nicotinamide ring and the N(5) — C(6) bond was possible. While the results of Charlton *et al.* (1979) do not determine the order of the reduction steps for folate, the observed stereospecificity and retention of deuterium labels suggest initial 7,8-reduction: unless an initial 5,6-reduction product remained bound to the enzyme for a subsequent 7,8-reduction step, rapid isomerization in solution to 7,8-DHF would result in loss of any isotope label from an initial reduction at C(6).

Stereospecificity for hydride transfer from the A side of NADPH has been demonstrated for DHFR from chicken liver, mouse leukemic cells (Pastore and Friedkin, 1962), *S. faecium* (Blakley *et al.*, 1963), *E. coli* (Pastore and Williamson, 1968; Poe and Hoogsteen, 1974), and L1210 lymphoma cells (Gupta *et al.*, 1977). The X-ray results (Matthews *et al.*, 1978) confirm that the transferable hydride ion at C(4) of NADPH must come from the A side.

To return to the question of the mechanism for proton addition, some general considerations may provide insight: it is assumed here that normal solution-site protonation of folates in the enzyme complexes has not been established by the UV spectral difference experiments (Section III,B,1) and also that the calorimetric experiments (Subramanian and Kaufman, 1978) have indicated no net proton transfer on formation of the substrate binary complexes. First, during enzyme evolution structural constraints at the active site may have precluded development of a residue side chain donor capable of directly protonating both N(5) and N(8)—assuming folate-reducing and DHF-reducing capabilities arose in very similar DHFRs. Another aspect is that while N(5) in free 7,8-DHF is the most basic atom, N(8) and N(5) in free folate are only the third and second most basic atoms (Section III,A,2): therefore the N(1) and N(5) environments in bound folate would both need to be very hydrophobic before N(8) could be effectively protonated before reduction. In view of these difficulties it is pertinent to examine why preprotonation is thought to be necessary for the enzyme-catalyzed reaction. By analogy with solution reactions of the pteridines initial protonation may be expected to enhance the ease of hydride transfer: it will increase the overall reaction rate only if it is not rate-limiting. The particular environment of the enzyme-bound substrate pyrazine ring in the ternary complex (i.e., water excluded, specific interactions with the ring etc.) together with the entropic advantage due to the proximity of the hydride donor may make preliminary protonation unnecessary. Matthews *et al.* (1978) have noted the possibility that preprotonation elsewhere in the pteridine—specifically in the area accessible by the Asp-29 side chain—followed either by a proton jump within the pteridine ring, or proton rearrangement mediated by water either during the reaction or after release of products may be a possibility. Such a mechanism would probably have developed, however, only if a substantial enhancement of hydride transfer at C(6) or C(7) were produced. The other obvious possibilities are that the proton is simply abstracted from water directly by N(5) or N(8) after or (less likely) during the hydride transfer step. Which of these numerous alternatives is correct will have an important influence on the intermediate stages in folate reduction—i.e., whether the initial product dissociates and/or rearranges before the second reduction step—and, hence, has a bearing on the unresolved question of the mechanism of formation of the substrates ternary complexes (random or sequential; Section III,C).

Blakley (1969) presented data indicating the ability of DHFR to reduce a variety of folate derivatives: as previously noted, lack of information on the solution redox potentials of most of these compounds precludes judgment on whether their relative substrate activities are due soley to different binding affinities or interference with the reduction process. This point does not seem to have gained sufficient attention in the course of the search for *in vivo* reduced inhibitors of thymidylate synthetase (Section IV). Folate derivatives with an alkyl substituent at C(7) cannot act as substrates for DHFR (Blakley, 1969): this may be generally accounted for by steric hindrance to formation of an active ternary complex. The close fit of the pyrimidine ring in the active site region provides a simple explanation for loss of binding and substrate properties of a number of compounds altered in this region [e.g., N^2,N^2-dimethylfolate (Baker, 1967; Blakley, 1969)] but the rationalization of loss of substrate activity for compounds such as 2-desaminofolate (Baker, 1967) and 4-amino-4-deoxy folate is not so obvious.

It was suggested some time ago (Hitchings and Burchall, 1965) that production of a tetrahedral carbon atom at C(6) (and destruction of ring planarity) by 7,8-DHF reduction would assist disengagement of THF from the enzyme.

IV. Biochemical Aspects

A. Alterations to the C(9) — N(10) Bridge Region

Interest in the C(9) — N(10) bridge region of MTX has focused largely on developing compounds which retain the strong inhibitory power of MTX on DHFR but exhibit altered transport properties which may overcome the difficulties presented by MTX-resistant tumours. At the same time, similar modifications of folate derivatives have proceeded with the aim of producing compounds that are substrates of DHFR but inhibitors of thymidylate synthetase (or serine hydroxymethyltransferase) or which block the transport of folates. As the complexity and variability of the folate and MTX transport mechanisms have only fairly recently been appreciated (Section V,B), some of the results of early work reported here may be nongeneral—particularly with regard to tests on folate- or nonfolate-requiring species. Also, although the binding of the C(9) — N(10) (and phenyl ring) region was thought to be relatively nonspecific (Baker, 1971; Neely, 1971) in binary complexes, steric considerations in the ternary complexes due to the superposition of NADPH may ultimately impose limits on the size of substituents etc. (see Section II,B,1). Structures of the major classes of compounds discussed in this section are given in Fig. 4.

The bridge region has indeed been shown to tolerate structural changes in the folates involving the presence of substituents such as methyl, ethyl, formyl, and nitroso groups at C(9) or N(10) (Plante *et al.*, 1967) or replacement of the heteroatom by a methylene group (Struck *et al.*, 1971), with substrate activity for DHFR still being maintained. Plante *et al.* (1967) have observed that elongation of the bridge region by one or more carbon units and the introduction of halogens at the ortho-positions in the phenyl ring of the folate, homofolate (IV), or bis(homofolate) (V) skeleton actually enhances binding to DHFR, and all the derivatives tested were found to be effectively reduced by L1210 DHFR. However, all these enzymatically produced tetrahydrohomofolates inhibited *E. coli* thymidylate synthetase to varying degrees. Kisliuk and Gaumont (1970) further investigated the effects of the tetrahydrohomofolates. They found that *dl*, L-tetrahydrohomofolate (where *dl* is a diastereoisomeric mixture of the natural *l*-configuration at C(6) and the artificial *d*-configuration) *could* substitute as a cofactor for *L. casei* thymidylate synthetase and *S. faecium* serine hydroxymethyltransferase. Only the *d*,L-tetrahydrohomofolate diastereoisomer was found to inhibit the growth of *S. faecium:* this effect was ascribed to the blocking of folate transport.

The inhibition of *S. faecium* and *L. casei* by isofolate (VI) (Nair and

$$-(CH_2)_n-\underset{\displaystyle R}{\underset{|}{X}}-(CH_2)_m-$$

FIG. 4. Structural changes to the C(9)—N(10) bridge region of folate (or aminopterin or MTX). R ≡ H for folate or aminopterin, ≡ CH_3 for MTX. (III) $n = 1, m = 0, X =$ N[folate]; (IV) $n = 2, m = 0, X =$ N[homofolate]; (V) $n = 3, m = 0, X =$ N [bis(homofolate)]; (VI) $n = 0, m = 1, X =$ N [isofolate]; (VII) $n = 1, m = 1, X =$ N [isohomofolate]; (VIII) $n = 1$, $m = 1$, X deleted [N^{10}-deazafolate]; (IX) $n = 1, m = 0, X =$ O (R deleted) [10-oxafolate]; (X) $n = 1, m = 0, X =$ S (R deleted) [10-thiafolate]; (XI) $n = 1, X =$ N, $(CH_2)_m =$ NH [11-azahomofolate].

Baugh, 1974) and isoaminopterin (Nair *et al.,* 1974) was found to be similar to that of MTX. Interestingly, isopteroic acid did not inhibit *L. casei* even at five orders of magnitude higher concentration than required to inhibit *S. faecium:* it is suggested by Nair and Baugh (1974) that isopteroic acid might have use as an antibacterial since those organisms such as man and *L. casei* incapable of the biosynthetic attachment of the glutamyl residue would not be affected. Dihydroisofolic acid was not a substrate for the DHFR and isofolic acid was only weakly inhibitory (Nair *et al.,* 1974). Isoaminopterin was somewhat less inhibitory for the DHFR than aminopterin itself (Nair *et al.,* 1974).

Slavik *et al.* (1972) synthesized and tested isohomofolic acid (VII) and isohomoaminopterin. Both compounds inhibited the growth of *L. casei, S. faecium,* and HeLa and Sarcoma 180 cells in tissue culture, the latter compound being a considerably better inhibitor. Both compounds were competitive inhibitors but not substrates of DHFR, the inhibition by isohomoaminopterin being two orders of magnitude greater than that by isohomofolate. Results indicated active uptake of isohomoaminopterin. Nair *et al.* (1978) recently extended this work to the N^{10}-tosyl derivatives in order to study the effect of introducing bulky substituents at the N(10) position. N^{10}-tosylisohomoaminopterin—but not the folate analog—was a relatively poor inhibitor of *L. casei* DHFR. Neither compound was a substrate for the DHFR. Both compounds could be transported by the 5-methyl-THF transport system.

de Graw *et al.* (1974) found that N^{10}-deazaaminopterin and its dihydro and tetrahydro derivatives were strong inhibitors of the growth of *S. faecium* and *L. casei*–comparable with or stronger inhibitors than aminopterin. However, these compounds were considerably weaker inhibitors of DHFR than aminopterin and very weak inhibitors of thymidylate synthetase. N^{10}-deazapteroic acid (de Graw *et al.,* 1971; Struck *et al.,* 1971), N^{10}-deazafolic acid (VIII), and the 9,10-dehydro-derivatives of the two acids (Struck *et al.,* 1971) have been tested against *S. faecium:* antifolate activity was limited for the pteroic acid analogs and 9,10-deazafolic acid but strong for the folic acid analog itself. 7,8-Dihydro-N^{10}-deazafolic acid was a substrate for pigeon liver DHFR but the unreduced acid was mildly inhibitory and not a substrate (Struck *et al.,* 1971).

Nair and Baugh (1976) synthesised the 10-thia derivatives of folic acid (X) and aminopterin and compared their biological activities against those of isofolic acid and isoaminopterin. All four compounds were powerful inhibitors of the growth of *S. faecium* and *L. casei* but only the aminopterin derivatives inhibited DHFR, 10-thiaaminopterin being a stronger inhibitor than isoaminopterin and as strong as aminopterin. 7,8-Dihydro-10-thiafolic acid showed ~25% substrate activity compared with DHF (dihydroisofolic acid is not a substrate: see this section). On the basis of these results the above authors suggest that location of the heteroatom at least one carbon unit from the C(6) pteridine moiety is essential for proper enzyme–substrate/inhibitor interaction. Similar results for the 10-thia derivatives are reported by Mautner *et al.* (1976) who note in addition that neither the folate nor aminopterin derivative is a good inhibitor of thymidylate synthetase.

The 10-oxa derivatives of folic acid (IX) and aminopterin were studied by Nair and Campbell (1976). Both compounds were potent inhibitors of the growth of *S. faecium* and *L. casei* but while the aminopterin derivative was almost as strong an inhibitor of DHFR as aminopterin, the folate analog did not display enzyme inhibition. 7,8-Dihydro-10-oxafolic acid showed no substrate activity: comparison of this result with the substrate behavior of 7,8-DHF, 7,8-dihydrohomofolic acid, and 7,8-dihydro-10-thiafolic acid led the authors to postulate that substituents less electronegative than either sulfur or oxygen might elicit better substrate activity in this series.

The inhibitory effects of the 10-oxa and 10-thia derivatives have been further investigated in a detailed study of the transport behavior in HeLa cells (Rosemond-Hornbeak and Nair, 1978). HeLa cells have distinct transport systems for folate and MTX. 10-Oxaaminopterin inhibited both folate and MTX uptake whereas 10-thiaaminopterin selectively inhibited only MTX uptake. The thia- and oxa-analogs of folic acid effectively inhibited folate transport but not MTX uptake. The potential of using 10-oxaaminopterin in the treatment of MTX-resistant forms of cancer is discussed.

10-Formylfolate was discovered by d'Urso-Scott *et al.* (1974) during investigations of folate biosynthesis in rat liver. It is the most potent natural inhibitor of DHFR known and the authors suggested it might perform a regulatory function in the cell.

The 11-azahomo-derivatives of folate (XI) and aminopterin were studied by Slavik *et al.* (1969). Neither showed significant inhibitory effects on HeLa cells in tissue culture. The aminopterin derivative was a two-order of magnitude weaker inhibitor of DHFR from mouse liver than aminopterin and the folate derivative was not a substrate.

Finally in this section we note the results of Suster *et al.* (1974) on the effect of changing the position of attachment of the C(9) — N(10) bridge region to the pteridine ring to C(7) instead of C(6). The altered MTX derivative showed markedly decreased effectiveness against rat and mouse leukemias.

B. Alterations to the Glutamate Side Chain

Studies of the importance of the glutamate side chain on the biological activity of folate and MTX derivatives have investigated several features:

the influence of the optically active center of the glutamate, the effect of substituting other amino acid residues, the properties of polyglutamyl and other poly (amino acid) derivatives, and the effect of esterifying the carboxylate group(s). These studies have dealt with both the effects on binding to DHFR and other folate-dependent enzymes, and also with the effect on cellular uptake as the glutamate side chain is thought to be involved in the active transport processes for folate and MTX analogs (Section V,B). Baker (1971) notes that analogs with a dianionic glutamate side chain cannot enter cells by passive diffusion.

The D-form of DHF is reduced at only about half the rate of L-DHF in tissue extracts of murine cancer cells (Plante *et al.*, 1967). Lee *et al.* (1974) found that the D-form of MTX was a considerably less effective inhibitor of DHFR compared with the L-form.

In view of the X-ray results (Section II,B,2) showing a conserved interaction of DHFR with the α-carboxyl group but not the γ-group of the glutamate portion of MTX, it is interesting to analyze the experimental work incorporating changes in one or more of these regions. Thus Plante *et al.* (1967) found that methylation of the α-carbon resulted in a decreased rate of reduction of DHF while β- and γ-methylation caused little change; these results could be rationalized in terms of steric hindrance to the α-carboxyl binding interaction. Similarly Suster *et al.* (1978a) studied the effect by substituting amino acids containing either an α- or a γ-carboxyl group into MTX: they found that the α-COOH appears to be relatively more important in assisting binding to DHFR than the γ-COOH group. Rosowsky *et al.* (1978) studied the *in vivo* differences between α- and γ-monomethyl, ethyl, and butylesters of MTX: although the γ-monoesters were more active growth inhibitors than the isomeric α-monoesters, problems in the transport of esters (this section) do not allow a direct inference concerning the relative merits of α- versus γ-binding to DHFR.

Studies of amino acid substitution of the glutamate residue have clearly differentiated binding from transport effects. Lee *et al.* (1974) prepared MTX derivatives with L-glutamate replaced by D-glutamate, glutaric acid, and L-lysine: while all were inhibitors of DHFR only the D-glutamate derivative showed activity against L1210 mouse leukemia. Similarly the nine monobasic amino acid derivatives studied by Suster *et al.* (1978a) showed insignificant activity against L1210 leukemia *in vivo*. In another study Suster *et al.* (1978b) investigated whether a terminal glutamate is necessary for biological activity by synthesizing a number of dipeptides of MTX containing an initial neutral amino acid and either aspartate or glutamate as the terminal residue. Insertion of the extra amino acid between the *p*-aminobenzoyl and glutamate moieties gave compounds with borderline activity against L1210 cells while only one compound, the glycyl aspartate analog, exhibited moderate activity against both L1210 leukemia and W256 carcinosarcoma.

Early work on amino acid substitution in DHF and dihydrohomofolate by Plante *et al.* (1967) suggested that thymidylate synthetase was comparatively more sensitive to side chain changes than DHFR. Thus all the dihydro-derivatives studied were efficiently reduced by L1210 DHFR while only certain tetrahydro-analogs showed cofactor activity with *E. coli* thymidylate synthetase. The tetrahydrohomofolates inhibited the thymidylate synthetase to varying degrees, depending on the nature of the amino acid.

Interest has recently been shown in the polyglutamates of MTX because of growing evidence for a larger role in the clinical pharmacology. Thus it has been independently established (Baugh *et al.*, 1973; Brown *et al.*, 1974; Shin *et al.*, 1974; Whitehead *et al.*, 1975) that monoglutamate, MTX (G_1), and diglutamate, MTX (G_2), adducts of MTX accumulate in the liver and kidneys of animals treated with MTX. The structures of MTX (G_1) and MTX (G_2) have been established by chemical synthesis (Nair and Baugh, 1973). Both MTX (G_1) and MTX (G_2) are active inhibitors of DHFR and MTX (G_1) is about as effective as MTX in inhibiting the growth of L1210 leukemia cells *in vitro* and *in vivo* (Jacobs *et al.*, 1975; Whitehead, 1977). Surprisingly higher polyglutamates of MTX are not produced in measurable amounts in mammalian tissues although higher polyglutamates of reduced folates have been found to exhibit some important biological properties in both animal and bacterial cells (Coward *et al.*, 1974, 1975; Kisliuk *et al.*, 1974; Cheng *et al.*, 1975; Friedkin *et al.*, 1975; Plante *et al.*, 1976; Moran *et al.*, 1976). Baggott and Krumdieck (1979) have presented evidence supporting the hypothesis that regulation of one-carbon metabolism of folate-dependent pathways is achieved by enzyme-cosubstrate specificity mediated by alterations in the poly-γ-glutamyl chain length.

Other studies have focused on preparing poly-amino acid derivatives of folates or homofolates (Section IV,A) which would be substrates for DHFR but inhibitors of thymidylate synthetase. Plante *et al.* (1976) synthesized a series of N^{ϵ}-poly-α-glutamyl and N^{α}-polylysyl derivatives of N^{α}-pteroyllysine and N^{α}-homopteroyllysine: several of the compounds were up to 3.5 times as active as DHF as substrates for L1210 murine leukemia DHFR but none of the enzymatically prepared N^{α}-tetrahydropteroyllysine derivatives was as active as THF as a substrate for *E. coli* thymidylate synthetase. None of the enzymatically prepared tetrahydrohomopteroyl derivatives tested was as active as tetrahydrohomofolate as an inhibitor of thymidylate synthetase, although all were substrates for DHFR. It is noteworthy that substrate activity for DHFR is retained in spite of the positively charged poly (amino acid) side chain: this implies that the side chain extends into the solution and interacts little with the protein (note X-ray studies, Section II,B,2). This study complements an earlier series on single acidic or neutral amino acid replacements of the glutamate moiety of DHF or dihydrohomofolate, which gave qualitatively similar results (Plante *et al.*, 1967).

A large number of studies have dealt with the biological properties of esters of MTX (Rosowsky *et al.*, 1978, plus references therein). The underlying rationale was that lipophilic derivatives might enter cells by passive diffusion instead of active transport and therefore might be effective against MTX-resistant tumors. However, it was recognized that the derivatives might also act as prodrugs with free MTX being released as a result of cleavage by nonspecific esterases in the plasma. Although initial studies—mostly on rodents—indicated the latter effect was predominant, later work has established that the prodrug effect shows considerable species and organ variation with a partly inherent effect being involved in systems such as human lymphoblastic leukemia cells (Rosowsky *et al.*, 1978).

The polyglutamate derivative studies of MTX have also been extended to cover various esters. Rosowsky (1975) found that the monosodium salt of MTX (G_1) diethyl ester showed considerable activity against L1210 leukemia *in vivo*. Studies on the MTX-γ-L-glutamate diethyl ester, the isomeric α-derivative, and MTX-α,γ-bis(L-glutamate tetraethyl ester) showed less activity than MTX itself, with the γ-monoadduct being 10 times more active than the α-monoadduct (Rosowsky and Yu, 1978). This result is also consistent with the earlier observations in this section on the importance of α-carboxyl versus γ-carboxyl binding to DHFR. Rosowsky and Yu (1978) point out the potential adverse effects on antitumor activity of partial side chain racemization of MTX conjugates by enzymic or chemical hydrolysis *in vivo*, citing the previously mentioned results of Lee *et al.* (1974) on the effectiveness of the D-enantiomer of MTX.

C. Macromolecular Complexes of Methotrexate

Efforts aimed at enhancing the cellular specificity and/or ensuring a persistent concentration of unmetabolized drug at the enzyme target site have led to the synthesis of covalent complexes of MTX with soluble starch (Whiteley, 1971; Harding, 1971), serum albumins (Harding, 1971; Jacobs *et al.*, 1971; Chu and Whiteley, 1977), and immunoglobulins (Robinson *et al.*, 1973). Possible mechanisms for the cellular uptake of the drug—pinocytosis or active transport of the whole macromolecule, or cleavage of the MTX moiety at the cell membrane followed by active transport of MTX—are discussed by Harding (1971) and Robinson *et al.* (1973). The macromolecule may be attached to MTX either by a carboxamide link to the α-carboxyl group of the glutamyl side chain or by reactions of diazonium salts of the 2,4-diaminopyrimidine ring. The latter route would be expected to destroy the cytotoxic properties: however, the results of Robinson *et al.* (1973) did not seem to bear this out. The immunoglobulin and serum derivatives are effective in increasing survival time of mice injected with L1210 tumor cells, but the dextran derivatives are ineffective (Robinson *et al.*, 1973; Chu and Whiteley, 1977).

V. Folate Biochemistry

A. Relevance to Pharmacology

During the 1970s a large number of studies on aspects of folate biochemistry other than properties of isolated DHFR have contributed greatly to the understanding of the pharmacologic action of antifolate agents and, in particular, uncovered a variety of mechanisms whereby cells develop resistance to particular drugs. The most important aspects in the latter regard are impaired drug transport across cell membranes, alterations in the rate of synthesis of DHFR, and changes in the binding affinity of the enzyme for the drug. A valuable spin-off of the transport studies has been the recognition of the possibilities for developing a new type of antifolate agent which selectively blocks folate transport and may or may not also inhibit DHFR: the rationale is discussed in general in Section V,B while specific studies were noted in Section IV.

The importance of studying drug activity in intact cells is emphasized by recent studies (Goldman, 1975; Sirotnak and Donsbach, 1973) which show that although DHFRs bind MTX almost stoichiometrically (and, hence, are inhibited by *nanomolar* concentrations of MTX), intracellular drug levels considerably higher than that of the enzyme are required to suppress DNA synthesis to the point where cell replication is prevented. There are indications (White *et al.*, 1975; Flintoff *et al.*, 1976) that in the intracellular state, the enzyme may exist in high—and low—affinity forms with respect to interaction with the drug.

B. Folate Transport

Major features of folate transport pertinent to chemotherapy are summarized in this section. A comprehensive review of transport in bacterial and mammalian cells has been published recently by Huennekens *et al.* (1978); earlier reviews are by Goldman (1971, 1973), Huennekens *et al.* (1974), and Huennekens and Henderson (1976).

The studies of Huennekens *et al.* (1974) on the energy requirements, substrate saturability, pH and temperature dependence, and concentrative ability (about 200-fold) of folate uptake by *L. casei* cells indicated an active carrier-mediated process. A membrane-associated folate-binding protein was later isolated from *L. casei* (Henderson *et al.*, 1976); its properties and indirect evidence for a role in transport are described by Henderson *et al.* (1977). Although the evidence for *L. casei* suggests a single system for transport of a variety of folate compounds, there is great variability in the ability of other bacteria to transport folates—for example, *Pediococcus cerevisiae* does not readily transport folate and *S. faecium* is impermeable to both 5-methyl-THF and MTX (Huennekens *et al.*, 1978). The substrate specificity of bacterial transport systems may also be altered by mutation, and acquired resistance to MTX is usually due in part to a defective transport system. Bacterial transport systems also vary in their stereospecificity for THF derivatives: wild-type *P. cerevisiae* transports only the *l*-diastereomer of 5-methyl-THF whereas a mutant and also *L. casei* take up both *d*- and *l*-forms (Huennekens *et al.*, 1978). Although folate derivatives such as DHF, THF, aminopterin, and also their polyglutamates can serve as substrates for the *L. casei* transport system, fragments of the folate molecules cannot (Huennekens *et al.*, 1978). *L. casei,* and probably other bacteria, are able to regulate the transport of folate compounds by varying the amount or possibly state of activity of the transport binding protein (Huennekens *et al.*, 1978). In line with other transport studies on malignant cells, L1210 cells have their folate transport systems under the control of cyclic nucleotides (Huennekens *et al.*, 1978).

In contrast with bacterial cells some mammalian cells have two separate transport systems with varying specificities toward folate compounds. Thus for L1210 cells Nahas *et al.* (1972) found that MTX but not folate inhibited the uptake of 5-methyl THF or 5-formyl THF, but that neither MTX nor the two reduced compounds inhibited folate uptake: other examples are summarized by Huennekens *et al.* (1978). Further evidence for multiple transport systems is provided by studies of mutant sublines of L1210 and WI-L2 cells showing resistance to MTX (Jackson *et al.*, 1975; Niethammer and Jackson, 1975): thus the degree of impairment of MTX transport paralleled that for 5-methyl THF while folate transport was unaffected by the mutations. Very recent work by Suresh *et al.* (1979) indicates that folate uptake in L1210 cells is mediated by a transport system whose primary substrate is adenine. The relatively low affinity of this system for folate is explained by the authors in terms of its secondary importance to the system which transports 5-methyl THF, the principal form of the vitamin in the circulation of animals.

The above results for mammalian systems indicate that some folate antagonists have an extracellular target in addition to the intracellular enzyme, namely, the transport system for reduced folates. The success in cancer chemotherapy of "high-dose MTX" regimens used in conjunction with 5-methyl THF "rescue" can be rationalized in terms of blocking the uptake of the major vitamin, 5-methyl THF.

The uptake of 5-methyl THF in freshly isolated hepatocytes from rat liver was found by Horne *et al.* (1978) to be a complex process consisting of a primary saturable component inhibited by MTX, 5-formyl THF, and to a lesser extent folic acid, and a secondary nonsaturable component unaffected by high concentrations of these compounds. These active transport process(es) are composed of sodium-independent and sodium-dependent components and the efflux may also be an energy-dependent process.

Studies of folate-binding proteins from rat intestinal epithelial cells and rabbit choroid plexus are discussed by Huennekens *et al.* (1978): evidence for a direct implication in the transport process is not available, however. Huennekens *et al.* (1978) note the technical problems which have hampered the attempts to solubilize folate-binding proteins from L1210 cells. Work has recently been reported by Yang *et al.* (1979) with isolated membrane vesicles of L1210 cells showing intact transport systems for folate/folate analog uptake.

Mammalian and bacterial folate transport systems are sensitive to a variety of nonfolate analog inhibitors (references in Huennekens *et al.*, 1978) although most of these effects are attributed to inhibition of the energy-supplying system rather than specific components of the transport system. Some inhibitors can actually enhance the steady-state concentration of MTX in eukaryotic cells (references in Huennekens *et al.*, 1978); attempts at exploiting this effect in cancer chemotherapy by coadministration of nontoxic compounds with MTX have been reported (Bender *et al.*, 1975). Maintenance of a sufficiently high and constant intracellular concentration of MTX is a common problem in clinical chemotherapy although in some cases—for example, Ehrlich ascites tumor cells (Goldman, 1971)—sufficient concentrations of MTX can accumulate intracellularly to saturate DHFR and begin to inhibit thymidylate synthetase. Efforts to increase the effective concentration of intracellular drug by retarding its breakdown in animals are described in Section IV,C.

A general conclusion from the transport studies is that the molecular configuration of the folates necessary for binding to DHFR is distinct from the site that determines the affinity for the transport system. Thus, for L1210 cells the affinity of DHFR for 5-formyl THF is several orders of magnitude lower than that for MTX but the transport carrier appears to have an equally high affinity for both (Goldman, 1971). This finding has led to interest in the development of new folate analogs which retain a high affinity for DHFR but move across cell membrances at an increased velocity. In this respect attention has focused on the C(9) — N(10) bridge region and glutamate side chain of folates as discussed in Section IV. There have also been attempts to circumvent the active transport systems entirely using lipophilic folate derivatives designed to cross cell membranes by passive diffusion (Section IV,B).

C. Alteration to the Rate of DHFR Synthesis

A number of studies have been performed in order to elucidate the underlying mechanism for increased DHFR levels in MTX- or other drug-resistant cell lines. The results suggest a variety of causes for different bacterial and mammalian species.

It has been shown (Alt *et al.*, 1976; Hänggi and Littlefield, 1976) in MTX-resistant murine cell lines derived by progessively increasing the concentration of MTX in the growth medium that the consequent elevation in the levels of DHFR is due to an increase in the rate of synthesis. This increase is accompanied by a corresponding increase in translatable DHFR mRNA (Kellems *et al.*, 1976; Chang and Littlefield, 1976) and also a proportionate increase in the number of DHFR genes (Alt *et al.*, 1978; Nunberg *et al.*, 1978; Schimke *et al.*, 1978). Two general types of DHFR overproducing lines have been identified (references in Kaufman *et al.*, 1978)—those which retain their elevated levels of DHFR and MTX resistance when cultured in the absence of MTX and those which rapidly lose the elevated DHFR levels when cultured in the absence of the drug: Alt *et al.* (1978) and Schimke *et al.* (1978) have demonstrated that DHFR gene multiplication occurs in both stable and unstable resistant lines. Alt *et al.* (1978) advance arguments in support of a selective, but not a direct, mutagenic effect by MTX.

Kaufman *et al.* (1978) have extended these studies by use of a fluorescein derivative of MTX coupled with a fluorescence-activated cell sorter technique which allowed them to measure DHFR levels in individual cells in MTX-sensitive, -resistant, and -revertant mouse Sarcoma 180 cell lines. Most of the cell lines studied showed a linear relationship between cellular fluorescence intensity and both DHFR specific activity and rates of DHFR synthesis indicating little contribution from resistance mechanisms involving DHFR with low affinity for the MTX-derivative or alterations in MTX transport. The clinical possibilities for using the fluorescence-activated cell sorter technique in determining MTX sensitivities of cancer cells is noted by Kaufman *et al.* (1978).

Mechanisms other than gene multiplication have also been implicated in studies of increased DHFR synthesis in other species. On the basis of results obtained with *Diplococcus pneumoniae,* Goldberger (1974) suggested that DHFR regulates its own synthesis by modulating the gene specifying its protein structure. On the basis of results on *E. coli* DHFR regulatory mutants Sheldon (1977) has proposed that alteration of the levels of DHFR in different *E. coli* mutants is due to differences in efficiency of translational initiation of mRNA. Kaufman *et al.* (1978) have noted preliminary indications of DHFR synthesis induced by viral infection and in response to other promoters of DNA synthesis.

D. R-Plasmid Enzyme

Another mechanism of drug resistance that has been characterized is that of R-plasmid determined trimethoprim resistance in *E. coli* and *Citrobacter* sp. (Sköld and Widh, 1974; Amyes and Smith, 1974, 1976; Pattishall *et al.,* 1977). Two distinct types of R-plasmid DHFR have now been identified (Pattishall *et al.,* 1977) which show little difference from the chromosomal enzyme in the binding of DHF, NADPH, folic acid, or 2,4-diaminopyrimidine. However, these type I and II enzymes are several thousand-fold to hundred-thousand-fold less sensitive to MTX, aminopterin, and trimethoprim than the chromosomal enzyme, the type II enzyme being almost completely insensitive to these inhibitors.

E. Enzyme Polymorphism

There are several reported instances for DHFR polymorphism: in most cases a physiological role has not been discovered for the diversity. In the case of *L. casei* (Gundersen *et al.,* 1972), chicken liver (Huennekens *et al.,* 1971), and L1210 cells (Perkins *et al.,* 1967) the two forms observed by column chromatography and electrophoresis were identified as the free enzyme and enzyme—NADPH binary complex. Multiple forms of DHFR isolated from various strains of *S. faecium* have been shown to be genetically determined isozymes with different physical and kinetic properties (Nixon and Blakley, 1968; Albrecht *et al.,* 1969); their physiological role is ascribed to separate functions as folate and DHF reductases. The occurrence of polymorphism in hamster kidney cells (Hänggi and Littlefield, 1974), *D. pneumoniae* (Sirotnak, 1973), and bovine liver (Kaufman and Kemerer, 1976; Bauman and Wilson, 1975) has been established but the functional role is not understood. Baccanari *et al.* (1977) have isolated and studied the properties of two similar but noninterconvertible forms of DHFR from a trimethoprim-resistant strain of *E. coli* B (RT500). Interconvertible forms of DHFR from *E. coli* B (RT500) which differ in their binding affinities for trimethoprim and pyrimethamine in binary and ternary complexes have been studied by Pattishall *et al.* (1976).

F. Folate-Binding Proteins

It is appropriate to simply note some recent studies on soluble folate binding proteins in the liver, kidneys, and intestines of rats (Zamierowski and Wagner, 1976) and serum and milk (Waxman and Schreiber, 1977) although they *may* not be particularly important for an understanding of folate pharmacology. They have been implicated in intracellular storage of folates—possibly in a polyglutamate form. A recent review is given by Waxman (1976).

VI. Antifolate Pharmacology

A. General

The relationship between inhibition of DHFR and subsequent blockage of thymidylate formation was stressed in Section I and has been expanded on in subsequent sections. The relationship between DHFR and thymidylate synthetase was discussed by Dunlap *et al.* (1971) and a review of thymidylate synthetase as a target enzyme in cancer chemotherapy has recently appeared (Danenberg, 1977). Also the first sequence of the enzyme (for *L. casei*) has just been published (Maley *et al.,* 1979).

However, as also noted in Section I, the folate coenzymes are involved in a number of other 1-carbon transfer and reduction reactions in purine and pyrimidine, amino acid, protein, and lipid metabolism (Blakley, 1969; Silber and Mansouri, 1971; Rader and Huennekens, 1973; Taylor and Weissbach, 1973). Blakley (1969) noted that administration of folate analogs may have a number of metabolic effects many of which closely resemble nutritional folate deficiency. However, in assessing the experimental evidence as to which effects were responsible for the toxicity of folate analogs, Blakley (1969) concluded that blockage of DNA synthesis was the key factor: consequently the greatest damage in animals is in rapidly proliferating tissues such as intestinal mucosa and the hemopoietic system.

One particular aspect that should be mentioned is that MTX administration may produce neurological effects (references in Turner *et al.,* 1974): the roles of folate and pteridine derivatives in neurotransmitter metabolism are receiving increasing attention in the study of mental illness (Turner, 1977). As it was thought that brain contains very little DHFR (Makulu *et al.,* 1973) attention was directed to possible inhibition of dihydropteridine reductase which is involved in supply of the reduced pterin cofactor for the primary and rate-limiting step in the synthesis of catecholamines—the conversion of tyrosine to 3,4-dihydroxyphenylalanine (DOPA) by tyrosine hydroxylase (Musacchio *et al.*, 1971). The pterin cofactors are also required by the reactions catalyzed by phenylalanine and tryptophan (to produce serotonins) hydroxylases. Turner *et al.* (1974) confirmed that MTX inhibits dihydropteridine reductase from rat brain but also noted negative results by some other authors. Recently, however, Spector *et al.* (1977) isolated DHFR from rabbit brain: although its role in brain is unclear it was speculated that it might reduce 7,8-dihydrobiopterin to tetrahydrobiopterin, also a cofactor for brain tyrosine and tryptophan hydroxylases.

This article has described only the action of classical inhibitors in detail although very many other classes of compounds have been tested on DHFRs, particularly in search for new antibacterial or antimalarial agents. Baker (1967) systematized the results of his experiments in accord with his approach for rational drug design: references and analyses of Baker's and other workers' results may be found in the recent reports of Hansch and co-workers noted in Section I. In particular, there has been a great deal of interest in the quinazoline (5,8-deazapteridine ring) series (Hynes *et al.*, 1974; McCormack, 1976; Elslager *et al.*, 1978) including alterations to the C(9) — N(10) bridge region (Hynes *et al.*, 1977) and other alterations to the heteroatom structure of the pteridine ring (e.g., Lin *et al.*, 1979).

B. Conclusions

Most of the work reported here represents systematic biochemical and physicochemical studies on DHFR and its complexes, much of it performed with the direct aim of elucidating the pharmacological action of inhibitors at the molecular level. Associated problems of drug transport and acquired drug resistance have also been studied recently at a fundamental level. Although many physicochemical differences—in addition to shared conserved properties—between DHFRs from a number of organisms have been characterized, this information has not been translated into a form that would readily assist the design of species-specific inhibitors. Of particular interest are the differences between mammalian and bacterial DHFRs: basic information is already available from the amino acid sequences (Fig. 3) and insight into how these differences are reflected in the secondary and tertiary structures of the mammalian enzymes would be very useful.

A few concluding remarks regarding rational drug design are apt as the aim of much of the type of work reported here is to facilitate development of new inhibitors through a detailed understanding of the binding of substrates and known inhibitors. The study of classical inhibitors is central in the rational approach because it aims to "anchor" part of the inhibitor molecule in an analogous binding site to that of the corresponding portion of the substrate and then to explore and develop species-specific or stronger binding properties by modification or extension of other parts of the inhibitor molecule. (The search for new compounds that would be substrates of DHFR but inhibitors of thymidylate synthetase represents a variation of this theme.) It is likely that the most immediate benefits of the approach will result from systems displaying the substrate/inhibitor binding characteristics noted as points 1 and 2 in Section III,B—i.e., where binding differences are fairly straightforward reflections of the properties of the isolated molecules. In the "inverted-pteridine-ring" hypothesis (Section III,B,3) the choice between orientations is presumably a fairly subtle energetic one rather than a simple one of geometrical fitting: this type of phenomenon is very difficult to predict and detect using currently available theoretical and experimental techniques.

Acknowledgments

I am thankful for conversations and correspondence with Prof. A. Albert and Drs. A. L. Fink, W. G. Richards, and G. C. K. Roberts. Financial support from the Nuffield Foundation is gratefully acknowledged.

References

Albert, A. (1967). *Angew. Chem.* (Int. ed.) **6,** 919–928.

Albert, A. (1976). *Adv. Heterocycl. Chem.* **20,** 117–143.

Albrecht, A., Pearce, F. K., Suling, W. J., and Hutchison, D. J. (1969). *Biochem.* **8,** 960–967.

Alt, F. W., Kellems, R. E., and Schimke, R. T. (1976). *J. Biol Chem.* **251,** 3063–3074.

Alt, F. W., Kellems, R. E., Bertino, J. R., and Schimke, R. T. (1978). *J. Biol. Chem.* **253,** 1357–1370.

Amyes, S. G. B., and Smith, J. T. (1974). *Biochem. Biophys. Res. Commun.* **58,** 412–418.

Amyes, S. G. B., and Smith, J. T. (1976). *Eur. J. Biochem.* **61,** 597–603.

Archer, M. C., Vonderschmitt, D. J., and Scrimgeour, K. G., (1972). *Can. J. Biochem.* **50,** 1174–1182.

Baccanari, D. P., Averett, D., Briggs, C., and Burchall, J. (1977). *Biochemistry* **16,** 3566–3572.

Baggott, J. E., and Krumdieck, C. L. (1979). *Biochemistry* **18,** 1036–1041.

Baker, B. R. (1959). *Cancer Chemother. Rep.* **4,** 1.

Baker, B. R. (1967). "Design of Active-Site-Directed Irreversible Enzyme Inhibitors." Wiley, New York.

Baker, B. R. (1971). *Ann. N.Y. Acad. Sci.* **186,** 214–266.

Baker, B. R., and Ho, B. T. (1964). *J. Pharm. Sci.* **53,** 1457–1466.

Baker, B. R., and Shapiro, H. S. (1966). *J. Pharm. Sci.* **55,** 308–317.

Batley, K. E., and Morris, H. R. (1977). *Biochem. Biophys. Res. Commun.* **75,** 1010–1014.

Baugh, C. M., Krumdieck, C. L., and Nair, M. G. (1973). *Biochem. Biophys. Res. Commun.* **52,** 27–34.

Bauman, H., and Wilson, K. J. (1975). *Eur. J. Biochem.* **60,** 9–15.

Bender, R., Bleyer, W. A., Frisby, S.A., and Oliverio, V. T. (1975). *Cancer Res.* **35,** 1305–1308.

Bennett, C. D. (1974a). *Nature (London)* **248,** 67–68.

Bennett, C. D. (1974b). *Nature (London)* **252,** 511–512.

Bennett, C. D., Rodkey, J. A., Sondey, J. M., and Hirschmann, R. (1978). *Biochemistry* **11,** 1328–1337.

Bertino, J. R., ed. (1971). "Folate Antagonists as Chemotherapeutic Agents" (Ann. N.Y. Acad. Sci., Vol. 186).

Bieri, J. H. (1976). *In* "Chemistry and Biology of Pteridines" (W. Pfleiderer, ed.), pp. 721–724. De Gruyter, Berlin.

Bieri, J. H. (1977). *Helv. Chim. Acta* **60,** 2303–2308.

Bieri, J. H., and Visconti, M. (1974). *Helv. Chim. Acta* **57,** 1651–1657.

Bieri, J. H., and Visconti, M. (1977a). *Helv. Chim. Acta* **60,** 447–453.

Bieri, J. H., and Visconti, M. (1977b). *Helv. Chim. Acta* **60,** 1926–1931.

Bieri, J. H., Hummel, W.-P., and Visconti, M. (1976). *Helv. Chim. Acta* **59,** 2374–2379.

Birdsall, B., Griffiths, D. V., Roberts, G. C. K., Feeney, J., and Burgen, A. S. V. (1977a). *Proc. R. Soc. B* **196,** 251–265.

Birdsall, B., Roberts, G. C. K., Feeney, J., and Burgen, A. S. V. (1977b). *FEBS Lett.* **80,** 313–316.

Birdsall, B., Burgen, A. S. V., Rodriguez de Miranda, J., and Roberts, G. C. K. (1978). *Biochemistry* **17,** 2102–2110.

Bitar, K. G., Blankenship, D. T., Walsh, K. A., Dunlap, R. B., Reddy, A. V., and Freisheim, J. H. (1977). *FEBS Lett.* **80,** 119–122.

Blakley, R. L. (1969). "The Biochemistry of Folic Acid and Related Pteridines" (Frontiers in Biology, Vol. 13). North-Holland Publ., Amsterdam.

Blakley, R. L., Ramasastri, B. V., and McDougall, B. M. (1963). *J. Biol. Chem.* **238,** 3075–3079.

Blakley, R. L., Schrock, M., Sommer, K., and Nixon, P. F. (1971). *Ann. N.Y. Acad. Sci.* **186,** 119–130.

Blakley, R. L., Cocco, L., London, R. E., Walker, T. E., and Matwiyoff, N. A. (1978). *Biochemistry* **17,** 2284–2293.

Blaney, J. M., Dietrich, S. W., Reynolds, M. A., and Hansch, C. (1979). *J. Med. Chem.* **22,** 614–617.

Brown, J. P., Davidson, G. E., Weir, D. G., and Scott, J. M. (1974). *Int. J. Biochem.* **5,** 727–733.

Burchall, J. J. (1971). *Ann. N.Y. Acad. Sci.* **186,** 143–152.

Burchall, J. J. (1973). *J. Infect. Dis.* **128,** S437–S441.

Burchall, J. J., and Hitchings, G. H. (1965). *Mol. Pharmacol.* **1,** 126–136.

Camerman, A., Smith, H. W., and Camerman, N. (1978). *Biochem. Biophys. Res. Commun.* **83,** 87–93.

Cayley, P. J., Albrand, J. P., Feeney, J., Roberts, G. C. K., Piper, E. A., and Burgen, A. S. V. (1979). *Biochemistry* **18,** 3886–3894.

Chang, S., and Littlefield, J. W. (1976). Cell **7,** 391–396.

Charlton, P. A., Young, D. W., Birdstall, B., Feeney, J., and Roberts, G. C. K. (1979). *Chem. Commun.* 922–924.

Cheng, F. W., Shane, B., and Stokstad, E. L. R. (1975).*Can. J. Biochem.* **53,** 1020–1027.

Chu, B. C. F., and Whiteley, J. M. (1977). *Mol. Pharmacol.* **13,** 80–88.

Cocco, L., Blakley, R. L., Walker, T. E., London, R. E., and Matwiyoff, N. A. (1977). *Biochem. Biophys. Res. Commun.* **76,** 183–188.

Cocco, L., Blakley, R. L., Walker, T. E., London, R. E., and Matwiyoff, N. A. (1978). *Biochemistry* **17,** 4285–4290.

Collin, R., and Pullman, B. (1964). *Biochim. Biophys. Acta* **89,** 232–241.

Coward, J. K., Parameswaran, K. N., Cashmore, A. R., and Bertino, J. R. (1974). *Biochemistry* **13,** 3899–3903.

Coward, J. K., Chello, P. L., Cashmore, A. R., Parameswaran, K. N., DeAngelis, L. M., and Bertino, J. R. (1975). *Biochemistry* **14,** 1548–1552.

Dalziel, K. (1975). *In* "The Enzymes" (P. D. Boyer, ed.), 3rd ed., Vol. XI, pp. 1–60. Academic Press, New York.

Danenberg, P. V. (1977). *Biochim. Biophys. Acta* **473,** 73–92.

Dann, J. G., Ostler, G., Bjur, R. A., King R. W., Scudder, P., Turner, P. C., Roberts, G. C. K., and Burgen, A. S. V. (1976). *Biochem. J.* **157,** 559–571.

de Graw, J. I., Tsakotellis, P., Kisliuk, R. L., and Gaumont, Y. (1971). *J. Heterocycl. Chem.* **8,** 105–110.

de Graw, J. I., Kisliuk, R. L., Gaumont, Y., Baugh, C. M., and Nair, M. G. (1974). *J. Med. Chem.* **17,** 552–553.

Dieffenbacher, A., and von Philipsborn, W. (1969). *Helv. Chim. Acta* **52,** 743–763.

Dieffenbacher, A., Mondelli, R., and von Philipsborn, W. (1966). *Helv. Chim. Acta* **49,** 1355–1376.

Dietrich, S. W., Smith, R. N., Fukunaga, J. Y., Olney, M., and Hansch, C. (1979a). *Arch. Biochem. Biophys.* **194,** 600–611.

Dietrich, S. W., Smith, R. N., Brendler, S., and Hansch, C. (1979b). *Arch. Biochem. Biophys.* **194,** 612–619.

D'Souza, L., and Freisheim, J. H. (1972). *Biochemistry* **11,** 3770–3774.

Dunlap, R. B., Harding, N. G. L., and Huennekens, F. M. (1971). *Ann. N.Y. Acad. Sci.* **186,** 153–165.

Dunn, S. M. J., Batchelor, J. G., and King, R. W. (1978). *Biochemistry* **17,** 2356–2364.

d'Urso-Scott, M., Uhoch, J., and Bertino, J. R. (1974). *Proc. Natl. Acad. Sci. U.S.A.* **71,** 2736–2739.

Elguero, J., Marzin, C., Katritzky, A. R., and Linda, P. (1976). "The Tautomerism of Heterocycles" (Adv. Heterocyclic Chem. Suppl. 1). Academic Press, New York.

Elslager, E. F., Jacob, P., Johnson, J., Werbel, L. M., Worth, D. F., and Rane, L. (1978). *J. Med. Chem.* **21,** 1059–1070.

Erickson, J. S., and Mathews, C. K. (1972). *J. Biol. Chem.* **247,** 5661–5667.

Everse, J., Berger, R. L., and Kaplan, N. O. (1972). *In* "Structure and Function of Oxidation-Reduction Enzymes" (A. Akeson and A. Ehrenberg, eds.), pp. 691–708. Pergamon, New York.

Ewers, U., Günther, H., and Jaenicke, L. (1973). *Chem. Ber.* **106,** 3951–3961.

Ewers, U., Günther, H., and Jaenicke, L. (1974). *Chem. Ber.* **107,** 3275–3286.

Ewers, U., Gronenborn, A., Günther, H., and Jaenicke, L. (1976). *In* "Chemistry and Biology of Pteridines" (W. Pfleiderer, ed.), pp. 687–692. De Gruyter, Berlin.

Farber, S., Diamond, L. K., Mercer, R. D., Sylvester, R. J., Jr., and Wolff, J. A. (1948). *New Engl. J. Med.* **238,** 787.

Feeney, J., Birdsall, B., Roberts, G. C. K., and Burgen, A. S. V. (1975). *Nature (London)* **257,** 564–566.

Feeney, J., Roberts, G. C. K., Birdsall, B., Griffiths, D. V., King, R. W., Scudder, P., and Burgen, A. S. V. (1977a). *Proc. R. Soc. B* **196,** 267–290.

Feeney, J., Birdsall, B., Roberts, G. C. K., and Burgen, A. S. V. (1977b). *In* "NMR in Biol-

ogy" (R. A. Dwek, I. D. Campbell, R. E. Richards, and R. J. P. Williams, eds.), pp. 111–124. Academic Press, New York.
Fink, A. L. (1979). Private communication.
Flintoff, W. F., Davidson, S. V., and Siminovitch, L. (1976). *Som. Cell. Genet.* **2,** 245–261.
Fontecilla-Camps, J. C., Bugg, C. E., Temple, C., Rose, J. D., Montgomery, J. A., and Kisliuk, R. L. (1979). *J. Am. Chem. Soc.* **101,** 6114–6115.
Freisheim, J. H., and D'Souza, L. (1971). *Biochem. Biophys. Res. Commun.* **45,** 803–808.
Freisheim, J. H., and Huennekens, F. M. (1969). *Biochemistry* **8,** 2271–2276.
Freisheim, J. H., Ericsson, L. H., Bitar, K. G., Dunlap, R. B., and Reddy, A. V. (1977). *Arch. Biochem. Biophys.* **180,** 310–317.
Freisheim, J. H., Bitar, K. G., Reddy, A. V., and Blankenship, D. T. (1978). *J. Biol. Chem.* **253,** 6437–6444.
Freisheim, J. H., Kumar, A. A., Blankenship, D. T., and Kaufman, B. T. (1979). *In* "Chemistry and Biology of Pteridines" (R. L. Kisliuk and G. M. Brown, eds.), pp. 419–424. Elsevier, Amsterdam.
Frick, W. (1976). *In* "Chemistry and Biology of Pteridines" (W. Pfleiderer, ed.), pp. 695–702. De Gruyter, Berlin.
Frick, W., Weber, R., and Visconti, M. (1974). *Helv. Chim. Acta* **57,** 2658–2661.
Friedkin, M., Plante, L. T., Crawford, E. J., and Crumm, M. (1975). *J. Biol. Chem.* **250,** 5614–5621.
Fukunaga, J. Y., Hansch, C., and Steller, E. E. (1976). *J. Med. Chem.* **19,** 605–611.
Furrer, H.-J., Bieri, J. H., and Visconti, M. (1978). *Helv. Chim. Acta* **61,** 2744–2751.
Futterman, S. (1957). *J. Biol. Chem.* **228,** 1031–1038.
Gleisner, J. M., and Blakley, R. L. (1975a). *J. Biol. Chem.* **250,** 1580–1587.
Gleisner, J. M., and Blakely, R. L. (1975b). *Eur. J. Biochem.* **55,** 141–146.
Gleisner, J. M., Peterson, D. L., and Blakley, R. L. (1974). *Proc. Natl. Acad. Sci. U.S.A.* **71,** 3001–3005.
Goldberger, R. F. (1974). Science **183,** 810–816.
Goldman, I. D. (1971). *Ann. N.Y. Acad. Sci.* **186,** 400–422.
Goldman, I. D. (1973). *In* "Drug Resistance and Selectivity: Biochemical and Cellular Basis" (E. Mihich, ed.), pp. 229–358. Academic Press, New York.
Goldman, I. D. (1975). *Cancer Chemother. Rep.* **6,** 51–61.
Greenfield, N. J. (1974). *Biochemistry* **13,** 4494–4500.
Greenfield, N. J. (1975). *Biochem. Biophys. Acta* **403,** 32–46.
Greenfield, N. J., Williams, M. N., Poe, M., and Hoogsteen, K. (1972). *Biochemistry* **11,** 4706–4711.
Gund, P., Poe, M., and Hoogsteen, K. H. (1977). *Mol. Pharmacol.* **13,** 1111–1115.
Gundersen, L. E., Dunlap, R. B., Harding, N. G. L., Freisheim, J. H., Otting, F., and Huennekens, F. M. (1972). *Biochemistry* **11,** 1018–1023.
Gupta, S. V., Greenfield, N. J., Poe, M., Makulu, D. R., Williams, M. N., Moroson, B. A., and Bertino, J. R. (1977). *Biochemistry* **16,** 3073–3079.
Hañggi, U. J., and Littlefield, J. W. (1974). *J. Biol. Chem.* **249,** 1390–1397.
Hañggi, U. J., and Littlefield, J. W. (1976). *J. Biol. Chem.* **251,** 3075–3080.
Hansch, C., and Silipo, C. (1974). *J. Med. Chem.* **17,** 661–667.
Hansch, C., Silipo, C., and Steller, E. E. (1975). *J. Pharm. Sci.* **64,** 1186–1191.
Hansch, C., Fukunaga, J. Y., Jow, P. Y. C., and Hynes, J. B. (1977). *J. Med. Chem.* **20,** 96–102.
Harding, N. G. L. (1971). *Ann. N.Y. Acad. Sci.* **186,** 270–283.
Henderson, G. B., Zevely, E. M., and Huennekens, F. M. (1976). *Biochem. Biophys. Res. Commun.* **68,** 712–717.

Henderson, G. B., Zevely, E. M., and Huennekens, F. M. (1977). *J. Biol. Chem.* **252,** 3760–3765.

Hitchings, G. H., and Burchall, J. J. (1965). *Adv. Enzymol.* **27,** 417–468.

Hol, W. G. J., van Duynen, P. T., and Berendsen, H. J. C. (1978). *Nature* (*London*) **273,** 443–446.

Holbrook, J. J., Liljas, A., Steindel, S. J., and Rossmann, M. G. (1975). *In* "The Enzymes" (P. D. Boyer, ed.), 3rd ed., Vol. XI, pp. 191–292. Academic Press, New York.

Hood, K., and Roberts, G. C. K. (1978). *Biochem. J.* **171,** 357–366.

Hood, K., Bayley, P. M., and Roberts, G. C. K. (1979). *Biochem. J.* **177,** 425–432.

Horne, D. W., Briggs, W. T., and Wagner, C. (1978). *J. Biol. Chem.* **253,** 3529–3535.

Huennekens, F. M. (1968). *In* "Biological Oxidations" (T. P. Singer, ed.), pp. 439–509. Wiley (Interscience), New York.

Huennekens, F. M., and Henderson, G. B. (1976). *In* "Chemistry and Biology of Pteridines" (W. Pfleiderer, ed.), pp. 179–195. De Gruyter, Berlin.

Huennekens, F. M., and Scrimgeour, K. G. (1964). *In* "Pteridine Chemistry" (W. Pfleiderer and E. C. Taylor, eds.), pp. 355–376. Pergamon, New York.

Huennekens, F. M., Dunlap, R. B., Freisheim, J. H., Gundersen, L. E., Harding, N. G. L., Levison, S. A., and Mell. G. P. (1971). *Ann. N.Y. Acad. Sci.* **186,** 85–99.

Huennekens, F. M., Di Girolamo, P. M., Fujii, K., Henderson, G. B., Jacobsen, D. W., Neef, V. G., and Rader, J. I. (1974). *Adv. Enzyme Reg.* **12,** 131–153.

Huennekens, F. M., Vitols, K. S., and Henderson, G. B. (1978). *Adv. Enzymol.* **47,** 313–346.

Hynes, J. B., Ashton, W. T., Bryansmith, D., and Freisheim, J. H. (1974). *J. Med. Chem.* **17,** 1023–1025.

Hynes, J. B., Eason, D. E., Garrett, C. M., Colvin, P. L., Jr., Shores K. E., and Freisheim, J. H. (1977). *J. Med. Chem.* **20,** 588–591.

Iwai, K., Akino, M., Goto, M., and Iwanami, Y., eds. (1970). "Chemistry and Biology of Pteridines" (Proc. 4th Int. Symp. 1969). International Academic Printing Co., Tokyo.

Jackson, R. C., Niethammer, O., and Huennekens, F. M. (1975). *Cancer Biochem. Biophys.* **1,** 151–155.

Jacobs, S. A., d'Urso-Scott, M., and Bertino, J. R. (1971). *Ann. N.Y. Acad. Sci.* **186,** 284–286.

Jacobs, S. A., Adamson, R. H., Chabner, B. A., Derr, C. J., and Johns, D. G. (1975). *Biochem. Biophys. Res. Commun.* **63,** 692–698.

Kapoor, K. L. (1973). *Int. J. Quant. Chem.* **7,** 27–34.

Kaufman, B. T., and Kemerer, U. F. (1976). *Arch. Biochem. Biophys.* **112,** 289–300.

Kaufman, R. J., Bertino, J. R., and Schimke, R. T. (1978). *J. Biol. Chem.* **253,** 5852–5860.

Kellems, R. E., Alt, F. W., and Schimke, R. T. (1976). *J. Biol. Chem.* **251,** 6987–6993.

Khalifa, E., Bieri, J. H., and Visconti, M. (1979). *Helv. Chim. Acta* **62,** 1340–1344.

Kimber, B. J., Griffiths, D. V., Birdsall, B., King, R. W., Scudder, P., Feeney, J., Roberts, G. C. K., and Burgen, A. S. V. (1977). *Biochemistry* **16,** 3492–3500.

Kimber, B. J., Feeney, J., Roberts, G. C. K., Birdsall, B., Griffiths, D. V., Burgen, A. S. V., and Sykes, B. D. (1978). *Nature* (*London*) **271,** 184–185.

Kisliuk, R. L., and Brown, G. M., eds. (1979). "Chemistry and Biology of Pteridines" (Proc. 6th Int. Symp. 1978). Elsevier, Amsterdam.

Kisliuk, R. L., and Gaumont, Y. (1970). *In* "Chemistry and Biology of Pteridines" (K. Iwai, M. Akino, M. Goto, and Y. Iwanami, eds.), pp. 357–364. International Academic Printing Co., Tokyo.

Kisliuk, R. L., and Levine, M. D. (1964). *J. Biol. Chem.* **239,** 1900–1904.

Kisliuk, R. L., Gaumont, Y., and Baugh, C. M. (1974). *J. Biol. Chem.* **249,** 4100–4103.

Konrad, G., and Pfleiderer, W. (1970). *Chem. Ber.* **103,** 722–729.

Kretzschmar, K., and Jaenicke, W. (1971). *Z. Naturforsch.* **26b,** 225–228.
Lee, W. W., Martinez, A. P., and Goodman, L. (1974). *J. Med. Chem.* **17,** 326–330.
Lin, S.-C., Holmes, G. P., Dunn, D. L., and Skinner, C. G. (1979). *J. Med. Chem.* **22,** 741–743.
Liu, J. K., and Dunlap, R. B. (1974). *Biochemistry* **13,** 1807–1814.
London, R. E., and Avitabile, J. (1979). *J. Am. Chem. Soc.* **100,** 7159–7165.
London, R. E., Groff, J. P., and Blakley, R. L. (1979). *Biochem. Biophys. Res. Commun.* **86,** 779–786.
Lorenson, M. Y., Maley, G. F., and Maley, F. (1967). *J. Biol. Chem.* **242,** 3332–3344.
Lund, H. (1976). *In* "Chemistry and Biology of Pteridines" (W. Pfleiderer, ed.), pp. 645–667. De Gruyter, Berlin.
McCormack, J. J. (1976). *In* "Chemistry and Biology of Pteridines" (W. Pfleiderer, ed.), pp. 125–131. De Gruyter, Berlin.
McCullough, J. L., Nixon, P. F., and Bertino, J. R. (1971). *Ann. N.Y. Acad. Sci.* **186,** 131–142.
Makulu, D. R., Smith, E. F., and Bertino. J. R. (1973). *J. Neurochem.* **21,** 241–245.
Maley, G. F., Bellisario, R. L., Guarino, D. U., and Maley, F. (1979). *J. Biol. Chem.* **254,** 1288–1295, 1296–1300, 1301–1304.
Matthews, D. A. (1979). *Biochemistry* **18,** 1602–1610.
Matthews, D. A., Alden, R. A., Bolin, J. T., Freer, S. T., Hamlin, R., Xuong, N., Kraut, J., Poe, M., Williams, M., and Hoogsteen, K. (1977). *Science* **197,** 452–455.
Matthews, D. A., Alden, R. A., Bolin, J. T., Filman, D. J., Freer, S. T., Hamlin, R., Hol, W. G. J., Kisliuk, R. L., Pastore, E. J., Plante, L. T., Xuong, N.-H., and Kraut, J. (1978). *J. Biol. Chem.* **253,** 6946–6954.
Matthews, D. A., Alden, R. A., Freer, S. T., Xuong, N., and Kraut, J. (1979). *J. Biol. Chem.* **254,** 4144–4151.
Mautner, H. G., Kim, Y. H., Gaumont, Y., and Kisliuk, R. L. (1976). *In* "Chemistry and Biology of Pteridines" (W. Pfleiderer, ed.), pp. 515–522. De Gruyter, Berlin.
Moran, R. G., Werkheiser, W. C., and Zakrzewski, S. F. (1976). *J. Biol. Chem.* **251,** 3569–3575.
Morris, H. R., Batley, K. E., Harding, N. G. L., Bjur, R. A., Dann, J. G., and King R. W. (1974). *Biochem. J.* **131,** 409–411.
Müller, G., and von Philipsborn, W. (1973). *Helv. Chim. Acta* **56,** 2680–2687.
Musacchio, J. M., D'Angelo, G. L., and McQueen, C. A. (1971). *Proc. Natl. Acad. Sci. U.S.A.* **68,** 2087–2091.
Nahas, A., Nixon, P. F., and Bertino, J. R. (1972). *Cancer Res.* **32,** 1416–1421.
Nair, M. G., and Baugh, C. M. (1973). *Biochemistry* **12,** 3923–3927.
Nair, M. G., and Baugh, C. M. (1974). *J. Med. Chem.* **17,** 223–226.
Nair, M. G., and Baugh, C. M. (1976). *In* "Chemistry and Biology of Pteridines" (W. Pfleiderer, ed.), pp. 503–512. De Gruyter, Berlin.
Nair, M. G., and Campbell, P. T. (1976). *J. Med. Chem.* **19,** 825–829.
Nair, M. G., Mercer, L. P., and Baugh, C. M. (1974). *J. Med. Chem.* **17,** 1268–1272.
Nair, M. G., O'Neal, P. C., Baugh, C. M., Kisliuk, R. L., Gaumont, Y., and Rodman, M. (1978). *J. Med. Chem.* **21,** 673–677.
Neef, V. G., and Huennekens, F. M. (1975). *Arch. Biochem. Biophys.* **171,** 435–443.
Neely, W. B. (1967). *Mol. Pharmacol.* **3,** 108–112.
Neely, W. B. (1971). *Ann. N.Y. Acad. Sci.* **186,** 248–255.
Niethammer, D., and Jackson, R. C. (1975). *Eur. J. Cancer* **11,** 845–854.
Nixon, P. F., and Blakley, R. L. (1968). *J. Biol. Chem.* **243,** 4722–4731.
Nunberg, J. H., Kaufman, R. J., Schimke, R. T., Urlaub, G., and Chasin, L. A. (1978). *Proc. Natl. Acad. Sci. U.S.A.* **75,** 5553–5556.

Osborn, M. J., Freeman, M., and Huennekens, F. M. (1958). *Proc. Soc. Exp. Biol. Med.* **97,** 429–431.

Pastore, E. J. (1971). *Ann. N.Y. Acad. Sci.* **186,** 43–54.

Pastore, E. J., and Friedkin, M. (1962). *J. Biol. Chem.* **237,** 3802–3810.

Pastore, E. J., and Williamson, K. L. (1968). *Fed. Proc.* **27,** 764.

Pastore, E. J., Kisliuk, R. L., Plante, L. T., Wright, J. M., and Kaplan, N. O. (1974a). *Proc. Natl. Acad. Sci. U.S.A.* **71,** 3849–3853.

Pastore, E. J., Plante, L. T., and Kisliuk, R. L. (1974b). *Methods Enzymol.* **34,** 281–288.

Pastore, E. J., Plante, L. T., Wright, J. M., Kisliuk, R. L., and Kaplan, N. O. (1976) *Biochem. Biophys. Res. Commun.* **68,** 471–475.

Pattishall, K. H., Burchall, J. J., and Harvey, R. J. (1976). *J. Biol. Chem.* **251,** 7011–7020.

Pattishall, K. H., Acar, J., Burchall, J. J., Goldstein, F. W., and Harvey, R. J. (1977). *J. Biol. Chem.* **252,** 2319–2323.

Perault, A.-M., and Pullman, B. (1960). *Biochim. Biophys. Acta* **44,** 251–262.

Perault, A.-M., and Pullman, B. (1961). *Biochim. Biophys. Acta* **52,** 266–280.

Perkins, J. P., Hillcoat, B. L., and Bertino, J. R. (1967). *J. Biol. Chem.* **242,** 4771–4776.

Peterson, D. L., Gleisner, J. M., and Blakley, R. L. (1975a). *J. Biol. Chem.* **250,** 4945–4954.

Peterson, D. L., Gleisner, J. M., and Blakley, R. L. (1975b). *Biochemistry* **14,** 5261–5267.

Pfleiderer, W., ed. (1976). "Chemistry and Biology of Pteridines" (Proc. 5th Int. Symp. 1975). De Gruyter, Berlin.

Plante, L. T., Crawford, E. J., and Friedkin, M. (1967). *J. Biol. Chem.* **242,** 1466–1476.

Plante, L. T., Crawford, E. J., and Friedkin, M. (1976). *J. Med. Chem.* **19,** 1295–1299.

Poe, M. (1973). *J. Biol. Chem.* **248,** 7025–7032.

Poe, M. (1977). *J. Biol. Chem.* **252,** 3724–3728.

Poe, M., and Hoogsteen, K. (1974). *Fed. Proc.* **33,** 1382.

Poe, M., and Hoogsteen, K. (1978). *J. Biol. Chem.* **253,** 543–546, 4499.

Poe, M., Greenfield, N. J., Hirshfield, J. M., and Hoogsteen, K. (1974a). *Cancer Biochem. Biophys.* **1,** 7–11.

Poe, M., Greenfield, N. J., and Williams, M. N. (1974b). *J. Biol. Chem.* **249,** 2710–2716.

Poe, M., Williams, M. N., Greenfield, N. J., and Hoogsteen, K. (1975). *Biochem. Biophys. Res. Commun.* **67,** 240–247.

Poe, M., Bennett, C. D., Donoghue, D., Hirshfield, J. M., Williams, M. N., and Hoogsteen, K. (1976). *In* "Chemistry and Biology of Pteridines" (W. Pfleiderer, ed.), pp. 51–58. De Gruyter, Berlin.

Poe, M., Breeze, A. S., Wu, J. K., Short, C. R., Jr., and Hoogsteen, K. (1979). *J. Biol. Chem.* **254,** 1799–1805.

Rader, J. I., and Huennekens, F. M. (1973). *In* "The Enzymes" (B. D. Boyer, ed.), 3rd ed., Vol. IX, pp. 197–223. Academic Press, New York.

Reddy, V. A., and Rao, N. A. (1977). *Arch. Biochem. Biophys.* **183,** 90–97.

Reddy, A. V., Behnke, W. D., and Freisheim, J. H. (1978). *Biochim. Biophys. Acta* **533,** 415–427.

Roberts, G. C. K. (1977). *In* "Drug Action at the Molecular Level" (G. C. K. Roberts, ed.), pp. 127–150. Macmillan, New York.

Roberts, G. C. K. (1978). Private communication.

Roberts, G. C. K. (1979). Private communication.

Roberts, G. C. K., Feeney, J., Burgen, A. S. V., Yuferov, V., Dann, J. G., and Bjur, R. (1974). *Biochemistry* **13,** 5351–5357.

Roberts, G. C. K., Feeney, J., Birdsall, B., Kimber, B., Griffiths, D. V., King, R. W., and Burgen, A. S. V. (1977). *In* "NMR in Biology" (R. A. Dwek, I. D. Campbell, R. E. Richards, and R. J. P. Williams, eds.), pp. 95–109. Academic Press, New York.

Robinson, D. A., Whiteley, J. M., and Harding, N. G. L. (1973). *Biochem. Soc. Trans.* **1,** 722–726.

Rodkey, J. A., and Bennett, C. D. (1976). *Biochem. Biophys. Res. Commun.* **72,** 1407–1413.

Rosemond-Hornbeak, H., and Nair, M. G. (1978). *Mol. Pharmocol.* **14,** 299–305.

Rosowsky, A. (1975). *Proc. Am. Assoc. Cancer Res.* **16,** 144.

Rosowsky, A., and Yu, C.-S. (1978). *J. Med. Chem.* **21,** 170–175.

Rosowsky, A., Beardsley, G. P., Ensminger, W. D., Lazarus, H., and Yu, C.-S. (1978). *J. Med. Chem.* **21,** 380–386.

Rothman, S. W., Kisliuk, R. L., and Langerman, N. (1973). *J. Biol. Chem.* **248,** 7845–7851.

Saperstein, D. D., Rein, A. J., Poe, M., and Leahy, M. F. (1978). *J. Am. Chem. Soc.* **100,** 4296–4300.

Schimke, R. T., Alt, F. W., Kellems, R. E., Kaufman, R. J., and Bertino, J. R. (1978). *Cold Spring Harbor Symp. Quant. Biol.* **42,** 649–657.

Schircks, B., Bieri, J. H., and Visconti, M. (1976). *Helv. Chim. Acta* **59,** 248–252.

Scrimgeour, K. G. (1976). *In* "Chemistry and Biology of Pteridines" (W. Pfleiderer, ed.), pp. 731–751. De Gruyter, Berlin.

Schwotzer, W., Bieri, J. H., Visconti, M., and von Philipsborn, W. (1978). *Helv. Chim. Acta* **61,** 2108–2115.

Seeger, D. R., Smith, J. M., Jr., and Hultiquist, M. E. (1947). *J. Am. Chem. Soc.* **69,** 2567.

Sheldon, R. (1977). *Mol. Gen. Genet.* **147,** 91–97.

Shin, Y. S., Buehring, K. U., and Stokstad, E. L. R. (1974). *J. Biol. Chem.* **249,** 5772–5777.

Shirrell, C. D., and Williams, D. E. (1975). *J. C. S. Perkin* **II,** 40–43.

Silber, R., and Mansouri, A. (1971). *Ann. N.Y. Acad. Sci.* **186,** 55–69.

Silipo, C., and Hansch, C. (1975). *J. Am. Chem. Soc.* **97,** 6849–6861.

Silipo, C., and Hansch, C. (1976). *J. Med. Chem.* **19,** 62–71.

Simon, Z., Badilescu, I., and Racovitan, T. (1977). *J. Theor. Biol.* **66,** 485–495.

Sirotnak, F. M. (1973). *Biochim. Biophys. Acta* **312,** 426–432.

Sirotnak, F. M., and Donsbach, R. C. (1973). *Cancer Res.* **33,** 1290–1294.

Sköld, O., and Widh, A. (1974). *J. Biol. Chem.* **249,** 4324–4325.

Slavik, K., Slavikova, V., Motycka, K., Hermanova, E., Soucek, J., Tomsova, Z., Spundova, M., and Novakova, E. (1969). *Mol. Pharmacol.* **5,** 137–147.

Slavik, K., Cihar, R., Soucek, J., Hermanova, E., Pristoupilova, K., and Slavikova, V. (1972). *Mol. Pharmacol.* **8,** 740–750.

Spector, R., Levy, P., and Abelson, H. T. (1977). *Biochem. Pharmacol.* **26,** 1507–1511.

Stone, D., and Phillips, A. W. (1977). *FEBS Lett.* **74,** 85–87.

Stone, D., Phillips, A. W., and Burchall, J. J. (1977). *Eur. J. Biochem.* **72,** 613–624.

Stone, D., Paterson, S. J., Raper, J. H., and Phillips, A. W. (1979). *J. Biol. Chem.* **254,** 480–488.

Struck, R. F., Shealy, Y. F., and Montgomery, J. A. (1971). *J. Med. Chem.* **14,** 693–698.

Subramanian, S., and Kaufman, B. T. (1978). *Proc. Natl. Acad. Sci. U.S.A.* **75,** 3201–3205.

Suresh, M. R., Henderson, G. B., and Huennekens, F. M. (1979). *Biochem. Biophys. Res. Commun.* **87,** 135–139.

Suster, D. C., Feyns, L. V., Ciustea, G., Botez, G., Dobre, V., Bick, R., and Niculescu-Duvăz, I. (1974). *J. Med. Chem.* **17,** 758–760.

Suster, D. C., Tărnăuceanu, Botez, G., Dobre, V., and Niculescu-Duvăz, I. (1978b). *J. J. Med. Chem.* **21,** 1162–1165.

Suster, D. C. Tărnăuceanu, E., Botez, G., Dobre, V., and Niculescu-Duvăz, I. (1978b). *J. Med. Chem.* **21**, 1165–1167.

Taylor, R. T., and Weissbach, H. (1973). *In* "The Enzymes" (B. D. Boyer, ed.), 3rd ed., Vol. IX, pp. 121–165. Academic Press, New York.

Turner, A. J. (1977). *Biochem. Pharmacol.* **26**, 1009–1014.

Turner, A. J., Ponzio, F., and Alger, S. (1974). *Brain Res.* **70**, 553–558.

Vehar, G. A., and Freisheim, J. A. (1976). *Biochem. Biophys. Res. Commun.* **68**, 937–941.

Vehar, G. A., Reddy, A. V., and Freisheim, J. H. (1976). *Biochemistry* **15**, 2512–2518.

Warwick, P. E., and Freisheim, J. H. (1975). *Biochemistry* **14**, 664–668.

Warwick, P. E., D'Souza, L., and Freisheim, J. H. (1972). *Biochemistry* **11**, 3775–3779.

Waxman, S. (1976). *In* "Chemistry and Biology of Pteridines" (W. Pfleiderer, ed.), pp. 165–177. De Gruyter, Berlin.

Waxman, S., and Schreiber, C. (1977). *Adv. Nutr. Res.* **1**, 55–76.

Way, J. L., Birdsall, B., Feeney, J., Roberts, G. C. K., and Burgen, A. S. V. (1975). *Biochemistry* **14**, 3470–3475.

Weber, R. (1976). *In* "Chemistry and Biology of Pteridines" (W. Pfleiderer, ed.), pp. 705–708. De Gruyter, Berlin.

Weber, R., and Visconti, M. (1975). *Helv. Chim. Acta* **58**, 1772–1780.

Weber, R., and Visconti, M. (1976). *Helv. Chim. Acta* **59**, 2379–2382.

White, J. C., Loftfield, S., and Goldman, I. D. (1975). *Mol. Pharmacol.* **11**, 287–297.

Whitehead, V. M. (1977). *Cancer Res.* **37**, 408–412.

Whitehead, V. M., Perrault, M. M., and Stelcner, S. (1976). *In* "Chemistry and Biology of Pteridines" (W. Pfleiderer, ed.), pp. 475–482. De Gruyter, Berlin.

Whiteley, J. M. (1971). *Ann. N. Y. Acad. Sci.* **186**, 29–42.

Williams, M. N. (1975). *J. Biol. Chem.* **250**, 322–330.

Williams, M. N., and Bennett, C. D. (1977). *J. Biol. Chem.* **252**, 6871–6877.

Williams, T. J., Lee, T. K., and Dunlap, R. B. (1977). *Arch. Biochem. Biophys.* **181**, 569–579.

Williams, J. W., Morrison, J. F., and Duggleby, R. D. (1979). *Biochemistry* **18**, 2567–2573.

Wood, H. C. S. (1976). *In* "Chemistry and Biology of Pteridines" (W. Pfleiderer, ed.), pp. 27–47. De Gruyter, Berlin.

Yang, C. H., Peterson, R. H. F., Sirotnak, F. M., and Chello, P. L. (1979). *J. Biol. Chem.* **254**, 1402–1407.

Yoshimoto, M., and Hansch, C. (1976). *J. Med. Chem.* **19**, 71–98.

Zakrzewski, S. F. (1963). *J. Biol. Chem.* **238**, 1485–1490.

Zakrzewski, S. F. (1966). *J. Biol. Chem.* **241**, 2962–2967.

Zakrzewski, S. F., and Nichol, C. A. (1958). *Biochim. Biophys. Acta* **27**, 425–426.

Zakrzewski, S. F., Hakala, M. T., and Nichol, C. A. (1962). *Biochemistry* **1**, 842–846.

Zamierowski, M., and Wagner, C. (1976). *In* "Chemistry and Biology of Pteridines" (W. Pfleiderer, ed.), pp. 209–215. De Gruyter, Berlin.

Distribution and Classification of Airway Histamine Receptors: The Physiological Significance of Histamine H_2-Receptors

N. CHAND

Department of Physiology
Downstate Medical Center
State University of New York
Brooklyn, New York

I. Introduction

Lung is one of the most important target organs of immediate hypersensitivity (allergic) reactions in guinea pig and man (Piper, 1977; Chand, 1979a–c; Mitchell and Denborough, 1979; Yen and Kruetner, 1979b), rabbit (Halonen *et al.*, 1979), rat (Stotland and Share, 1974; Church, 1975), calf and sheep (Chand and Eyre, 1977a; Eyre and Burka, 1978), horse (Eyre, 1972, 1976), cat (Lulich *et al.*, 1976; Chand and Eyre, 1977b; Mitchell and Sparrow, 1977), dog (Krell and Chakrin, 1977; Krell, 1978b; Barnett *et al.*, 1978), swine (Wells *et al.*, 1974), chicken (Chand, 1979d), and monkey (Chakrin *et al.*, 1974a,b; Krell, 1976; Michoud *et al.*, 1979). Mast cells in the lung are located around the pulmonary blood vessels and in the submucosa of the airways (Meyers *et al.*, 1973; Staub, 1975). Mast cells and basophils are the primary target cells in allergic inflammatory conditions. They contain several highly potent pharmacologically active

ISBN 0-12-032917-4

substances like biogenic amines (histamine, 5-HT, dopamine), eosinophil chemotactic factor of anaphylaxis (ECF-A), proteolytic enzymes, etc. (Sadavongvivad, 1970; Orr, 1973; Austen and Orange, 1975; Goth and Johnson, 1975; Piper, 1977; Chand, 1979c,d; Henderson and Kaliner, 1979). The immunological (allergic) release of histamine along with several other chemical mediators of immediate hypersensitivity has frequently been demonstrated from the sensitized lung tissues on appropriate antigen challenge (Austen and Orange, 1975; Piper, 1977; Holroyde *et al.*, 1977).

Histamine produces bronchospasm, dilates capillaries, and increases capillary permeability, gastrointestinal motility, and secretions. Histamine-induced bronchospasm is easily blocked by "traditional" H_1-antihistamines (Altura and Altura, 1974; Chand, 1979d; Hirschowitz, 1979). However H_1-antihistaminics have little or no beneficial effects in allergic respiratory diseases (Karlin, 1972; Eyre, 1976; Chand and Eyre, 1977a; Casterline and Evans, 1977; Nogrady *et al.*, 1978; Svedmyr and Simonsson, 1978; Eyre and Burka, 1978; Krell, 1978b; Chand, 1979a,b,c; Chand and DeRoth, 1980; Mitchell and Denborough, 1979; Adams and Lichtenstein, 1977, 1979). Other chemical mediators like slow-reacting substance of anaphylaxis (SRS-A), and possibly endoperoxides (PGG_2, PGH_2) and thromboxanes play a more important role in the pathogenesis of allergic respiratory diseases (Hamberg *et al.*, 1976; Piper, 1977; Wasserman and Griffin, 1977; Chand, 1979b,c; Yen and Kruetner, 1979b; Everitt *et al.*, 1979; Sirois, 1979). Before the discovery of the selective H_1- and H_2-receptor agonists and antagonists (Fig. 1) (Black *et al.*, 1972, 1973; Brimblecombe *et al.*, 1975; Chand and Eyre, 1975; Durant *et al.*, 1975, 1977, 1978; Parsons *et al.*, 1977, Buck *et al.*, 1979; Yellin *et al.*, 1979), histamine was only perceived as a chemical mediator of anaphylaxis (Austen and Orange, 1975; Piper, 1977). Recently histamine has been shown to play a more important autoregulatory role in the immunological release of histamine itself (Lichtenstein and Gillespie, 1973, 1975; Chand and Eyre, 1975; Holroyde *et al.*, 1977; Schleimer, 1978; Plaut, 1979), and of other chemical mediators, e.g., SRS-A (Chakrin *et al.*, 1974a,b; Burka and Eyre, 1976), prostaglandins (Yen *et al.*, 1976), and lysosomal enzymes (Busse and Sosman, 1975, 1977; Bush *et al.*, 1978; Busse *et al.*, 1979). Histamine also modulates the pathophysiological events in the lung during allergic reactions, e.g., bronchodilatation/constriction (Dunlop and Smith, 1977; Drazen *et al.*, 1978b; Chand, 1979a), and vasoconstriction/dilatation in pulmonary vascular beds (Eyre and Wells, 1973; Chand and Eyre, 1975; Eyre 1976; Owen, 1977; Chand and DeRoth, 1980). These modulatory actions of histamine also operate via histamine H_2-receptors (Chand and Eyre, 1975; Halevy and Altura, 1977; Schleimer, 1978; Plaut, 1979; Hirschowitz, 1979).

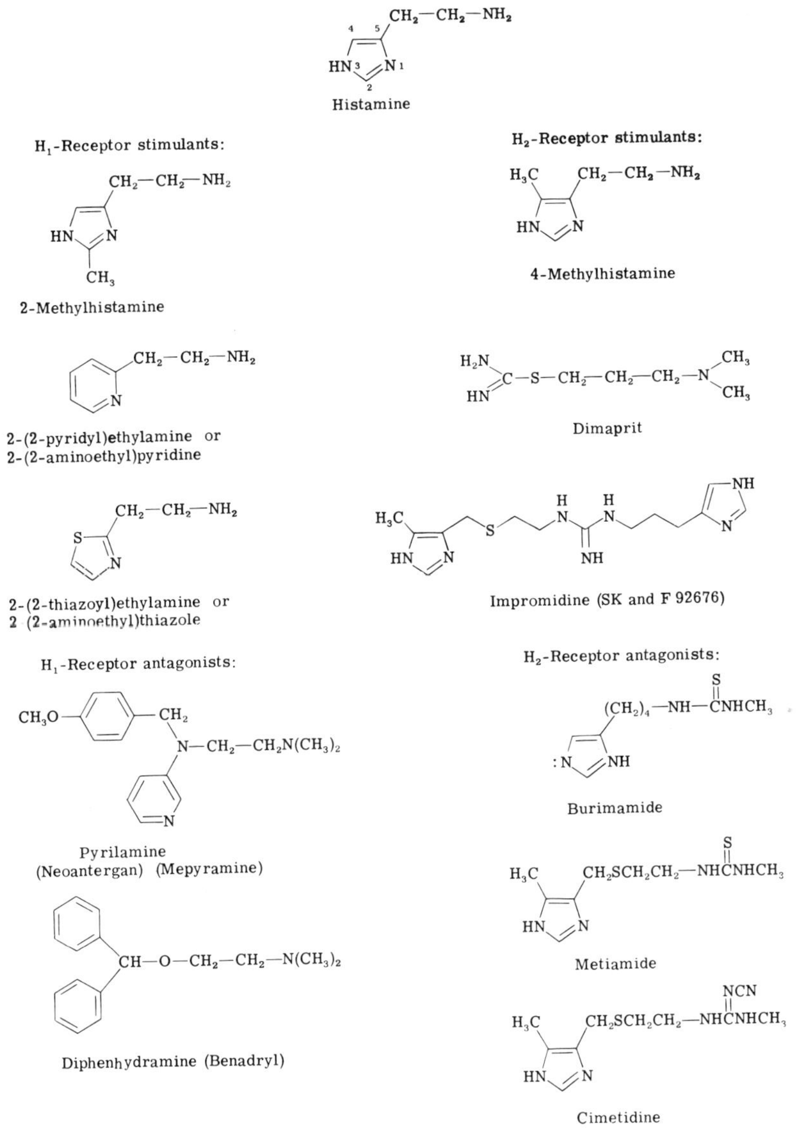

Histamine

H_1-Receptor stimulants:

2-Methylhistamine

2-(2-pyridyl)ethylamine or
2-(2-aminoethyl)pyridine

2-(2-thiazoyl)ethylamine or
2-(2-aminoethyl)thiazole

H_2-Receptor stimulants:

4-Methylhistamine

Dimaprit

Impromidine (SK and F 92676)

H_1-Receptor antagonists:

Pyrilamine
(Neoantergan) (Mepyramine)

Diphenhydramine (Benadryl)

H_2-Receptor antagonists:

Burimamide

Metiamide

Cimetidine

FIG. 1. The chemical structures of histamine, H_1- and H_2-receptor agonists, and antagonists

Soon after the introduction of the specific H_1- and H_2-receptor agonists and antagonists (Fig. 1), it has become firmly established that histamine commonly exhibits a dual mode of action (Chand and Eyre, 1975; Owen, 1977; Hirschowitz, 1979), In guinea pig, cat, and dog, mepyramine (a specific H_1-antagonist (Ash and Schild, 1966) blocks histamine-induced pulmonary arterial pressor response, converting it to a depressor response, which in turn is blocked by burimamide and metiamide (specific H_2-antagonists) (Chand and Eyre, 1975; Owen, 1977; Tucker *et al.*, 1975, 1976, 1977a,b; Hoffman *et al.*, 1975, 1977; Barer *et al.*, 1976, 1978). These reports have established a dual mode of action of histamine in the pulmonary microvasculature. Furthermore, dual actions of histamine in the gastrointestinal tract and cardiovascular system (the heart itself, renal and other peripheral vessels) have frequently been documented (Chand and Eyre, 1975; Owen, 1977; Bareica and Rocha e Silva, 1976; Ercan and Turker, 1977; Hakanson *et al.*, 1978; Chand and DeRoth, 1978a; Fjalland, 1979).

Histamine is well known to produce airway constrictions in several mammalian species. However, there are a number of reports describing the spasmolytic actions of histamine on the airway smooth muscles (Akçasu, 1952, 1959; Main, 1964; Maengwyn-Davies, 1968; Eyre, 1969, 1973; Fleisch and Calkins, 1976; Chand and Eyre, 1977b–f, 1978a–d, 1979; Chand and DeRoth, 1978b–d, 1979a–g, Chand *et al.*, 1979a–e, 1980a–c; Yen, 1978; Yen and Kruetner, 1979a) (Table I). Recently a "dual" mode of action of histamine on airway smooth muscles of man (Dunlop and Smith, 1977), horse (Chand and Eyre, 1977c,f, 1978a), guinea pig (Okpako *et al.*, 1978; Chand and DeRoth, 1979c,d; Drazen *et al.*, 1978a, 1979b; Chand, 1979a), swine (Chand and DeRoth, 1978b,d), and monkey (Chand and Altura, 1979; Chakrin *et al.*, 1979; Chand *et al.*, 1980a–c) has been reported. Therefore, it was considered timely and important to summarize briefly the distribution and classification of airway histamine receptors and also to review briefly the modulatory (autoregulatory) role(s) of histamine H_2-receptors in the pathophysiological conditions.

II. Airway Histamine Receptor Distribution and Classification

In 1910, Dale and Laidlaw were first to observe bronchoconstriction to histamine in the guinea pig. Subsequent *in vitro* studies have revealed that histamine produces highly variable effects on the respiratory smooth muscles depending upon the tone, region of the airways, and species (Table I). Factors like age (Altura and Altura, 1977; Schneider *et al.*, 1978; Newman

TABLE I

SPECIES AND REGIONAL DIFFERENCES IN THE RESPONSIVENESS OF THE AIRWAY SMOOTH MUSCLE TO HISTAMINE

Species	Region of the airways		
	Trachea	Bronchus	Lung strip (bronchioalveolar ducts)
Rat	Unresponsive (Jamieson, 1962; Burns and Doe, 1978) Contraction (Brocklehurst, 1958) *Relaxation*[a] (Chand and Eyre, 1978c; Eyre and Besner, 1979)	Unresponsive (Burns and Doe, 1978) Contraction (Brocklehurst, 1978)	Unresponsive (Burns and Doe, 1978; Chand, 1979f)
Ferret	Contraction (Main, 1964; Chand and Eyre, 1978c) *Relaxation* (Chand and Eyre, 1978c)	Contraction (Chand and Eyre, 1978c) Relaxation (Chand and Eyre, 1978c)	Contraction (unpublished observation)
Rabbit	Unresponsive (Main, 1964) *Relaxation* (Fleisch and Calkin, 1976; Chand *et al.*, 1979d)	*Contraction* (Fleisch and Calkins, 1976; Chand and Eyre, 1977c)	*Contraction* (Chand and DeRoth, 1979b)
Cat	Unresponsive (Lulich *et al.*, 1976) Contraction (Brocklehurst, 1958) *Relaxation* (Maengwyn-Davies, 1968)	Unresponsive (Mitchell and Sparrow, 1975) Contraction (Brocklehurst, 1958) Relaxation (Chand and Eyre, 1977d)	*Contraction* (Lulich *et al.*, 1976; Chand and DeRoth, 1979e)
Rhesus monkey	Unresponsive (Main, 1964) Contraction (Brocklehurst, 1958) *Relaxation* (Chand and Altura, 1979)	Contraction (Brocklehurst, 1958) *Relaxation* (Chand and Altura, 1979a)	*Contraction* (Chand *et al.*, 1980a)
Swine	Unresponsive (Main, 1969) Contraction (Chand and DeRoth, 1978b,d) *Relaxation*	Contraction (Chand and DeRoth, 1978b,d)	*Contraction* (unpublished observation)
Sheep	*Contraction* (Eyre, 1969; Chand and Eyre, 1977c)	Primary: contraction (Eyre, 1969) Intermediate: *Relaxation* (Eyre, 1973; Chand, 1979e) Terminal: Relaxation	*Contraction* (Chand, 1979e)

[a] Italics indicate the predominant effect.

et al., 1978, 1979; Chand and DeRoth, 1978b, 1979a), sex (Altura, 1972), the state of the health of man and experimental animals (Chand and Altura, 1979), storage of the tissues at low temperatures (Kenakin *et al.*, 1974), especially tissues obtained at lung surgery or autopsies, method of euthanasia–anesthesia, season, temperature, pH, and composition of the physiological solutions (Spilker and Minatoya, 1975), the nature and type of the spasmogen used to induce tone for recording relaxant responses (Fig. 2a) (Akçasu, 1952; Chand and Eyre, 1978a), doses of histamine used (Brocklehurst, 1958; Main, 1964), loading tensions (no tension to 5 gm), and the extent of H_1- or H_2-receptor blockade by antagonists or by disease processes may possibly explain in part the bewildering and often contradictory responses of the airway smooth muscles to histamine (Table I).

Histamine relaxes trachea of cat, rabbit, and rat, which are partially contracted by acetylcholine but is inactive on tissues contracted by potassium chloride (KCl) (Akçasu, 1952). Histamine reduces contractile response to acetylcholine and KCl and KCl-induced rhythmic movements as well as spontaneous movements in the trachea of cat, rabbit, and rat (Akcasu, 1952, 1959). Histamine [10 to 100 $\mu g\ ml^{-1}$] often antagonizes acetylcholine responses on the trachea of swine, rhesus monkey, cat, and rabbit (Main, 1964). These reports were the first to describe the spasmolytic (inhibitory) actions of histamine on the airway smooth muscles, beside its well-known spasmogenic (excitatory) actions on the airways of several mammalian species (Castillo and deBeer, 1947; Castillo, 1948; Hawkins *et al.*, 1951; McDouglas and West, 1953; Brocklehurst, 1958; Eyre, 1969, 1973; Mathé *et al.*, 1971; Joiner *et al.*, 1975; Fleisch and Calkins, 1976; Persson and Ekman, 1976; Yamatake *et al.*, 1978; Krell, 1978a; Drazen and Schneider, 1978; Chand and Eyre, 1977c,f, 1978a–d; Martin and Fertel, 1978; Drazen *et al.*, 1978a, 1979a; Antonissen *et al.*, 1978a,b; Chand and DeRoth, 1978b–d, 1979g; Eyre and Chand, 1978, 1979; Anderson *et al*; 1979a,b; Chand 1979a,b,e; Chand and Altura, 1979; Chand *et al.*, 1979a–e, 1980a–c; DeRoth and Chand 1979a–g; Dixon *et al.*, 1979).

Histamine does not readily leave smooth muscle resulting in tachyphylaxis in the airways, especially if tested at frequent intervals (Akçasu, 1959; Chand, unpublished observations). The development of the rapid tachyphylaxis in the airway smooth muscles (especially in the canine tracheal muscle) is attributed to the increased synthesis and release of PGE_2 (Anderson *et al.*, 1979a,b).

The distribution and classification of airway histamine receptors have been summarized in Table II. In general, there is a preponderance of H_1-receptors mediating constrictions in the tracheobronchial smooth muscles of dog, horse, man, guinea pig, and langur, the trachea and primary bronchus of sheep, and the bronchus of rabbit and lung strips (peripheral air-

TABLE II

CLASSIFICATION AND DISTRIBUTION OF THE HISTAMINE RECEPTORS IN THE RESPIRATORY SMOOTH MUSCLES[a]

Species	Respiratory smooth muscle		
	Tracheal	Bronchial	Peripheral airways (lung strip) bronchioalveolar ducts
Guinea pig	H_1[b](Drazen *et al.*, 1979b)	H_1[b] (Okpako *et al.*, 1978)	H_1[b] (Chand and DeRoth, 1978c, 1979d; Yen and Kruetner, 1979a; Drazen *et al.*, 1979b)
	H_2 (Drazen *et al.*, 1979b)	H_2 (Okpako *et al.*, 1978)	H_2
Horse	H_1[b] (Chand and Eyre, 1977c,f, 1978a)	H_1[b] (Chand and Eyre, 1978a)	H_1[b] (Chand and DeRoth, 1979c)
	H_2, H_3? (Chand and Eyre, 1977c,f, 1978a)	H_2 (Chand and Eyre, 1978a)	
Man	H_1?	H_1[b] (Dunlop and Smith, 1977)	H_1?
	H_2?	H_2 (Dunlop and Smith, 1977)	
Rhesus monkey	H_1	H_1	H_1[b] (Chand and Altura, 1979, 1980a,c)
	H_2[b]	H_2[b]	
Langur monkey	H_1[b]	H_1[b]	H_1[b] (Chand *et al.*, 1980b)
	H_2	H_2	
Swine	H_1[b] (Chand and DeRoth, 1978d)	H_1[b] (Chand and DeRoth, 1978a)	H_1[b] (Chand, unpublished)
	H_2 (Chand and DeRoth, 1978d)	H_2 (Chand and DeRoth, 1978a)	
Neonatal piglet	H_1 (DeRoth and Chand, 1979)	H_1 (Chand and DeRoth, 1979a)	H_1 (Chand *et al.*, 1979c)
	H_2 (DeRoth and Chand, 1979)	H_2 (Chand and DeRoth, 1979a)	
Rabbit	H_1 (Fleisch and Calkins, 1979; Eyre and Chand, 1979)	H_1 (Fleisch and Calkins, 1976)	H_1 (Chand and DeRoth, 1979b)
	H_2, H_3?		

(*continued*)

TABLE II (*continued*)

Species	Respiratory smooth muscle		
	Tracheal	Bronchial	Peripheral airways (lung strip) bronchioalveolar ducts
Dog	H_1[b] (Persson and Ekman, 1976)	H_1[b] (Chand and Eyre, 1977c) H_2, H_3? (Eyre and Chand, 1979)	H_1[b] (Chand *et al.*, 1979a; Kleinstiver and Eyre, 1978, 1979)
Cat	H_1 (Chand and Eyre, 1977c) H_2[b] (Eyre, 1973; Chand and Eyre, 1977c)	H_2, H_3? (Chand and Eyre, 1977d)	H_1[b] (Lulich *et al.*, 1976; Chand and DeRoth, 1979e)
Rat	H_2, H_3? (Chand and Eyre, 1978c; Eyre and Besner, 1979)		
Ferret	H_1[b] H_2, H_3?	H_1[b] (Chand and Eyre, 1978c) H_2	H_1[b] (unpublished observation)
Chicken		H_1[b] (Chand and Eyre, 1978b) H_2	H_1[b] (unpublished)
Sheep	H_1[b] (Eyre, 1969) H_2	H_1 (Eyre, 1969, 1973; Chand and Eyre, 1977c) H_2[b] (Eyre, 1969, 1973; Chand and Eyre, 1977c)	H_1[b] (Chand, 1979e)
Goat	H_1[b] (Chand *et al.*, 1979b) H_2	H_1[b] H_2	H_1[b] (Chand and Altura, 1979)
Cattle	H_1[b]	H_1[b] (Chand *et al.*, 1979e) H_2, H_3?	H_1[b] (Kleinstiver and Eyre, 1978, 1979)

[a] H_1 = contraction; H_2, H_3? = relaxation.
[b] The preponderance of histamine receptor subtype.

ways) of all the species studied (Table II) (Hawkins *et al.*, 1951; Eyre, 1969; Fleisch and Calkins, 1976; Dunlop and Smith, 1977; Persson and Ekman, 1976; Martin and Fertel, 1978; Lulich *et al.*, 1978; Chand and Eyre, 1977c,e,f, 1978a–d; Drazen *et al.*, 1978a, 1979b; Chand and DeRoth, 1978b,c,d, 1979a–e; Chand and Altura, 1979).

The airway smooth muscles of the neonatal swine, dog, and calf are relatively insensitive to histamine, which is not related to the presence of H_2-receptors in these tissues. These observations probably suggest that either H_1-receptors are not present in these tissues or their functional maturation takes place later during the postnatal life (Schneider *et al.*, 1978; Chand and DeRoth, 1978b, 1979a; DeRoth and Chand, 1979; Chand *et al.*, 1979e; Kleinstiver and Eyre, 1979).

The H_2-receptor antagonists (metiamide, cimetidine) (Black *et al.*, 1973; Brimblecombe *et al.*, 1975) potentiate contractile responses to histamine on the tracheobronchial smooth muscles of man (Dunlop and Smith, 1977), horse (Chand and Eyre, 1977c,f, 1978a), and guinea pig (Okpako *et al.*, 1978; Drazen *et al.*, 1978a). Furthermore after H_1-receptor blockade, carbachol precontracted tracheobronchial smooth muscle preparations of horse (Fig. 2), swine, man, rhesus monkey, and chicken respond with relaxations of varying magnitudes to histamine, 4-methylhistamine, impromidine, and dimaprit (H_2 agonists). These relaxations are subsequently antagonized by H_2-antagonists (Dunlop and Smith, 1977; Chand and Eyre, 1977c,f, 1978a,b; Chand and DeRoth, 1978b,d; Chakrin *et al.*, 1979; Chand and Altura, 1979; Chand *et al.*, 1980a,c). Thus a "dual" histamine receptor mechanism appears to operate in the tracheobronchial smooth muscles of guinea pig, man, rhesus monkey, swine, horse, and chicken.

Cat trachea partially contracted to carbachol or acetylcholine relaxes to histamine (Akçasu, 1952, 1959; Maengwyn-Davies, 1968; Eyre, 1973; Turker and Ercan, 1976; Chand and Eyre, 1977b,c). This relaxation is attenuated by mepyramine, pronethalol (Maengwyn-Davies, 1968), propranolol (Eyre, 1973), or catecholamine depletion by reserpine. These observations seems to suggest the release of catecholamines by histamine in this tissue (Maengwyn-Davis, 1968). Later, burimamide (Eyre, 1973), metiamide (Turker and Ercan, 1976), and cimetidine (Chand and Eyre, 1977c) were shown to antagonize histamine-induced relaxation on cat trachea. Histamine, 2-methylhistamine, 2-pyridylethylamine (H_1-agonists), 4-methylhistamine, impromidine, and dimaprit (H_2-agonists) all relax cat trachea (Chand and Eyre, 1977b). These relaxations are strongly antagonized by cimetidine and metiamide but only weakly by mepyramine (Chand, unpublished observations). The relaxations to histamine on sheep terminal-intermediate bronchus (Eyre, 1969, 1973; Chand and Eyre, 1977c; Chand, 1979e) and tracheobronchial smooth muscles of rhe-

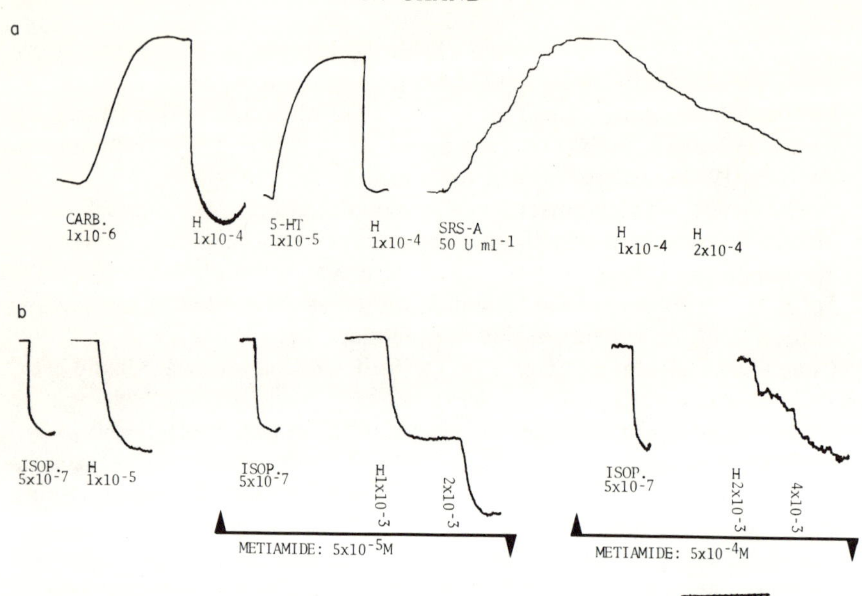

FIG. 2. Responses of the horse airway smooth muscle in Krebs–Henseleit solution gassed with 5% CO_2 in O_2, at 37°C in the presence of mepyramine (5×10^{-5} *M*) and indomethacin (5×10^{-6} *M*). Resting tension = 3 *g*. Contractions are taken from rest. Relaxations are taken from partial contraction (50 ± 10% maximum) to carbachol. (a) Secondary bronchus: histamine (H)-induced relaxation on the bronchus contracted to carbachol (10^{-6} *M*), 5-HT (10^{-5} *M*), or SRS-A. (b) Primary bronchus: metiamide (5×10^{-5} *M*) blocked H-induced relaxations (dose-ratio = 100) without interfering with isoprenaline (Isop.). Higher concentration of metiamide (5×10^{-4} *M*) further antagonized histamine specifically (dose-ratio = 600). From Chand and Eyre (1978a). Courtesy of *Agents Actions*.

sus monkey (Chand and Altura, 1979; Chand *et al.*, 1980a,c; Chakrin *et al.*, 1979) are blocked by H_2-antagonists (burimamide, metiamide, and cimetidine) showing the preponderance of histamine H_2- (inhibitory) receptors in these tissues.

Lung parenchymal strip has been introduced to study the autonomic and autacoid pharmacology of the peripheral airways (bronchioles and bronchioalveolar ducts) (Mitchell and Sparrow, 1975; Lulich *et al.*, 1976; Drazen and Schneider, 1978; Drazen *et al.*, 1978a, 1979a,b; Burns and Doe, 1978; Chand and DeRoth, 1978b,c, 1979b–f; Chand *et al.*, 1979a, 1980a–c; Chand, 1979a,b; Kleinstiver and Eyre, 1978, 1979; Chand and Altura, 1979). The lung strips of guinea pig respond with relaxations to impromidine, dimaprit (Fig. 3a), and low doses of histamine and 4-methylhistamine (Chand and DeRoth, 1978c, 1979d; Yen, 1978; Drazen *et al.*, 1979b; Yen and Kruetner, 1979a). Guinea pig lung strips respond with

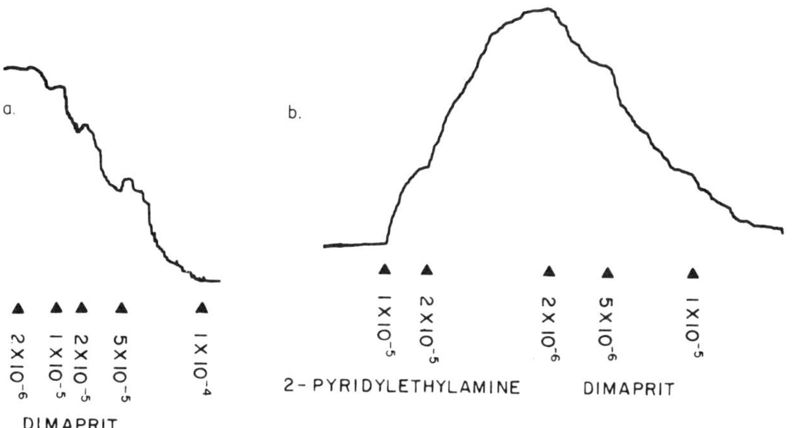

FIG. 3. Isolated guinea pig lung parenchymal strips (a, b) in Krebs–Henseleit solution gassed with 5% CO_2 in O_2, 37°C. Resting tension = 2 *g*. Relaxant responses to dimaprit under resting tone (a) and partial contraction to 2-pyridylethylamine (H_1-agonist) (about 40% of histamine max.) (b). From Chand and DeRoth (1979d). Courtesy of *Pharmacology*.

dose-related contractions to histamine, 2-methylhistamine, carbachol, and 2-pyridylethylamine. Guinea pig lung strips which were partially contracted by carbachol or H_1-agonists (2-methylhistamine or 2-pyridylethylamine) also react with relaxations to impromidine and dimaprit (Fig. 3b) (Chand and DeRoth, 1978c, 1979d). Metiamide antagonizes relaxations to low doses of histamine and enhances its contractile responses (Chand and DeRoth, 1978c, 1979d; Yen, 1978; Yen and Kruetner, 1979a; Drazen *et al.*, 1978a). Thus guinea pig peripheral airways seem to possess both histamine H_1- and H_2-receptors, respectively, producing contraction and relaxation. With the exception of guinea pig, the lung strips of cat, rabbit, horse, sheep, rhesus and langur monkey, goat, dog, neonatal swine, and cattle seem to have only H_1-receptors producing peripheral airway contractions (Lulich *et al.*, 1976; Chand and DeRoth, 1978b, 1979b,c,e; Chand *et al.*, 1979a,c, 1980a–c; Chand and Altura, 1979; Kleinstiver and Eyre, 1978, 1979).

After H_1-receptor blockade, high doses of histamine also relax carbachol-contracted bronchus of cat and dog, and trachea of horse, and rabbit, rat, and ferret. This relaxation is relatively resistant to propranolol, indomethacin, and H_2-antagonists (Fleisch and Calkins, 1976; Chand and Eyre, 1977c,d,e,f, 1978a,c; Chand *et al.*, 1979d; Eyre and Chand, 1978, 1979; Eyre and Besner, 1979). These observations possibly exclude the histamine-induced release of catecholamines (Staszewska-Barczak and Vane, 1965; Maengwyn-Davies, 1968; Colebatch, 1970; Tozzi, 1973;

Verma and McNeil, 1976), prostaglandins (Bakhle and Smith, 1972; Orehek *et al.*, 1973, 1975; Grondzinska *et al.*, 1975; Yen *et al.*, 1976), and thromboxanes (Berti *et al.*, 1979) in these tissues. For the interpretation of such "unusual" or "atypical" responses to histamine, several possibilities are offered: (1) a "nonspecific" spasmolytic effect to relatively high doses of histamine; (2) the release of a "nonadrenergic/and nonprostaglandinergic" mediator, e.g., adenosine or ATP (Burnstock, 1971; Ohhubo *et al.*, 1975; Kamakawa and Shimo, 1976), and (3) the existence of another type of histamine receptor (H_3- or H_2-isoreceptor) (Fleisch and Calkins, 1976; Eyre and Chand, 1979; Fjalland, 1979). In view of the existence of β_1- and β_2-adrenoceptors (Lands *et al.*, 1967), the latter could occur in the trachea of rabbit, ferret, and rat and the bronchus of dog and cat (Fleisch and Calkins, 1976; Chand and Eyre, 1977c,d,f, 1978a; Chand and DeRoth, 1978a; Chand *et al.*, 1979d; Eyre and Chand, 1978, 1979; Eyre and Besner, 1979) and would also account for the chemoattractant activity of histamine on human eosinophils (Clark *et al.*, 1977). Obviously much remains to be learned about the existence of another type of histamine H_2-receptor (H_2-isoreceptors; H_3?) in the biological tissues. The physiopharmacological significance of such receptors in the airways is not yet clear.

III. Mechanisms of Action of Histamine on Airway Smooth Muscles

The multiple sites of action of histamine in the airways are schematically presented in Fig. 4. It may be generalized that histamine produces

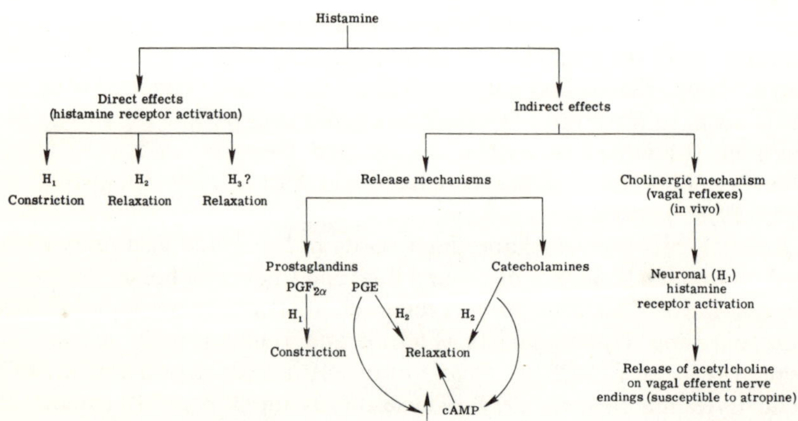

FIG. 4. A scheme of the possible mechanisms of action of histamine on the airway smooth muscles.

one or more of the following effects on the airways: (1) constriction involving the activation of both muscular (Maconochie *et al.*, 1979) (Table I) and neuronal histamine H_1-receptors (Gold, 1977; Vidruk and Sampson, 1978; Irvin and Dempsey, 1978; Dixon *et al.*, 1979); (2) relaxation mediated via histamine H_2-receptors in the airway smooth muscles (Table I); and (3) the release of catecholamines, prostaglandins, and thromboxanes in the lungs may be operating via both H_1- and H_2-receptors (Staszewska-Barczak and Vane, 1965; Maengwyn-Davies, 1968; Eyre 1973; Yen *et al.*, 1976; Verma and McNeil, 1976; Berti *et al.*, 1979).

IV. Modulatory Roles of Histamine H_2-Receptors

A. Hypoxic Pulmonary Vasoconstriction

The exact mechanism of induction of hypoxic pulmonary vasoconstriction is not yet clearly understood (Bergofsky, 1974; Howard *et al.*, 1975; Fishman, 1976). Rats suffering from chronic hypoxia exhibit pulmonary mast-cell hyperplasia (Kay *et al.*, 1974; Mungall, 1976; Martin *et al.*, 1978). Mast cells contain large amounts of histamine (Adams and Lichtenstein, 1977). Histamine produces pulmonary vasodilatation during hypoxia in calf, rat, dog, cat, and ferret (Hauge and Melmon, 1969; Shaw, 1971; Silove and Simcha, 1973; Thompson *et al.*, 1976; Tucker *et al.*, 1976, 1977; Hoffman *et al.*, 1977; Barer *et al.*, 1978). Views on the release of histamine from the pulmonary mast cells during chronic hypoxia are still controversial (Haas and Bergofsky, 1972; Kay *et al.*, 1974; Mungall, 1976; McMurty *et al.*, 1977). It is suggested that under chronic hypoxic conditions, mast cell hyperplasia in the lung may be opposing hypoxic pulmonary vasoconstriction (Martin *et al.*, 1978) possibly by activating H_2-receptors, which mediate pulmonary vasodilation in several mammalian species (Chand and Eyre, 1975; Owen, 1977; Hoffman *et al.*, 1975, 1977; Tucker *et al.*, 1975, 1976, 1977a,b; Barer *et al.*, 1978).

Compound 48/80 (a potent releaser of mast cell histamine) abolishes the hypoxic pulmonary vasoconstrictor response in the cat (Barer and McCurrie, 1969; Hauge and Staub, 1969; Dawson *et al.*, 1974). H_1-antagonists attenuate the pulmonary hypoxic response in cat and dog (Duke, 1969; Shaw, 1971; Susmano and Carleton, 1971). Based on these experimental observations, some investigators have suggested that histamine may be a chemical mediator of pulmonary vasoconstrictor response to hypoxia (Hauge and Melmon, 1968; Shaw, 1971; Bergofsky, 1974). However, others were unable to demonstrate any suppressing effects of H_1-blockers on pulmonary hypoxic response in cat and dog (Barer, 1966; Barer *et al.*, 1969, 1978; Hoffman *et al.*, 1975, 1977; Tucker *et al.*, 1976, 1977b). Furthermore, H_2-antagonists enhance hypoxic pulmonary vasoconstriction in dogs and cats (Hoffman *et al.*, 1975, 1977; Tucker *et al.*, 1976, 1977b; Barer *et al.*, 1978). Therefore, based on these experimental observations histamine is proposed as a modulator of hypoxic pulmonary vasoconstriction operating via H_2-receptors (Hoffman *et al.*, 1975, 1977; Tucker *et al.*, 1976, 1976b; Barer *et al.*, 1978). It is evident that the effects of H_1- and H_2-antagonists on pulmonary vasoconstrictor response to hypoxia vary considerably from species to species. Therefore, either the effects of histamine H_1-antagonists and histamine releasers occur through some nonspecific mechanism(s) rather than via histamine receptors, or histamine acts as a mediator in some species and a modulator in others.

B. Immediate Hypersensitivity Reactions

The autoregulatory (modulatory) functions of histamine in the light of immunopathophysiology have been reviewed earlier (Chand and Eyre, 1975; Holroyde *et al.*, 1977; Schleimer, 1978; Plaut, 1979) and are briefly summarized in Table III. The effects of H_2-receptor antagonists on the allergic release of chemical mediators of immediate hypersensitivity are presented in Table IV. H_2-blockers inhibit the histamine-induced inhibition of the release of histamine (Lichtenstein and Gillespie, 1973, 1975), lysosomal enzymes (Busse and Sosman, 1975, 1977; Bush *et al.*, 1978; Busse *et al.*, 1979), and prostaglandins of E series (Yen *et al.*, 1976) and thus block the "protective" negative feedback mechanisms on the basophils (mast cells), polymorphonuclear cells, and eosinophils (Fig. 5).

Burimamide and metiamide enhance pulmonary anaphylactic response in guinea pig (Fig. 6a), while 4-methylhistamine (H_2-agonist) partially inhibits this response (Fig. 6b) (Drazen *et al.*, 1978b). Dimaprit and impromidine (highly selective H_2-stimulants) (Durant *et al.*, 1977, 1978) reverse

TABLE III

Modulatory (Autoregulatory) Functions of Histamine H_2-Receptors

1. Inhibition of histamine release from human basophils (Lichtenstein and Gillespie, 1973, 1975; Chand and Eyre, 1975; Holyroyde *et al.*, 1977)
2. Inhibition of lysosomal enzyme release from human neutrophils (Busse and Sosman, 1975, 1977; Bush *et al.*, 1978; Busse *et al.*, 1979)
3. Inhibition of lymphocyte (T)-mediated cytotoxicity (Chand and Eyre, 1975; Plaut *et al.*, 1975)
4. Inhibition of lymphocyte activation (Beets and Dale, 1978) and antibody production by lymphocytes (Weinstein and Melmon, 1976; Schleimer, 1978)
5. Inhibition of eosinophil migration (Clark *et al.*, 1977)
6. Inhibition of lymphocyte (T)-mediated migration inhibitory factor (MIF) production and proliferation (Rocklin, 1976, 1977)

TABLE IV

THE EFFECTS OF H_2-RECEPTOR ANTAGONISTS ON THE IMMUNOLOGICAL RELEASE OF PHARMACOLOGICAL MEDIATORS OF IMMEDIATE HYPERSENSITIVITY

Species	Tissue or cells	H_2-blocker	Effect on chemical mediator release
Man (Allergic patients)	Basophils	Burimamide Metiamide	Block histamine-induced inhibition of histamine-release (Lichtenstein and Gillespie, 1973, 1975; Holyroyde *et al.*, 1978)
Monkey	Passively sensitized lung; skin	Metiamide (SK&F 92058)	Enhance histamine and SRS-A release (Chakrin *et al.*, 1974a,b)
Rat	Passively sensitized lung	Metiamide	Slight (no) enhancement of histamine release (Chakrin *et al.*, 1974a,b)
Dog	Passively sensitized lung	Metiamide	Enhance histamine (but not SRS-A) (Krell and Chakrin, 1977)
Calf	Actively sensitized lung	Burimamide	Enhance SRS-A release (Burka and Eyre, 1976)

in vitro Schultz–Dale anaphylactic contractions (Chand and Eyre, 1978e) in the isolated guinea pig peripheral airways (lung strips) (Fig. 7a). Metiamide enhances and mepyramine partially inhibits this reaction (Fig. 7b) (Chand, 1979a). The potentiation of *in vitro* allergic bronchoconstriction in man (Dunlop and Smith, 1977), pulmonary anaphylactic response in guinea pig (Drazen *et al.*, 1978b; Dulabh and Vickers, 1978; Chand, 1979a), and systemic anaphylaxis in calf (Eyre and Wells, 1973), horse (Eyre, 1976) and domestic fowl (Chand and DeRoth, 1980) by H_2-antagonists could possibly be attributed to the blockade of H_2-receptors on the mast cells and basophils leading to enhancement of the chemical mediators (Lichtenstein and Gillespie, 1973, 1975; Chakrin *et al.*, 1974a,b, 1979; Burka and Eyre, 1976; Krell and Chakrin, 1977) and also in the airway smooth muscles resulting in enhanced airway constrictions.

C. PRELIMINARY EVIDENCE FOR THE H_2-RECEPTOR DEFICIENCY THEORY OF ASTHMA

Escherichia coli endotoxin enhances bronchoconstrictions by phenylephrine and histamine in man (Svedmyr, 1970, 1971; Simonsson *et al.*, 1972) possibly by producing blockage of the β-adrenoceptors (Szenti-

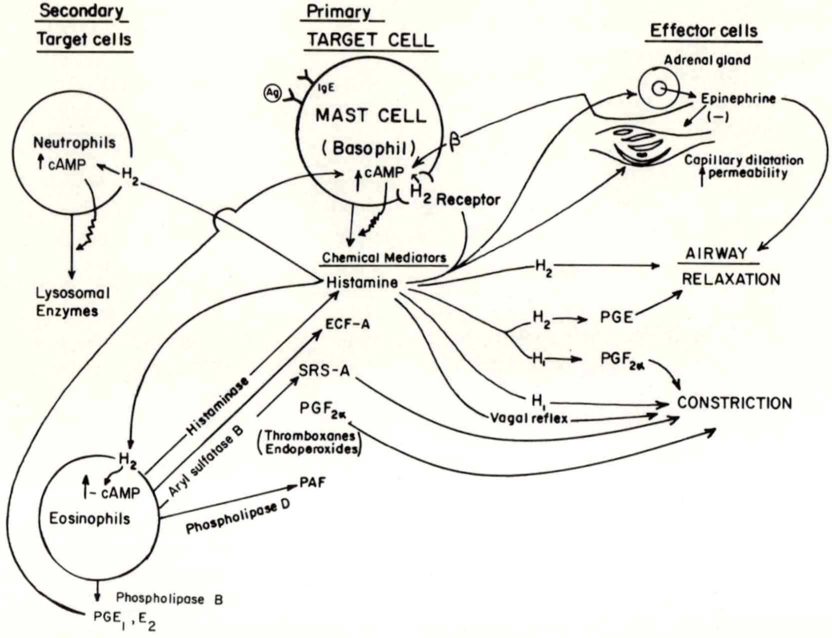

FIG. 5. A scheme for the autoregulatory (modulatory) functions of histamine H_2-receptors. Histamine released during allergic reactions acts on target organs and produces airway constriction and capillary dilatation, and increases capillary permeability etc. Histamine performs possibly a more important modulatory role, i.e., it acts on primary (mast cells, basophils) and secondary (neutrophils and eosinophils) target cells and increases intracellular levels of cAMP via H_2-receptor activation and subsequently inhibits the further allergic release of histamine and SRS-A from mast cells and basophils, and lysosomal enzymes from neutrophils. At low concentrations, histamine acts as a chemoattractant for eosinophils, a response not mediated through H_1- or H_2-receptors. At high concentrations, it inhibits the migration of eosinophils, a response mediated via H_2-receptors. Eosinophils contain histaminase, arylsulfatase B, and phospholipase D etc.; these enzymes are released at the site of inflammation and respectively inactivate histamine, SRS-A, and PAF (platelet activating factor). Eosinophils also releases PGE_1 and E_2, which produce bronchodilatation and also inhibit the release of chemical mediators from the target cells. During systemic anaphylaxis, histamine releases adrenaline from the adrenal medulla, which also produces bronchorelaxation, counteracts the effect of histamine on capillaries, and inhibits the release of chemical mediators from mast cells and basophils by acting on the β_2-adrenoceptors.

vanyi, 1968). Human bronchus also contains a significant population of H_2-receptors which mediate relaxations (Dunlop and Smith, 1977). Therefore, it is possible that the enhancement of the histamine-induced bronchoconstriction in man by endotoxin (Svedmyr, 1970, 1971; Simonsson *et al.*, 1972) could have resulted from the H_2-receptor blockade. Similar

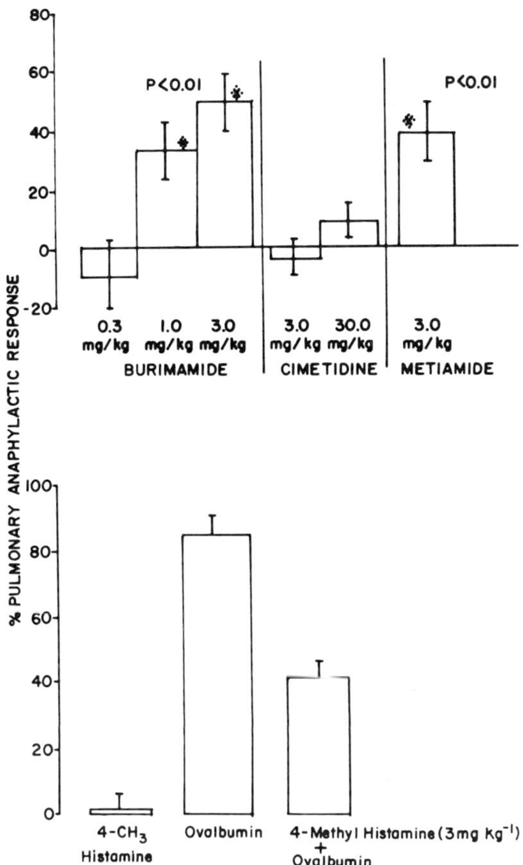

FIG. 6. (a) The potentiation of pulmonary anaphylactic response by H_2-antagonists (burimamide and metiamide) in guinea pigs. Cimetidine, another potent H_2-antagonist, is devoid of any effect on the severity of pulmonary anaphylactic response. (b) The inhibitory effect of 4-methylhistamine (3 mg kg^{-1}, injected intravenously 2 minutes before antigen challenge) on pulmonary anaphylactic response (percentage change in relaxation volume) in guinea pig. From Drazen *et al.* (1978b). Courtesy of the authors and *Am. Rev. Respir. Dis.*

mechanisms resulting from the blockade or induction of H_2-receptor deficiency by infectious agents or their by products (endotoxins) may play an important role in the pathogenesis of the airway diseases as well as in the induction of airway-hyperreactivity to histamine. Interestingly the tracheal preparations obtained from cats suffering from upper-respiratory viral infections (rhinotracheitis) exhibit little or no relaxations to histamine. Similarly the tracheobronchial smooth muscle preparations, ob-

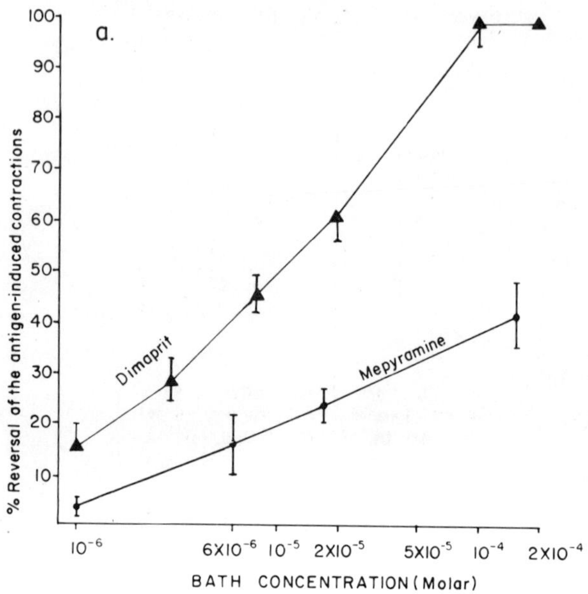

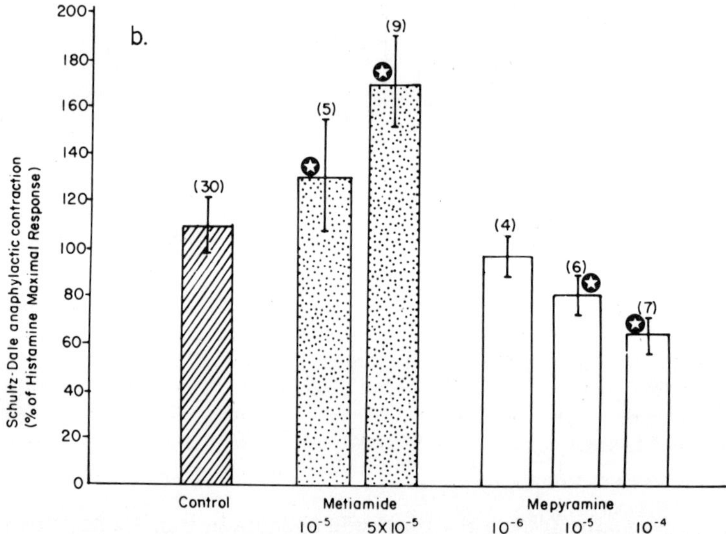

FIG. 7. (a) Reversal of the preexisting anaphylactic contractions to ovalbumin (5 μg ml^{-1}) by dimaprit (H_2-agonist) and mepyramine (H_1-antagonist) in isolated guinea pig lung parenchymal strips. Each point represents mean + SD of observations from 7 to 9 guinea pigs. (b) Effect of metiamide and mepyramine on antigen- (5 μg ml^{-1}) induced contraction (Schultz–Dale response) in guinea pig lung strips. Vertical bar indicates SD. Values in parenthesis show the number of observations. Asterisks indicate the significance ($p < 0.05$) calculated by the Student's t test. From Chand (1979a). Courtesy of *Eur. J. Pharmacol.*

tained from the moneky lungs showing the signs of naturally occurring respiratory infections, exhibit H_1-receptor-mediated strong contractile responses to histamine (Chand, unpublished observations). Normal monkey bronchus and trachea as well as cat trachea precontracted to carbachol relax to histamine (10^{-6} to 10^{-3} *M*) in dose-related fashion (Maengwyn-Davies, 1968; Eyre, 1973; Chand and Eyre, 1977c; Altura and Chand, 1979; Chand *et al.*, 1980a,c). These relaxations are markedly attenuated or absent in the trachea and bronchus obtained from the diseased lungs (Chand and Altura, 1979). Furthermore in some sensitized cats (Chand and Eyre, 1977b), trachea contracts to histamine (Brocklehurst, 1958) and this is antagonized by mepyramine (Chand and Eyre, 1977b). This is in complete contrast to its relaxant action on unsensitized (normal) cats (Maengwyn-Davies, 1968; Eyre, 1973; Tucker and Ercan, 1976; Chand and Eyre, 1977b,c; Eyre and Chand, 1978, 1979; Altura and Chand, 1979). The bronchorelaxant effect of dimaprit (H_2-agonist) is markedly attenuated or absent in the sensitized dogs (Chand and Eyre, 1979). The chicken bronchus which is relatively insensitive to histamine, becomes about 5 to 10 times more reactive to histamine in sensitized chickens (Chand and Eyre, 1978d). The histamine-induced increase in cAMP and inhibition of the release of lysosomal enzyme from neutrophils, responses mediated via H_2-receptors, are markedly suppressed in the granulocytes of asthmatics (Fig. 8) and of normal subjects with rhinoviral respiratory infections or immunized with live influenza vaccine (Busse and Sosman, 1975, 1977; Bush *et al.*, 1978; Busse *et al.*, 1979). The histamine-induced increase in the cAMP (Schmutzler *et al.*, 1973; Allouche *et al.*, 1977; Norn *et al.*, 1978; Barnett *et al.*, 1978) is significantly and consistently lowered in the sensitized guinea-pig lung (Schmutzler *et al.*, 1973; Mathé *et al.*, 1978). The H_2-receptor-mediated relaxation to low doses of histamine is markedly attenuated in the isolated lung strips of some sensitized guinea pigs (Chand, 1979a,b). Furthermore, in the sensitized guinea pig lung, histamine releases larger amounts of thromboxanes A_2, which is mediated via H_1-receptors (Berti *et al.*, 1979). These changes may be related to the process of sensitization or may in part be attributed to the conversion of H_2-inhibitory receptors to mainly H_1-excitatory receptors (Chand and Eyre, 1977b, 1979; Mathé *et al.*, 1978; Berti *et al.*, 1979). The histamine receptor population on leukocytes changes during the processes of proliferation, maturation, and sensitization to the antigen (Chand and Eyre, 1975; Plaut *et al.*, 1973, 1975; Schleimer, 1978). Much remains to be learned about the transmutation of histamine receptors in relation to the development of hypersensitivity and pathogenesis of the airway diseases. Conversion of H_2-receptors (inhibitory) to H_1-type (excitatory) during the hypersensitization in the central airways of some cats, monkeys, and dogs and in the peripheral airways of guinea pigs could con-

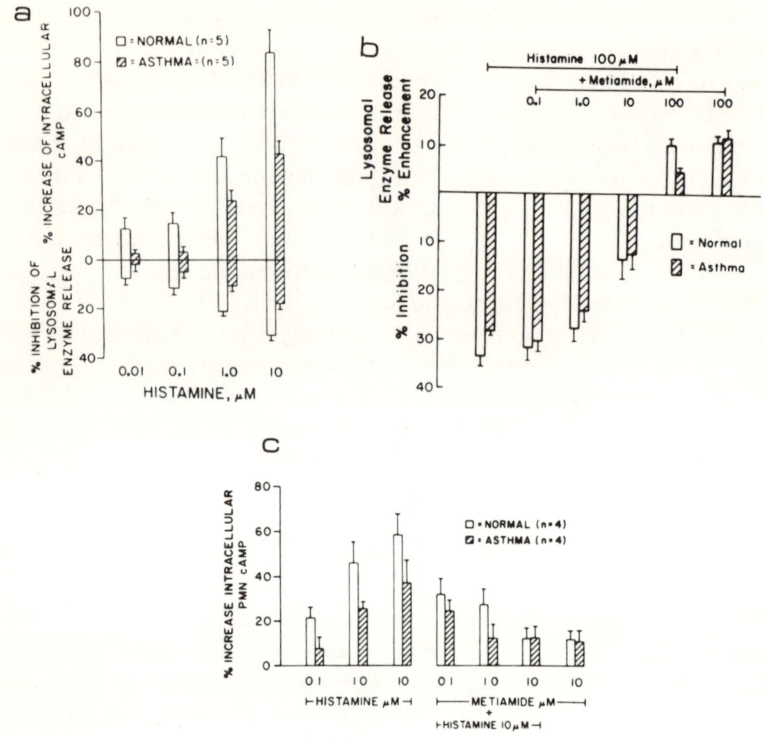

FIG. 8. Deficiency of H_2-histamine receptors on the neutrophils of asthmatic patients.(a) Histamine inhibits the serum-activated zymogen-induced release of lysosomal enzymes (β-glucuronidase) by increasing intracellular levels of cAMP. These responses are significantly decreased in the neutrophils of asthmatic patients as compared to the normal individuals. (b) Metiamide inhibits the histamine-induced inhibition of the release of lysosomal enzymes in concentration related manner, and even produces reversal of the enzyme release reaction at high concentrations. (c) The increase in intracellar levels of cAMP in neutrophils by histamine is blocked by metiamide. From Busse and Sosman (1977). Courtesy of the authors and *J. Clin. Invest.*

ceivably happen in man and animals to enhance airway obstruction (H_1-mediated bronchospasm) in immediate hypersensitivity reactions and other obstruction respiratory diseases. Based on the interesting experimental observations from several laboratories (Busse and Sosman, 1975, 1977; Bush *et al.*, 1978; Chand and Eyre, 1977b, 1979; Mathé *et al.*, 1978; Chand and Altura, 1979; Chand, 1979a,b; Berti *et al.*, 1979), the "theory" of histamine H_2-receptor deficiency in allergic diseases, i.e., physiological imbalance of H_1- and H_2-receptors, possibly comparable with the theory of β-adrenoceptor deficiency in asthma (Szentivanyi, 1968) is proposed.

This concept may partly explain the overall pulmonary "allergic" response and help to interpret the airway hyperreactivity to histamine in asthmatics (Curry, 1947; Obel and Schmitterlow, 1948; Herxheimer, 1951; Townley *et al*, 1965; Makino, 1966; Itkin, 1967; Spector and Farr, 1975; Krell, 1976; Cockcroft *et al.*, 1977; Spector *et al.*, 1979; Michoud *et al.*, 1979).

In clinical obstructive respiratory diseases such as "human asthma," respiratory smooth muscles are constricted by a variety of pharmacological mediators (for example SRS-A, $PGF_{2\alpha}$, thromboxanes, endoperoxides, and acetylcholine: vagal reflexes) (Austen and Orange, 1975; Gold, 1977). It seems possible that the treatment of the obstructive airway diseases with "conventional" H_1-antihistamines may lead to the "unmasking" of histamine H_2-receptors in the respiratory smooth muscles (Dunlop and Smith, 1977; Chand and Eyre, 1977c, 1978a; Yen and Kreutner, 1979a). Consequently, the further immunological (allergic) release of histamine in the lung (Piper, 1977) may serve a "protective" role by inhibiting the further release of chemical mediators from the mast cells and basophils and by relaxing airway smooth muscles via H_2-receptor activation. The aerosol administration of H_2-agonists (dimaprit and impromidine) combined with H_1-antagonists as therapeutic agents in "allergic" obstructive respiratory diseases offers an intriguing but strong possibility.

D. Other Miscellaneous Modulatory Functions of Histamine H_2-Receptors

Histamine produces neutrophil leukocytosis in dogs, an effect which is blocked by metiamide. Several possibilities were put forward to explain this effect: (1) metiamide may inhibit the release of leukotactic factor by histamine; (2) it may antagonize the action of histamine (or leukotactic factor) in the bone marrow; or (3) may have a nonspecific suppressive action on the release of neutrophils from bone marrow in dogs (Code, 1975). Metiamide and cimetidine therapy produces hematotoxicity (agranulocytosis) in man (Burland *et al.*, 1975; Posnett *et al.*, 1979), which may be related to the occurrence of histamine H_2-receptors in hematopoietic (pluripotent bone marrow) stem cell (Bryon, 1977; Posnett *et al.*, 1979).

Metiamide and burimamide inhibit the histamine-induced inhibition of lymphocyte activation by mitogens, tuberculin proteins, and tumor-specific antigens in guinea pig. Metiamide and burimamide in low doses enhance the lymphocyte activation possibly suggesting that locally released (endogenous) histamine may be acting as a chemical modulator of lymphocyte function operating via H_2-receptors in the intact animals (Beets and Dale, 1979).

Histamine suppresses the antigen-induced production and proliferation of migration inhibitory factor (MIF). This effect is again mediated through H_2-receptors (Rocklin, 1976, 1977). Histamine also diminishes the delayed hypersensitivity (cellular immune) response in guinea pig which is completely inhibited by burimamide (Rocklin, 1976). Rocklin (1976) has suggested that histamine released during immediate hypersensitivity reactions could subsequently modulate the expression of the delayed hypersensitivity (cellular-immune) reactions.

V. Summary and Conclusions

The overall effect of histamine on the airway smooth muscle is highly complex and depends on the algebraic sum of stimulatory and inhibitory actions of a mixed population of H_1- and H_2-receptors which in general act in opposite directions. The relative ratio of H_1- and H_2-receptors not only varies between species, but the ratio even differs considerably from one segment to another in the airways of the same species. Such is clearly the situation in the airways of cat, rabbit, and sheep. The striking species and regional differences in the reactivity of the airway smooth muscles to histamine and the proportional distribution of histamine H_1- and H_2-receptors (Table II) make extrapolation of the observations from one species to another extremely difficult and can be misleading, if not invalid.

In general, there is preponderance of histamine H_1-receptors mediating constrictions in the tracheobronchial smooth muscles of man, guinea pig, horse, goat, cattle, langur monkey, and dog, rabbit bronchus, sheep trachea, and peripheral airways (lung strips) of all the species investigated. Histamine H_2-receptors, which mediate airway relaxations, are present in the tracheobronchial smooth muscles of man, horse, swine, and guinea pig and also in the peripheral airways of guinea pig. Cat trachea and sheep intermediate bronchus and monkey tracheobronchial smooth muscle possess preponderance of H_2-receptors. The spasmolytic actions of histamine in the trachea of rabbit, ferret, and rat seem to be mediated via a different type of H_2-receptor.

Histamine inhibits the allergic release of chemical mediators (histamine and SRS-A) and lysosomal enzymes by activating H_2-receptors on the target cells of immediate hypersensitivity. Under experimental conditions, H_2-agonists (dimaprit, impromidine, etc.) partially inhibit or reverse respiratory allergic responses *in vitro* as well as *in vivo* in the guinea pig. On the other hand, H_2-antagonist (like burimamide and metiamide) in relatively high doses enhances the immunological release of histamine, SRS-A, and lysosomal enzymes, and potentiates pulmonary anaphylactic response in guinea pig and systemic anaphylaxis in horse, calf, and chicken. Thus H_2-receptors on basophils (mast cells), neutrophils, and eosinophils appear to play an important modulatory (autoregulatory) role via a negative "feedback" mechanism in the release of chemical mediators and lysosomal enzymes in the immediate hypersensitivity reactions. In general the autoregulatory functions of histamine appear to be associated with cAMP. The deficiency of H_2-receptors (or histamine-sensitive adenyl cyclase) on the mast cells (basophils) and in the airway smooth muscles in hypersensitive individuals (asthmatics) may be an important predisposing factor and may enhance overall respiratory allergic responses.

Aerosol administration of H_2-agonist (e.g., dimaprit and impromidine) combined with H_1-antagonist as therapeutic agents in "allergic" obstructive respiratory diseases is an intriguing but strong possibility. The H_2-receptors on lymphocytes seem to play an immunoregulatory role in their activation, proliferation, and production of migration inhibitory factor (MIF) and antibodies, and expression of cytotoxic and delayed hypersensitivity (cellular immune) reactions. Obviously much remains to be learned about the precise roles of H_2-receptors in pathophysiological conditions in man and animal.

References

Adams, G. K., and Lichtenstein, L. M. (1977). *Nature (London)* **270,** 255–257.

Adams, G. K., and Lichtenstein, L. (1979). *J. Immunol.* **122,** 555–562.

Akçasu, A. (1952). *J. Pharm. Pharmacol.* **4,** 671.

Akçasu, A. (1959). *Arch. Int. Pharmacodyn.* **122,** 201–207.

Allouche, G., Santais, M. C., Foussard, C., Ruff, F., and Parrot, J. L. (1977). *Agents Actions* **7,** 103–104.

Altura, B. M. (1972). *Eur. J. Pharmacol.* **20,** 261–265.

Altura, B. M., and Altura, B. T. (1974). *Anesthesiology* **41,** 197–214.

Altura, B. M., and Altura, B. T. (1977). *In* "Factors Influencing Vascular Reactivity" (O. Carrier, Jr. and S. Shibata, eds.), pp. 397–426. Igaku-Shoin, New York.

Anderson, W. H., Krzanowski, J. J., Polson, J. B., and Szentivanyi, A. (1979a). *Biochem. Pharmacol.* **28,** 2223–2226.

Anderson, W. H., Krzanowski, J. J., Polson, J. B., and Szentivanyi, a. (1979b). *Naunyn-Schmiedebergs Arch. Pharmacol.* **303,** 117–126.

Antonissen, L. A., Mitchell, R. W., Kroeger, E. A., and Stephens, N. L. (1978a). *Can. Fed. Biol. Soc.* **21,** 21.

Antonissen, L. A., Mitchell, R. W., Kroeger, E. A., and Stephens, N. L. (1978b). *Fed. Proc.* **37,** 639.

Ash, A. S. F., and Schild, H. O. (1966). *Br. J. Pharmacol. Chemother.* **27,** 427–439.

Austen, K. F., and Orange, R. P. (1975). *Am. Rev. Respir. Dis.* **112,** 423–436.

Bakhle, Y. S., and Smith, T. W., (1972). *Br. J. Pharmacol.* **46,** 543–544.

Bareica, I., and Rocha e Silva, M. (1976). *Gen. Pharmacol.* **7,** 103–106.

Barer, G. R. (1966). *Circ. Res.* **18,** 366–378.

Barer, G. R., and McCurrie, J. R. (1969). *Q. J. Exp. Physiol.* **54,** 156–173.

Barer, G. R., Emery, C. J., Mohammed, F. H., Mungall, I. P. F., and Thompson, B. (1976). *J. Physiol.* **259,** 41p.

Barer, G. R., Emery, C. J., Mohammed, F. H., and Mungall, I. P. F. (1978). *Q. J. Exp. Physiol.* **63,** 157–169.

Barnett, D. B., Chesrown, S. E., Zbinden, H. F., Nisam, M., Reed, B. R., Bourne, H. R., Melmon, K. H., and Gold, W. M. (1978). *Am. Rev. Respir. Dis.* **118,** 723–733.

Beets, J. L., and Dale, M. M. (1979). *Br. J. Pharmacol.* **66,** 365–372.

Bergofsky, E. H. (1974). *Am. J. Med.* **57,** 378–394.

Berti, F., Folco, G. C., Nicosia, S., Omini, C., and Pasargiklian, R. (1979). *Br. J. Pharmacol.* **65,** 629–633.

Black, J. W., Duncan, W. A. M., Durant, C. J., Ganellin, C. R., and Parsons, E. M. (1972). *Nature (London)* **236,** 385–390.

Black, J. W., Duncan, W. A. M., Emmett, J. C., Ganellin, C. R., Hesselbo, T., Parsons, M. E., and Wyllie, J. H. (1973). *Agents Actions* **3,** 133–137.

Brimblecombe, R. W., Duncan, G. J., Durant, J. C., Emmett, C. R., Ganellin, T., and Parsons, M. E. (1975). *J. Int. Med. Res.* **3,** 86–92.

Brocklehurst, W. (1958). *In* "5-Hydroxytryptamine" (G. P. Lewis, ed.), pp. 172–176. Pergamon, New York.

Buck, S. H., Yellin, T. O., and Mant, D. M. (1979). *Pharmacologist* **21,** 265.

Burka, J. F., and Eyre, P. (1976). *Int. Arch. Allergy Appl. Immunol.* **50,** 664–673.

Burland, W. L., Sharpe, P. C., Colin-Jones, D. C., Turnbull, P. R. G., and Bowskill, P. (1975). *Lancet* **11,** 1085.

Burns, J. W., and Doe, J. E. (1978). *Br. J. Pharmacol.* **64,** 71–74.

Burnstock, G. (1971). *Pharmacol. Rev.* **24,** 509–581.

Bush, R. K., Busse, W., Flaherty, D., Warshauer, D., Dick, E. C., and Reed, C. E. (1978). *J. Allergy. Clin. Immunol.* **61,** 80–87.

Busse, W. W., and Sosman, J. (1975). *Science* **194,** 737–738.

Busse, W. W., and Sosman, J. (1977). *J. Clin. Invest.* **59,** 1080–1287.

Busse, W. W., Cooper, W., Warshauer, D. M., Dick, E. C., Wallow, I. H. L., and Albrecht, R. (1979). *Am. Rev. Respir. Dis.* **119,** 561–569.

Byron, J. W. (1977). *Agents Actions* **7,** 209–213.

Castillo, J. C. (1948). *J. Pharmacol. Exp. Ther.* **94,** 412–415.

Castillo, J. C., and deBeer, E. J. (1947). *J. Pharmacol. Exp. Ther.* **90,** 104–109.

Casterline, C. L., and Evans, R. (1977). *J. Allergy Clin. Immunol.* **59,** 420–424.

Chakrin, L. W., Mengel, J., Young, D., Zaher, C., Krell, R. D., and Wardell, J. R. (1974a). *Fed. Proc.* **33,** 585.

Chakrin, L. W., Krell, R. D., Mengel, J., Young, D., Zaher, C., and Wardell, J. R. (1974b). *Agents Actions* **4,** 297–303.

Chakrin, L. W., Bostick, S., Hostelley, L., and Krell, R. D. (1979). *Pharmacologist* **21,** 266.

Chand, N. (1979a). *Eur. J. Pharmacol.* **55,** 337–339.

Chand, N. (1979b). *Lung* **156,** 271–277.

Chand, N. (1979c). *Agents Actions* **9,** 133–140.

Chand, N. (1979d). *J. Vet. Pharmacol. Ther.* **2,** 151–171.

Chand, N. (1979e). *J. Vet. Pharmacol. Ther.* **2,** 133–138.

Chand, N. (1979f). *Res. Commun. Chem. Pathol. Pharmacol.* **25,** 215–226.

Chand, N., and Altura, B. M. (1979). *J. Cell Biol.* **83** (Part II), 237a.

Chand, N., and DeRoth, L. (1978a). *Eur. J. Pharmacol.* **52,** 143–145.

Chand, N., and DeRoth, L. (1978b). *Physiologist* **21,** 19.

Chand, N., and DeRoth, L. (1978c). *Annu. Conf. Indian Pharmacol. Soc., XI, Dec., New Delhi.*

Chand, N., and DeRoth, L. (1978d). *Vet. Sci. Commun.* **2,** 151–155.

Chand, N., and DeRoth, L. (1979a). *Zbl. Vet. Med. A* **26,** 566–572.

Chand, N., and DeRoth, L. (1979b). *Res. Commun. Chem. Pathol. Pharmacol.* **23,** 223–232.

Chand, N., and DeRoth, L. (1979c). *J. Vet. Pharmacol. Ther.* **2,** 87–89.
Chand, N., and DeRoth, L. (1979d). *Pharmacology* **19,** 185–190.
Chand, N., and DeRoth, L. (1979e). *Vet. Human Toxicol.* (in press).
Chand, N., and DeRoth, L. (1979f). *J. Pharm. Pharmacol.* **31,** 712–714.
Chand, N., and DeRoth, L. (1979g). *Toxicon* **17,** 583–589.
Chand, N., and DeRoth, L. (1980). *Am. J. Vet. Res.* **41,** 101–105.
Chand, N., and Eyre, P. (1975). *Agents Actions* **5,** 277–295.
Chand, N., and Eyre, P. (1977a). *Can. J. Comp. Med.* **41,** 233–240.
Chand, N., and Eyre, P. (1977b). *Eur. J. Pharmacol.* **45,** 213–220.
Chand, N., and Eyre, P. (1977c). *Fed. Proc.* **36,** 1022.
Chand, N., and Eyre, P. (1977d). *Agents Actions* **7,** 183–190.
Chand, N., and Eyre, P. (1977e). *Annu. Conf. Indian Pharmacol. Soc., Xth* (Abstract No. 238).
Chand, N., and Eyre, P. (1977f). *Vet. Sci. Commun.* **1,** 85–90.
Chand, N., and Eyre, P. (1978a). *Agents Actions* **8,** 191–198.
Chand, N., and Eyre, P. (1978b). *Vet. Sci. Commun.* **2,** 77–82.
Chand, N., and Eyre, P. (1978c). *Res. Commun. Chem. Pathol. Pharmacol.* **21,** 55–66.
Chand, N., and Eyre, P. (1978d). *J. Pharm. Pharmacol.* **30,** 432–435.
Chand, N., and Eyre, P. (1978e). *Agents Actions* **8,** 171–184.
Chand, N., and Eyre, P. (1979). *Agents and Actions* **9,** 4–8.
Chand, N., DeRoth, L., and Eyre, P. (1979a). *Br. J. Pharmacol.* **66,** 511–556.
Chand, N., DeRoth, L., and Eyre, P. (1979b). *Br. J. Pharmacol.* **66,** 331–336. ·
Chand, N., DeRoth, L., and Phaneuf, L. P. (1979c). *Gen. Pharmacol.* **10,** 381–384.
Chand, N., Eyre, P., and DeRoth, L. (1979d). *Res. Commun. Chem. Pathol. Pharmacol.* **23,** 211–221.
Chand, N., Eyre, P., and DeRoth, L, (1979e). *Can. J. Comp. Med.* **43,** 384–391.
Chand, N., Dhawan, B. N., Srimal, R. C., Rahmani, N. H., Shukla, R., and Altura, B. M. (1980a). *J. Appl. Physiol.* (in press).
Chand., N., Dhawan, B. N., Srimal, R. C., Rahamani, N. H., Shukla, R., and Altura, B. M. (1980b). *J. Appl. Physiol.* (in press).
Chand, N., Srimal, R. C., Shukla, R., and Dhawan, B. N. (1980c). *Ind. J. Pharmacol. Soc.* **12** (in press).
Church, M. K. (1975). *Br. J. Pharmacol.* **55,** 423–431.
Clark, R. A. F., Sandler, J. A., Gallin, J. A., and Kaplan, A. P. (1977). *J. Immunol.* **118,** 137–145.
Cockcroft, D. W., Killian, D. N., Mellon, J. J. A., and Hargreave, F. F. (1977). *Clin. Allergy* **7,** 235–243.
Code, C. F. (1975). *J. Physiol.* **254,** 31–32P.
Colebatch, H. J. H. (1970). *Circ. Res.* **26,** 379–396.
Coleman, R. A., Kennedy, I., and Whelan, C. J. (1979). *Br. J. Pharmacol.* **66,** 83P.
Curry, J. J. (1974). *J. Clin. Invest.* **26,** 430–438.
Dale, H. H., and Laidlaw, P. O. (1910). *J. Physiol.* **41,** 318–344.
Dawson, C. A, Delano, F. A., Hamilton, L. H., and Stekeil, W. F. (1974). *J. Appl. Physiol.* **37,** 670–674.
DeRoth, L., and Chand, N. (1979). *Zbl. Vet. Med. A* **26,** 293–401.
Dixon, M., Jackson, D. M., and Richards, I. M. (1979). *Br. J. Pharmacol.* **66,** 203–209.
Drazen, J. M., and Schneider, M. W. (1978). *J. Clin. Invest* **61,** 1441–1447.
Drazen, J. M., Schneider, M. W., and Venugopalan, C. S. (1978a). *Physiologist* **21,** 31.
Drazen, J. M., Venugopalan, C. S., and Soter, N. S. (1978b). *Am. Rev. Respir. Dis.* **117,** 479–485.
Drazen, J. M., Lewis, R. A., Wasserman, S. I., and Orange, R. P. (1979a). *J. Clin. Invest.* **63,** 1–5.

Drazen, J. M., Schneider, M. W., and Venugopalan, C. S. (1979b). *Eur. J. Pharmacol.* **55,** 233–240.
Dulabh, R., and Vickers, M. R. (1978). *Agents Actions* **8,** 559–565.
Duke, H. N. (1969). *J. Physiol.* **200,** 133–135P.
Dunlop, L. S., and Smith, A. P. (1977). *Br. J. Pharmacol.* **59,** 475.
Durant, G. J., Ganellin, C. R., and Parsons, M. E. (1975). *J. Med. Chem.* **18,** 905–909.
Durant, G. J., Ganellin, C. R., and Parsons, M. E. (1977). *Agents Actions* **7,** 39–43.
Durant, G. J., Duncan, W. A. M., Ganellin, C. R., Parsons, M. E., Blakemore, R. C., and Rasmussen, A. C. (1978). *Nature (London)* **276,** 403–404.
Ercan, Z. S., and Turker, R. K. (1977). *Pharmacology* **15,** 18–126.
Everitt, B. J., Bentley, J. A., Spiegel, W. D., and Porter, M. A. (1979). *Pharmacologist* **21,** 153.
Eyre, P. (1969). *Br. J. Pharmacol.* **36,** 409–417.
Eyre, P. (1972). *Vet. Rec.* **91,** 134–140.
Eyre, P. (1973). *Br. J. Pharmacol.* **48,** 321–323.
Eyre, P. (1976). *Can. J. Comp. Med.* **40,** 149–152.
Eyre, P., and Besner, R. N. (1979). *Res. Commun. Chem. Pathol. Pharmacol.* **24,** 457–464.
Eyre, P., and Burka, J. F. (1978). *J. Vet. Pharmacol. Ther.* **1,** 97–109.
Eyre, P., and Chand, N. (1978). *Proc. Congr. Pharmacol., 7th, July, Paris.*
Eyre, P., and Chand, N. (1979). *Agents Actions* **9,** 1–3.
Eyre, P., and Wells, P. W. (1973). *Br. J. Pharmacol.* **49,** 364–367.
Fishman, A. P. (1976). *Circ. Res.* **38,** 221–231.
Fjalland, B. (1979). *J. Pharm. Pharmacol.* **31,** 50–51.
Fleisch, J. H., and Calkins, P. J. (1976). *J. Appl. Physiol.* **41,** 62–66.
Gold, W. M. (1977). *Am. Rev. Respir. Dis.* **115,** 127–137.
Goth, A., and Johnson, A. R. (1975). *Life Sci.* **16,** 1201–1214.
Grodzinska, L., Panczenko, B., and Gryglewski, R. J. (1975). *J. Pharm. Pharmcol.* **27,** 88–91.
Haas, F., and Bergofsky, E. H. (1972). *J. Clin. Invest.* **51,** 3254–3162.
Hakanson, R., Larssan, L. I., Leidberg, G., and Sundler, F. (1978). *J. Physiol.* **276,** 151–157.
Halevy, S., and Altura, B. M. (1977). *Proc. Soc. Exp. Biol. Med.* **154,** 453–456.
Halonen, M., Stanfield, M., and Palmer, J. D. (1979). *Fed. Proc.* **38,** 1415.
Hamberg, M., Svensson, J., Hedquist, P., Strandberg, K., and Samuelsson, B. (1976). *In* "Advances in Prostaglandin and Thromboxane Research" (B. Samuelsson and R. Paoletti, eds.), pp. 495–501. Raven, New York.
Hauge, A., and Melmon, K. L. (1968). *Circ. Res.* **22,** 385–392.
Hauge, A., and Staub, N. C. (1969). *J. Appl. Physiol.* **26,** 693–699.
Hawkins, D. F., Herxheimer, H., and Schild, H. O. (1951). *J. Physiol.* **113,** 26P.
Henderson, W. R., and Kaliner, M. (1979). *J. Immunol.* **122,** 1322–1328.
Herxheimer, H. (1951). *Int. Arch. Allergy* **2,** 27–39.
Hirschowitz, B. I. (1979). *Annu. Rev. Pharmacol. Toxicol.* **19,** 203–244.
Hoffman, E. A., Tucker, A., and Reeves, J. T. (1975). *Circulation* **52** (Suppl. 2), 196.
Hoffman, E. A., Munroe, M. L., Tucker, A., and Reeves, J. T. (1977). *Respir. Physiol.* **29,** 255–264.
Holroyde, M. C., Burka, J. F., and Eyre, P. (1977). *Agents Actions* **7,** 421–430.
Howard, P., Barer, G. R., Thompson, B., Warren, P. M., Abbott, C. J., and Mungall, I. P. F. (1975). *Respir. Physiol.* **24,** 325–345.
Irvin, C. G., and Dempsey, J. A (1978). *Respir. Physiol.* **35,** 161–176.
Itkin, I. H. (1967). *J. Allergy* **40,** 245–256.
Jamieson, D. (1962). *Br. J. Pharmacol. Chemother.* **19,** 286–294.

Joiner, P. D., Minor, L., Davis, L. B., Kadowitz, P. J., and Hyman, A. L. (1975). *Pharmacologist* **17,** 191.
Kamakawa, Y., and Shimo, Y. (1976). *J. Pharm. Pharmacol.* **28,** 854–855.
Karlin, J. M. (1972). *Ann. Allergy* **30,** 342–347.
Kay, J. M., Waymire, J. C., and Grover, R. F. (1974). *Am. J. Physiol.* **226,** 178–184.
Kenakin, T. P., Krueger, C. A., and Cook, D. A. (1974). *Nature (London)* **252,** 54–55.
Kleinstiver, P. W., and Eyre, P. (1978). *Can. Fed. Biol. Soc.* **21,** 81.
Kleinstiver, P. W., and Eyre, P. (1979). *J. Pharmacol. Methods* **2,** 175–185.
Krell, R. D. (1976). *Life Sci.* **19,** 1777–1782.
Krell, R. D. (1978a) *Eur. J. Pharmacol.* **49,** 151–155.
Krell, R. D.(1978b). *Br. J. Pharmacol.* **62,** 519–528.
Krell, R. D., and Chakrin, L. W. (1977). *Eur. J. Pharmacol.* **44,** 35–44.
Lands, A. M., Arnold, A., McAuliff, J. P., Uduena, F. P., and Brown, T. C. (1967). *Nature (London)* **214,** 597–598.
Lichtenstein, L. M., and Gillespie, E. (1973). *Nature (London)* **244,** 287–288.
Lichtenstein, L. M., and Gillespie, E. (1975). *J. Pharmacol. Exp. Ther.* **192,** 441–450.
Lulich, K. M., Mitchell, H. W., and Sparrow, M. P. (1976). *Br. J. Pharmacol.* **58,** 71–79.
McDouglas, M. D., and West, G. B. (1953). *Br. J. Pharmacol. Chemother.* **8,** 26–29.
McMurty, I. F., Dickey, D. W., and Souhrada, J. F. (1977). *Artery* **3,** 1–12.
Maconochie, J. G., Woodings, E. P., and Richards, D. A. (1979). *Br. J. Clin. Pharmacol.* **7,** 231–236.
Maengwyn-Davies, G. D. (1968). *J. Pharm. Pharmacol.* **20,** 572–573.
Main, I. H. M. (1964). *Br. J. Pharmacol. Chemother.* **22,** 511–519.
Makino, S. (1966). *J. Allergy.* **38,** 127–142.
Martin, G., and Fertel, R. H. (1978). *Fed. Proc.* **37,** 393.
Martin, L. F., Tucker, A., Munroe, M. L., and Reeves, J. T. (1978). *Respiration* **35,** 73–77.
Mathe, A. A., Astrom, A., and Persson, N. A. (1971). *J. Pharm. Pharmacol.* **23,** 905–910.
Mathe, A. A., Sohn, R. J., and Volicer, L. (1978). *Pharmacology* **16,** 30–36.
Meyers, J. L., Dain, D., Gold, W. M., Miller, R. L., and Bourne, H. R. (1973). *Physiologist* **16,** 396.
Michoud, M. C., Pare, P. D., Orange, R. P., and Hogg, J. C. (1979). *Am. Rev. Respir. Dis.* **119,** 419–424.
Mitchell, H. W., and Denborough, M. A. (1979). *Eur. J. Pharmacol.* **54,** 69–78.
Mitchell, H. W., and Sparrow, M. P. (1975). *Clin. Exp. Pharmacol. Physiol.* **2,** 427.
Mitchell, H. W., and Sparrow, M. P. (1977). *Br. J. Pharmacol.* **61,** 533–540.
Mungall, I. P. F. (1976). *Thorax* **31,** 94–100.
Newman, J. H., Souhrada, J. F., Reeves, J. T., Arroyave, C. M., Moore, L., and Grover, R. F. (1978). *Fed. Proc.* **37,** 458.
Newman, J. H., Souhrada, J. F., Reeves, J. T., Arroyave, C. M., and Grover, R. F. (1979). *Am. J. Physiol.* **237,** H76–H82.
Nogrady, S. G., Hartley, J. P., Handslip, P. D., and Hurst, N. P. (1978). *Thorax* **33,** 479–482.
Norn, S., Geisler, A., Klysner, R., and Stahl-Skov, P. (1978). *Agents Actions* **8,** 401.
Obel, N. J., and Schmitterlow, C. G. (1948). *Acta Pharmacol.* **4,** 71–80.
Ohhubo, H., Takayanagi, I., and Takagi, K. (1975). *Jap. J. Pharmacol.* **25,** 35P.
Okpako, D. T., Chand, N., and Eyre, P. (1978). *J. Pharm. Pharmacol.* **30,** 280–282.
Orehek, J., Douglas, J. S., Lewis, A. J., and Bouhuys, A. (1973). *Nature (London) New Biol.* **245,** 84–85.
Orehek, J., Douglas, J. S., and Bouhuys, A. (1975). *J. Pharmacol. Exp. Ther.* **194,** 554–564.
Orr, T. S. C. (1973). *Br. J. Dis. Chest* **67,** 87–105.
Owen, D. A. A. (1977). *Gen. Pharmacol.* **8,** 141–156.

Parsons, M. E., Owen, D. A. A., Ganellin, C. R., and Durant, G. J. (1977). *Agents Actions* **7,** 31–37.

Persson, C. G. A., and Ekman, M. (1976). *Agents Actions* **6,** 389–393.

Piper, P. J. (1977). *Pharmacol. Ther. B* **3,** 75–98.

Plaut, M. (1979). *J. Allergy Clin. Immunol.* **63,** 371–375.

Plaut, M., Lichtenstein, L. M., and Henney, C. S. (1973). *Nature* (*London*) **244,** 284–286.

Plaut, M., Lichtenstein, L. M., and Henney, C. S. (1975). *J. Clin. Invest.* **55,** 856–874.

Posnett, D. N., Stein, R. S., Graber, S. E., and Krantz, S. B. (1979). *Arch. Intern. Med.* **139,** 584–586.

Rocklin, R. E. (1976). *J. Clin. Invest.* **57,** 1051–1058.

Rocklin, R. E. (1977). *J. Immunol.* **118,** 1734–1738.

Sadavongvivad, C. (1970). *Br. J. Pharmacol.* **38,** 153–160.

Schleimer, R. (1978). *Proc. West Pharmacol. Soc.* **21,** 145–150.

Schmutzler, W., Poblete-Freundt, G., and Derwal, R. (1973). *Agents Actions* **3,** 192–193.

Schneider, W., Drazen, J. M., Snapper, J. R., Loring, S. H., and Ingram, R. H. (1978). *Fed. Proc.* **37,** 579.

Shaw, W. (1971). *J. Physiol.* **215,** 34–35P.

Silove, E. D., and Simcha, A. J. (1973). *J. Appl. Physiol.* **35,** 830–836.

Simonsson, B. G., Svedmyr, N., Skoogh, B. E., Anderson, R., and Bergh, N. P. (1972). *Scand. J. Respir. Dis.* **53,** 227–236.

Sirois, P. (1979). *Prostaglandins* **17,** 395–404.

Spector, S. L., and Farr, R. S. (1975). *J. Allergy Clin. Immunol.* **56,** 308–316.

Spector, S. L., Staudenmayer, H., Kinsman, R. A., Fukuhara, J., and Westmoreland, C. (1979). *Allergy* **34,** 167–173.

Spilker, B., and Minatoya, H. (1975). *Arch. Int. Pharmacol. Ther.* **217,** 201–217.

Staszewska-Barczak, J., and Vane, J. R. (1965). *Br. J. Pharmacol.* **25,** 728–742.

Staub, N. C. (1975). *Post Grad. Med. J.* **51,** 21–34.

Stotland, L. M., and Share, N. N. (1974). *Can. J. Physiol. Pharmacol.* **52,** 1119–1125.

Susmano, A., and Carleton, R. A. (1971). *J. Appl. Physiol.* **31,** 531–535.

Svedmyr, N. (1970). *Scand. J. Respir. Dis.* **74,** 15.

Svedmyr, N. (1971). *Post Grad. Med. J.* **747,** 120.

Svedmyr, N., and Simonsson, B. G. (1978). *Pharmacol. Ther. B* **3,** 397–440.

Szentivanyi, A. (1968). *J. Allergy* **42,** 203–232.

Thompson, B., Barer, G. R., and Shaw, J. W. (1976). *Clin. Exp. Pharmacol. Physiol.* **3,** 399–414.

Townley, R. G., Dennis, M., and Itken, I. H. (1965). *J. Allergy* **31,** 121–137.

Tozzi, S. (1973). *J. Pharmacol. Exp. Ther.* **187,** 511–517.

Tucker, A., Weir, E. K., Reeves, J. T., and Grover, R. F. (1975). *Am. J. Physiol.* **229,** 1008–1013.

Tucker, A., Weir, E. K., Reeves, J. T., and Grover, R. F. (1976). *J. Appl. Physiol.* **40,** 496–500.

Tucker, A., Hoffman, E. C., and Reeves, J. T. (1977a). *Eur. J. Pharmacol.* **45,** 73–77.

Tucker, A., Hoffman, E. A., and Weir, E. K. (1977b). *Chest* **71,** 261S–262S.

Turker, R. K., and Ercan, Z. S. (1976). *J. Pharm. Pharmacol.* **28,** 298–301.

Verma, S. C., and McNeill, J. H. (1976). *Res. Commun. Chem. Pathol. Pharmacol.* **13,** 55–64.

Vidruk, E. H., and Sampson, S. R. (1978). *Fed. Proc.* **37,** 689.

Wasserman, M. A., and Griffin, R. L. (1977). *Eur. J. Pharmacol.* **46,** 303–313.

Weinstein, Y., and Melmon, K. L. (1976). *Immunol. Commun.* **5,** 401–416.

Wells, P. W., Pass, D. A., and Eyre, P. (1974). *Res. Vet. Sci.* **16,** 347–350.

Yamatake, Y., Sasagawa, S., and Yanaura, S. (1978). *Chem. Pharm. Bull.* **26,** 318–320.
Yellin, T. O., Buck, S. H., Gilman, D. J., Jones, D. F., and Wardleworth, J. M. (1979). *Pharmacologist* **21,** 266.
Yen, S. S. (1978). *Fed. Proc.* **37,** 689.
Yen, S. S., and Kreutner, W. (1979a). *Life Sci.* **25,** 507–514.
Yen, S. S., and Kreutner, W. (1979b). *Pharmacologist* **21,** 154.
Yen, S. S., Mathe, A. A., and Dugan, J. J. (1976). *Prostaglandins* **11,** 227–239.

ADVANCES IN PHARMACOLOGY AND CHEMOTHERAPY, VOL. 17

In Vitro Methods to Predict for Patient Response to Chemotherapy

DANIEL D. VON HOFF

Department of Medicine
Division of Oncology
University of Texas Health Science Center at San Antonio
San Antonio, Texas

LARRY WEISENTHAL

Section of Hematology-Oncology
Veterans Administration Medical Center
Long Beach, California
and
Department of Medicine
University of California, Irvine
Irvine, California

I. Introduction

It has been the object of a great deal of investigation to find an *in vitro* test which would predict for response of an individual patient's tumor to a

ISBN 0-12-032917-4

specific anticancer drug (or combination of drugs). This type of tool would enable the oncologist to choose the appropriate chemotherapeutic agent for a particular patient's tumor much the way antibiotics are now chosen for a particular infection.

The concept of developing a predictive *in vitro* test for cancer chemotherapy is not a new concept. As early as 1954, there were attempts to correlate the effects of antineoplastics in *in vitro* systems with *in vivo* antitumor effects of the drugs.

The following discussion will deal with research and development of a variety of *in vitro* tests which have been used to predict for clinical response of a patient's tumor to a particular anticancer agent. Only trials which present clinical correlations will be discussed. The various systems used will be subdivided by general methodologies with short discussions of strengths and weaknesses of the methodologies. No attempt is made here to discuss *in vivo* predictive assay systems which involve measurement of antitumor effect in animal tumors. We will not discuss the effect of anticancer drugs on human tumors growing in an animal model such as the nude mouse. (Giovanella *et al.*, 1978). A number of these *in vivo* tests have appeared promising in early studies and are currently under continued development (Bevenbaum *et al*. 1974; Cobb and Mitchley, 1974; Bogden *et al.*, 1979; Smith *et al.*, 1976).

II. Requirements for *in Vitro* Systems

There are a number of conditions which should be met for an *in vitro* system to have some practical and clinical usefulness. Cline (1969) has considered these minimal conditions to be: (1) the drug must be active in the form in which it is added or must be converted to an active form by the constituents of the system; (2) the metabolism of the malignant cells *in vivo* and *in vitro* must be sufficiently similar so that drug effect under the two conditions are comparable; (3) there must be sufficient time for drug action to become manifest (but not so long that major changes in the "control" cell population takes place, relative to conditions *in vivo*); and (4) a representative sample of tumor must be obtained for testing.

In addition to the requirements expressed by Cline (1969) a few additional conditions would be desirable: the drug concentration used in the system must be realistically achievable in a patient; the test must be relatively inexpensive and must be technically fast, simple, and reproducible; and most importantly, the test must be a strong correlation between *in vitro* results and clinical results. Finally, it is important that an *in vitro* test be more sensitive than it is specific. Both sensitivity and specificity are desirable goals but for an *in vitro* test to exclude compounds that are useful *in vivo* is a more serious problem than for it occasionally to overpredict clinical usefulness.

III. General Technical Problems for *in Vitro* Systems

A. Selection of Culture Media

All cells growing *in vitro* require certain nutrients that must be supplied in the culture media. The nutrient requirements probably vary from cell to cell. These individual cell type requirements have been extensively reviewed elsewhere (Abaza *et al.*, 1978; Ham, 1974; Hayashi *et al.*, 1978; Hutchings and Sato, 1978; Kimball *et al.*, 1978; Leibovitz, 1975; Lickiss *et al.*, 1974; Mather and Sato, 1977; Mavligit *et al.*, 1975; Rizzino and Sato, 1978; Sato and Hayashi, 1976; Sherwin and Richters, 1975; Taylor, 1974; Waymouth, 1972, 1974, 1977; Wu and Sato, 1978). It is becoming increasingly clear that well-defined tissue culture media without the use of serum is a practical way for an investigator to understand what effects individual nutrients (such as hormones) are having on cell growth (Hayashi *et al.*, 1978; Hutchings and Sato, 1978; Mather and Sato, 1977; Rizzino and Sato, 1978; Sato and Hayashi, 1976; Wu and Sato, 1978).

There is a reason for being concerned about choosing the appropriate media. It is known that certain hormones appear necessary for growth of most cells but that the specific hormone requirements may be different for different cells (Hayashi *et al.*, 1978). Hormone-stimulated cell growth could conceivably alter a cell chemosensitivity pattern by stimulating the cell growth *in vitro* to a greater degree than the growth is affected *in vivo*. Therefore, in selecting the appropriate tissue culture media one must be chosen which allows the cells to grow but which also preserves, as closely as possible, the *in vivo* kinetics of cell growth.

B. Preparation of Single Cell Suspensions

Malignant pleural effusions, ascites, or tumor-containing bone marrow specimens are all good sources of single cell suspensions of both tumor and normal host cells. When biopsies of solid tumors are performed there is the major problem of making a single cell suspension from these biopsy specimens.

A number of techniques which will be discussed below have avoided the problem of making a single cell suspension by studying only whole pieces of the tumor biopsies. This approach presents several theoretical problems including contamination by a large number of nontumor elements which may adversely affect *in vitro* test results (i.e., *in vitro* results may reflect effect of antineoplastic agent on nontumor cells as opposed to tumor cells).

Another approach to avoid making a single cell suspension has involved growing tumor explants from a solid tumor biopsy. To accomplish this, a small piece of the biopsy is placed on glass coverslips (Morasca, 1976), metal mesh platforms (Lazons *et al.*, 1966; Beeby *et al.*, 1975), or a sponge matrix (Abaza *et al.*, 1978; Saez *et al.*, 1977). Tumor and other cells migrate or grow out away from the fragment. The effect of a drug on that phenomenon can be assessed.

To obtain true single cell suspensions a wide variety of techniques have been employed including mechanical disaggregation (Leibovitz, 1975; Mavligit *et al.*, 1973; Mattern *et al.*, 1976; Hamburger *et al.*, 1978), enzymes or chelating agents (Pretlow *et al.*, 1976, 1977; Rockwell, 1977), or combinations of mechanical disaggregations and enzymes or chelating agents (Leibovitz, 1975; Rous and Jones, 1916; Van Wezel *et al.*, 1972; Pretlow *et al.*, 1977; Lickiss *et al.*, 1974; Brattain *et al.*, 1977; Rockwell, 1977; Kimball *et al.*, 1978; Bose *et al.*, 1977; Pretlow *et al.*, 1975; Freshney, 1972). It is important to remember that these methods of producing single cell suspensions could lead to major changes in any *in vitro* chemosensitivity system and lead to incorrect interpretation of *in vitro* results (Leibovitz, 1975; Pretlow *et al.*, 1975; Hodges, 1976; Ham, 1974).

C. Eliminating Growth of Unwanted Cells

For an *in vitro* test to be relevant it is important that one assays tumor cells and not normal stromal cells (i.e., fibroblasts). To attempt to isolate tumor cells from other contaminating stromal cells both physical separation methods and selective media methods have been used.

Physical separation methods have the distinct advantage that they do not need an intervening period of growth in selective culture media. Physical separation methods used in the past include density gradient centrifugation which will separate different cell types into different zones (Pretlow *et al.*, 1975, 1976, 1977; Brittain *et al.*, 1977; Kimball *et al.*, 1978; Mavligit *et al.*, 1973, 1975; Wicha *et al.*, 1979) and removal of stromal cells by adherence (Pretlow *et al.*, 1975; Williams *et al.*, 1971; Bloom and Bennett, 1966; Agaki and Kimoto, 1976) and phagocytic cells by carbonyl iron phagocytosis (Hamburger *et al.*, 1978; Weisenthal and Ruddon, 1973).

Selective growth conditions have mainly been aimed at preventing growth of fibroblasts. Methods used to prevent the growth of fibroblasts have included the use of glucocorticoids, fibroblast-specific antibodies, and collagenase in the culture medium (Lasfargues and Moore, 1971). An ingenious method to prevent fibroblast growth was developed by Costachel *et al.* (1969) and utilized by Hamburger and Salmon (1977a,b) and a number of other authors. They used an agar underlayer to prevent attachment of the fibroblasts to the surface of the vessel. Normal fibroblasts do not seem to grow in these systems whether liquid is placed on the agar underlayer or an agar overlayer containing the cells is placed over the agar underlayer (Costachel *et al.*, 1969; Yuhas *et al.*, 1978; Hamburger and Salmon, 1977a,b; Hamburger *et al.*, 1978; Kimball *et al.*, 1978; Salmon *et al.*, 1978; McAllister and Reed, 1968). All of the two layer soft agar systems (cloning techniques) allow growth of selected tumor cell populations.

All of the above separation methods may be used to isolate the particular cells of interest. However it is important to keep in mind that this isolation may alter chemosensitivity spectrum of the tumor. It has now been demonstrated that removal of phagocytic cells from ovarian cancer cell preparations may decrease the plating efficiency of the tumor (Hamburger *et al.*, 1978), thus implying the phagocytic cells which were separated out actually encourage growth in some manner. Therefore, caution is needed whenever separation techniques are used to grow tumors *in vitro*.

D. Selection of Proper *in Vitro* Drug Concentrations and Exposure Times

This is a very complex and controversial area and has been extensively reviewed recently (Weisenthal *et al.*, 1980). Basically the effect of a drug on a patient's tumor would seem to depend on (1) the concentration of the drug at the site of the tumor; (2) the time during which an effective concentration of drug is present at the site of the tumor; and (3) the kinetics of the tumor at the time of drug exposure (i.e., nonproliferating versus proliferating cells).

The first problem is defining the concentration and time variables. At the present time information on the pharmacokinetics of commonly used antineoplastics is limited. Further complicating the situation is the fact that the level of drug achieved in plasma may not be achieved in the tumor, and there are 2 or 3 different rates of plasma decay *in vivo* representing distribution, metabolism, urinary excretion, and enterohepatic circulation. When one utilizes the available pharmacokinetic data and examines a number of published *in vitro* studies it is clear that a number of these studies have utilized levels of drugs and exposure times that would not be clinically achievable (Bender *et al.*, 1976; Lickiss *et al.*, 1974; Holmes and Little, 1974; Knock *et al.*, 1974; Wheeler *et al.*, 1974; Dendy *et al.*, 1970; Dickson and Suzge, 1976; Saez *et al.*, 1977; Kornblitz and Szypko, 1978; Durkin *et al.*, 1978). Obviously, determination of clinically valid and achievable exposure times and drug concentrations is an important consideration when analyzing a "predictive" chemosensitivity assay. It is very important to consider the kinetics of the cells at the time of drug exposure (Shackney *et al.*, 1978; Tannock, 1978).

It has been shown that cells in a nonproliferating state may be insensitive to S-phase specific agents while the same cells may be very sensitive to S-phase specific agents when the cells are in a proliferating state (Wilkoff *et al.*, 1967, 1972; Lloyd *et al.*, 1972). Ideally, then it would appear that an *in vitro* system would ensure that during the time of drug exposure, the kinetics of the *in vitro* tumor cells would be comparable to the tumor kinetics *in vivo*.

E. Additional Factors to Consider

Any methodology which utilizes several passages of cell lines must be analyzed in light of a study by Berry *et al.* (1975). They noted that there was an increase in chemosensitivity of monolayer cultures with serial passage. This finding was confirmed by Fuskova *et al.* (1977). This finding of increased chemosensitivity with serial passages indicates that it may be preferable to use primary cultures rather than passaged cultures to determine the chemosensitivity of a particular patient's tumor.

Other conditions during drug exposure may make a major difference in chemosensitivity spectrums of a tumor. Twentyman (1977) noted that cells exposed to bleomycin during the process of making a single cell suspension in Hank's balanced salt solution with trypsin were 3 orders of magnitude more sensitive to the drug than when the cells were exposed to bleomycin in complete medium following trypsin dispersion and washing. Thus careful study of these variables is very important for development of an *in vitro* predictive test for chemosensitivity of a patient's tumor.

IV. Specific *in Vitro* Predictive Tests

Over the past 25 years a large variety of *in vitro predictive* tests have emerged. These tests are basically several different methodologies to determine drug-induced cytotoxicity. Each one of these *in vitro* measurements is supposed to reflect the drug-induced elimination of the cell population which maintains tumor growth.

A. Tests Relying on Changes in Cell Morphology

These *in vitro* tests have relied on subjective inspection of cells to assay for drug-induced cytotoxicity. There have been several studies that have reported positive clinical correlations (Saez *et al.*, 1977; Dendy *et al.*, 1970; Waverius, 1976; Limburg and Heck, 1968). However one large study reported a very poor clinical correlation with subjective inspection of explant monolayer cultures 96 hours after drug exposure (Wright *et al.*, 1962). They found 45 instances in which antitumor activity was noted *in vitro* and none of the patients responded to treatment (*in vitro* false positives). Hurley and Yount (1965) using semiquantitative criteria for assessing cell damage, found that only 50% of 373 specimens used were satisfactory; among these, 35% showed a negative correlation (usually positive effect *in vitro* and no benefit *in vivo*). *In vitro* predictive tests which depend on the interpretation of morphologic changes in tumor cells, even when efforts are made to make such interpretations semiquantitative, do not appear promising (Lickiss *et al.*, 1974). There is always a subjective element, difficulty in determining which cells are tumor cells, which makes interpretation of changes technically demanding and requires experience, and clinical correlations to date have been disappointing. In addition, changes in cellular morphology may not reflect changes which render the cell reproductively sterile.

Most recently, Hittelman and Rao (1978) described an assay system for prediction of response in acute leukemia, based on a special kind of "morphologic change." It involved measurement of the fraction of prematurely condensed chromosomes apparent in bone marrow cells which have been fused with mitotic Chinese hamster ovary cells by the Sendai virus technique. This fraction, thought to represent those cells with proliferative potential (late G_1, S, and G_2), was decreased by chemotherapy *in vivo* among patients who were destined to achieve remission, and unaffected by such chemotherapy in nonresponders. Whether the technique could be applied to an *in vitro* exposure type of predictive system, or to a morphologically heterogeneous solid tumor system, remains to be determined.

B. Tests Relying on Measurements of Cell Viability

Drug-induced cytotoxicity has been measured by cell viability assays. Loss of cell viability has been assessed by a variety of techniques including failure to exclude vital dyes, ^{51}Cr release, and loss of adherence in monolayer cultures.

1. *Exclusion of Vital Dyes*

Cytotoxicity based on the ability of cells to exclude supravital stains such as trypan blue, eosin, and nigrosin has been in use for a number of years (Durkin *et al.*, 1978; Shrek, 1936; Hoskiss *et al.*, 1956; Tsukeda *et al.*, 1978; Eagle and Foley, 1956; Graff and Blakley, 1978; Burke *et al.*, 1978; Grunwald *et al.*, 1978; Yates and King, 1978; Bhuyan *et al.*, 1976).

One published study has reported *in vitro–in vivo* clinical correlations using trypan blue exclusion as a measure of cell survival (Durkin *et al.*, 1978). This study reports on only 7 patients with non-Hodgkin's lymphoma in which cells from lymph nodes were stained with trypan blue 48 hours after drug exposure.

On the other hand a number of preclinical studies have shown that the assesment of cytotoxicity by vital stains may not be a reliable measure of drug-induced cytotoxicity (Roper and Drewinko, 1976). As noted by Weisenthal *et al.* (1980), the timing of the vital stain viability may be important. In a cell system with a rapid proliferation rate, the "dead" cells may become diluted out by the multiplication of living cells during the 2 to 4 days required for the test to turn positive and the percentage of nonviable cells may be misleadingly low. In monolayer systems, nonviable cells tend to detach and may be washed away during the process of cell harvesting, leaving behind only viable cells to test with dye (Holmes and Little, 1974). Therefore until some of these technical problems are accounted for, it appears that, as an end-point for drug effect, loss of dye exclusion is too insensitive to provide the desired correlation with loss of reproductive potential.

2. ^{51}*Cr Release*

^{51}Cr has been used extensively in immunologic assays for cytotoxicity. It is thought that ^{51}Cr is covalently bound to basic amino acids of intracellular proteins (Ronai, 1969), which leak from the cell as a consequence of membrane damage. The extent of the target cell damage is therefore assessed as a function of ^{51}Cr release. There is little reported experience with the use of this assay as an indicator of drug effects from chemotherapy: the one available study (Roper and Drewinko, 1976) found that "the degree of release was so modest that this assay appeared completely insensitive in measuring the magnitude of injury caused by chemotherapeutic agents." Like dye exclusion tests, ^{51}Cr release assays are probably dependent on the loss of cell membrane integrity: although this may be a relatively early event in the interaction of tumor target cells and host killer cells, it probably is not a sensitive indicator of lethal drug damage.

3. *Loss of Adherence*

Loss of cell viability, as assessed by loss of monolayer adherence following 72 hours in culture in the presence of a drug, was used in a clinical correlation study by Holmes and Little (1974). They used mechanical techniques of cell dispersion and plated small cell numbers into small microculture wells. They employed multiple washings with Hanks' solution, both before and after exposure of cells to drug-containing medium, in an attempt to remove all grossly nonviable cells and debris. They reported a 70% success rate in establishing primary cultures from 152 tumor specimens. After 24 hours in culture, multiple test microcultures were incubated with drug-containing solutions for 72 hours, then both control and test cultures were washed and trypsinized to obtain cell suspensions, from which aliquots were reseeded into microculture wells. The subcultures were harvested in 3 to 8 weeks, the period necessary to obtain sufficient cell growth for comparison of treated vs control cell numbers. The authors considered a 40% difference between control and test cell population sizes at the time of harvest to represent significant drug effect, for reasons not fully discussed. In 13 cases from whom clinical correlation was available, $\frac{5}{5}$ who had response *in vitro* also responded clinically. Only $\frac{1}{8}$ nonresponders *in vitro* demonstrated clinical response (to chlorambucil, an agent which may not have been activated *in vitro*), for an overall correlation of 92%. In no case was an attempt made to influence the clinican's choice of drugs. It bears emphasis that Holmes and Little exposed human-derived tumor cells to chemotherapeutic agents at only 24 hours after they were placed in culture, that the period of exposure was relatively long (72 hours), and that only cells that then demonstrated viability by eosin-Y dye exclusion were replaced in culture for the ultimate assay. No follow-up clinical studies have been performed utilizing this interesting methodology.

C. *In Vitro* Tests Based on Primary Site of Action

In this category fall tests that measure the effect of a drug on a defined enzyme or metabolic pathway in isolated tumor cells, and compare this to its clinical effectiveness: examples are inhibition of asparagine synthesis in sensitive cells by L-asparaginase (Ho *et al.*, 1970), inhibition of dihydrofolate reductase by methotrexate (Hryniuk and Bertino, 1969), inhibition of *de novo* thymidine synthesis by 5-fluorouracil (5FU) (Wolberg, 1967), the ability of alkylating agents to produce cross-linkage of DNA strands (Erickson *et al.*, 1978), assays of levels of uridine kinase (Reichard *et al.*, 1962), as well as levels of deoxycytidine kinase which activates cytosine arabinoside (Smyth *et al.*, 1976; Creasey *et al.*, 1975), and determination of levels of cytidine deaminase which inactivates cytosine arabinoside (Stewart and Burke, 1971; Smyth *et al.*, 1976). Several clinical trials utilizing the above tests have proved disappointing (Bender *et al.*, 1976; Smyth *et al.*, 1976; Bertino *et al.*, 1971).

Chang *et al.* (1977) found no utility in the measurement of drug uptake or of intracellular activating enzymes for cytosine arabinoside or daunorubicin, or for measurement of the ratio of activating to degradative enzymes for cytosine arabinoside in predicting drug responsiveness of patients with acute leukemia.

The work of Kessel and others (Kessel *et al.*, 1968, 1969; Kessel and Hull, 1969; Kessel, 1971) with systems in which uptake of radiolabeled drug and phosphorylation of drug by tumor cells are the end-points deserves mention. Methotrexate, 5FU, 6MP, and cytosine arabinoside have each been studied, and some clinical correlation has been demonstrated with response of human acute leukemia to these agents. However, Smyth *et al.* (1976) found no correlation between uptake, deamination, or phosphorylation of cytosine arabinoside by leukemic blast cells and clinical response to a regimen containing that drug.

There are 2 major problems with tests based on the primary site of drug action. First, they usually involve cumbersome and somewhat difficult assay systems. Second, they are not applicable to drugs whose primary site of action is unknown, and may not be accurate if there are multiple primary sites of drug action, each of varying importance in individual tumor systems. Thus, although methotrexate and 5-fluorouracil have been the major candidates for this type of assay, there is some controversy over the primacy of a single enzyme system as the critical intracellular target in even these cases (McBurney and Whitemore, 1975).

The approaches outlined above are not easily adaptable to a generalized screening panel to individualize chemotherapy, as it would require a different type of test for each drug being screened. However, assays of resistance loci may yet prove to be of clinical value for specific drugs, as the mechanism of resistance in human tumors become better understood.

One major *in vitro* test that has been of clinical importance is the presence or absence of steroid hormone receptors in breast cancer specimens. Resistance of patients' tumors to endocrine therapy has been well correlated with low levels of estrogen receptors while presence of the estrogen receptor predicts for response in 50–70% of the patients (McGuire, 1978; Lippman and Allegra, 1978). Early work has also correlated resistance of leukemia cells to prednisone with low levels of glucocorticoid receptors in the leukemia cells (Lippman *et al.*, 1973). Continued work in the area of steroid receptors looks quite promising.

D. *In Vitro* Tests Measuring Inhibition of Cellular Metabolism

In vitro tests measuring inhibition of cellular metabolism have been extensively studied (Black and Speer, 1954; Saez *et al.*, 1977; Beeby *et al.*, 1975; Kondo, 1971). Tests which measure effects on oxygen consumption have fallen from favor, related both to technical difficulties of measurement and to the large amount of variation in this parameter in control cell populations (Dickson and Suzge, 1976). Those which measure effects of anticancer agents on carbohydrate metabolism (or cellular dehydrogenase activity) (Black and Speer, 1954; Knock *et al.*, 1974) usually depends on reduction of a dye marker, such as methylene blue. Failure to reduce the dye results in a zone of color around "sensitive" cells. Using such an assay system, Di Paolo (1971) reported a strong correlation of clinical results with ineffectiveness *in vitro:* 0 of 42 patients responded. Unfortunately, only 12 of 47 patients whose tumors were "sensitive" *in vitro* had clinical effect from the same drugs employed *in vivo*. Kondo (1971) reported similar overall results: a "correct" prediction of effectiveness of chemotherapy for solid tumors in 61–89% of cases, but with the best correlation lying in the prediction of nonresponse. A theoretical problem with this approach is that it may not distinguish between "injured" cells, destined to recover, and cells that are reproductively dead (Twentyman, 1978). This type of test also may not distinguish between tumor "stem" cells, tumor "nonstem" cells, and stromal cells. Still another concern is that this type of test was first reported to correlate with clinical response in 1954 (Black and Speer). One is left to wonder why assays of drug perturbation of cellular metabolism have not been introduced into clinical practice, since all the reported studies (Dickson and Suzge, 1976; Knock *et al.*, 1974; Di Paolo, 1971) have been positive.

E. *In Vitro* Tests Utilizing Measurements of Radioactive Precursor Incorporation

The use of radiolabeled nucleosides (uridine, deoxyuridine, thymidine) in the period coincident with or shortly after *in vitro* drug exposure has been the indirect method utilized to determine cytotoxicity by a number of investigators (Mattern *et al.*, 1976; Dendy *et al.*, 1970, 1976; Bender *et al.*, 1976; Bishun *et al.*, 1977; Beeby *et al.*, 1975; Roper and Drewinko, 1976; Knock *et al.*, 1974; Raich, 1978; Freshney, 1976; Bickis *et al.*, 1966; Wolberg, 1967, 1972; Kann, 1978). Weisenthal *et al.* (1980) has outlined the possible pitfalls of using labeled nucleosides to estimate RNA or DNA synthesis. For instance, the use of labeled nucleosides to estimate RNA or DNA synthesis may be subject to artifacts such as a drug-induced depression of labeled nucleoside tranport (but not true of RNA or DNA synthesis) (Nakata and Bader, 1969). Conversely, a spontaneously *increased* estimate of DNA synthesis may be suggested by increased "salvage" pathway deoxythymidylate synthesis in the presence of drugs that effectively inhibit the *de novo* pathway (Wolberg, 1972). Weisenthal *et al.* (1980) also suggest that a variety of antineoplastic agents including 6-mercaptopurine (Scholar *et al.*, 1972), aminopterin (Adams *et al.*, 1971), ara-C (Skoog and Nordeuskjold, 1971; Graham and Whitmore, 1970), and hydroxyurea (Skoog and Nordeuskjold, 1971) may all cause changes in the intracellular nucleotide pool sizes which could easily lead to false estimations of nucleic acid synthesis as measured by the incorporation of radiolabeled nucleosides which are converted to nucleotides prior to incorporation into nucleic acids. The possibility also exists that cells destined to recover from "potentially lethal damage" (Twentyman, 1978) may have temporarily depressed metabolism as suggested earlier and have misleadingly low early label incorporation. Another problem with using radionuclides is that they may be toxic to the cells being assayed and thus artifactually potentiate the results of a cytotoxicity assay. This potential effect is probably not a problem with short labeling periods, but some effort to determine how the conditions of labeling may affect the results should be made for cytotoxicity assays in which radionuclides are used.

Despite the above recognized problems, several investigators have reported good correlations between *in vitro* radiolabeled precursor incorporation and clinical response or lack of response.

Cline and Rosenbaum (1969) found that depression of [^{3}H]uridine incorporation by 50% into leukemic blasts, after *in vitro* exposure for approximately 24 hours to cortisol at concentrations of 5×10^{-5} *M*, or 90% inhibition with vincristine at 7×10^{-5} *M*, was highly correlated with *in vivo* cytotoxicity. Depression of thymidine incorporation appeared to correlate equally well with cortisol, but was not studied for vincristine. The drug concentrations which produced *in vitro* effects were much higher than those achievable pharmacologically. Bickiss *et al.* (1966) and Wolberg (1971) reported significant correlation of clinical response with depression of DNA synthesis *in vitro,* after 2 and 24 hour incubation with tumor cells, respectively, using fluorinated pyrimidines as well as other compounds. In the studies in which correlation rates are quoted (Raich, 1978; Bender *et al.*, 1976; Wolberg, 1971) there are cumulative totals of 29 true positives (+ *in vitro*/+ *in vivo*), 2 false positives (+ *in vitro*/− *in vivo*), 79 true negatives (− *in vitro*/− *in vivo*), and 2 false negatives (− *in vitro*/+ *in vivo*). In the study by Wolberg (1971) there are however a large number of equivocal *in vitro* results.

Overall, the weight of available evidence seems to favor use of a measure of depression of DNA synthesis over one of RNA synthesis, as an endpont for *in vitro* effects to correlate with clinical efficacy. At least for proliferating cells, it seems logical that depression of DNA synthesis should be a common manifestation of cell damage leading to loss of reproductive integrity, regardless of the primary mechanism of action. For most chemotherapeutic agents, proliferating cells are preferentially affected: thus a test which measures effects on DNA synthesis could be reasonably expected to correlate with drug efficacy, provided the other criteria for clinical usefulness are met. However, for the theoretical reasons mentioned in the first portion of this section all of these radiolabeling methodologies have theoretical problems. Additional work using these methodologies for clinical correlations is definitely needed.

F. Measurement of Labeling Index

The labeling index is a special case of radiolabeling in which autoradiography is used to determine the percentage of the total cell population which incorporates radioactive thymidine. This procedure is theoretically subject to the same problems of other radiolabeling procedures, such as reduced nucleoside transport out of proportion to the extent of drug-induced cytotoxicity. If labeling is delayed to allow recovery from the potential artifacts associated with drug exposure, then a misleading high labeling index may be obtained, as the cells truly killed by the drug may have undergone degeneration, leaving only undamaged cells to be recognized and enumerated.

There is a very poor correlation between labeling index of experimental tumors and the actual lethality of anticancer drugs for cells *in vitro* (Steel, 1975; Roper and Drewinko, 1976; Tannock, 1978). It may be that labeling index data are dominated by cells that are incapable of contributing to regrowth and that the cells with the regrowth potential (i.e., the tumor stem cells) may form a kinetically atypical minority (Steel, 1975).

The relationship between *pretreatment* labeling index of a patient's tumor and response to chemotherapy is a complex and controversial area. There was no correlation between pretreatment labeling index and response to therapy in a large number of patients with solid tumors treated with 5-fluorouracil (Wolberg and Ansfield, 1971). In adult acute leukemia the frequency of complete remissions was not found to correlate with pretreatment labeling index (Crowther *et al.*, 1975). On the other hand, there are some studies that show a correlation between pretreatment labeling index and a good response to chemotherapy in carcinoma of the breast (Sulkes *et al.*, 1976; Thirwell and Mansell, 1976), acute leukemia (Hart *et al.*, 1977; Zittoun *et al.*, 1975), and a variety of solid tumors (Hart *et al.*, 1977). Remissions have tended to be shorter in patients with high pretreatment labeling indices (Hart *et al.*, 1977; Crowther *et al.*, 1975). To date then, *pretreatment* measurement of labeling index is of controversial value only.

There is increasing evidence that although pretreatment labeling index is not a good prognostic parameter the labeling index of the tumor cells does indeed go down (DNA synthesis is depressed) following chemotherapy or hormone therapy (Skypeck, 1971). This depression of labeling index has been associated with tumor regression (Livingston *et al.*, 1977).

Similar data have been provided by Tubiana and Malaise showing that depression of thymidine labeling index of tumor cells after radiation therapy is associated with favorable response to radiotherapy and no depression is associated with failure (Tubiana and Malaise, 1976).

Clinical correlations utilizing the labeling index to predict for *in vivo* response to a drug have been performed by Skypeck (1971). In that study 6 true positives were noted (+ *in vitro*/+ *in vivo*), and 15 true negatives were also noted (− *in vitro*/− *in vivo*). There were two false positives in the study.

More recently Livingston (1979) used depression of thymidine labeling index to predict effects of chemotherapy. Tumor suspensions were incubated with autologous pretreatment plasma or plasma obtained 10 minutes after intravenous chemotherapy. Labeling indices were determined at 24, 48, 72, or 96 hours. Five true positives and 5 true negatives were noted. Depression of tumor labeling index by the drug containing plasma by $>$2-fold relative to control plasma was considered a positive *in vitro* response. This interesting *in vivo–in vitro* trial is continuing.

As a clinically useful predictor of response, the study of labeling index pre- and posttherapy has 2 serious drawbacks: (1) the tumor must be accessible to repeated biopsy; and (2) the patient must be committed to a course of treatment before its effect can be evaluated. In addition the investigator must be able to differentiate between labeled tumor cells and labeled stromal cells. The grain counting in this technique is also tedious.

H. *In Vitro* Measurement of Reproductive Capability

Probably the most appealing approach, in theory at least, involves the application of *in vitro* testing procedures which quantitatively measure loss of reproductive integrity. This, of course, involves having cells grow in tissue culture. Unfortunately, at least until quite recently, human solid tumors have been notoriously difficult to adapt to tissue culture: Fjelde (1955), for instance, reported good growth in only 21 of 138 (15%) tumors where culture was attempted. When one does succeed in adapting a human tumor to long-term culture, this usually results in very different behavior of the cell population from that obtained *in vivo,* both with regard to the growth fraction (which tends to be much higher) and with regard to tumor antigenicity (usually reduced). Ideally what is required is consistent establishment of primary cultures with chemosensitivity assays on those cultures.

1. *The Stem Cell Concept*

Work on the cell kinetics of normal tissues has led to the concept that for every renewal tissue in an adult there is a subpopulation of stem cells.

These stem cells are defined as cells that can reproduce themselves (capacity of self-renewal) and also give rise to a differentiating line of mature and functional cells (Steel, 1975). In many tissues the identity and properties of stem cells have not been elucidated but for the bone marrow and intestinal epithelium this had been an area of intense investigation (Steel, 1975; Pike and Robinson, 1970: Metcalf, 1977). It has been shown that the marrow stem cells make up a very small percentage (1%) of the marrow population (Pike and Robinson, 1970). Under normal circumstances they proliferate rather slowly. In intestinal epithelium, most of the cells in the crypts of Lieberkuhn proliferate, rapidly migrating as a sheet onto the intestinal villi. Under normal circumstances only cells near the base of the crypts are the "effective" stem cells because all of the progeny cells that are higher up on the villi are eventually lost by exfoliation (Steel, 1975). It is not known what proportion of the crypt cells are stem cells.

Bearing in mind that many tumors retain some of the structural and morphologic characteristics of the tissue of origin, it is possible to conceptualize that tumors may also have stem cell populations. The definition of a tumor stem cell is a cell which gives rise to large numbers of tumor-specific progeny cells and still has the ability to renew itself (make other stem cells). These tumor stem cells may be only a small proportion of the total number of tumor cells and they may be kinetically different from the majority of tumor cells (Steel, 1975).

It should be pointed out that at present the view that only a small proportion of cells in primary tumors are potential stem cells is only a hypothesis. However, it is an attractive hypothesis which is gaining some scientific basis.

2. *In Vitro Growth of Stem Cells*

Clonogenic or stem cells may be detected in animal tumors by a variety of transplantation techniques including the end-point dilution method (Hewitt and Wilson, 1959), the spleen colony or lung colony methods (Hill and Bush, 1969; Bruce *et al.*, 1966), regrowth assays (Wilcox *et al.*, 1965), and *in vitro* cloning (Brown and Carbone, 1971; Hermans and Barendsen, 1969). It is uncertain whether these various techniques measure the same population of cells (Steel, 1975). Because of recent developments outlined below, methods are now available to grow human tumor stem cells directly from biopsies in a clonogenic assay in semisolid media.

About 13 years ago Bruce and colleagues at the Ontario Cancer Institute demonstrated the potential for studying tumor stem cells from transplantable murine neoplasms by using a spleen colony assay (Bruce *et al.*, 1966). Subsequently, investigators from the same institute developed and tested an *in vitro* agar colony assay for transplantable BALB/c mouse myeloma which used irradiated tumor-inoculated spleen cells as a feeder layer (Park *et al.*, 1971). They further showed that the results obtained for drug assays against the tumor *in vitro* were predictive for *in vivo* results (ogawa *et al.*, 1973).

Unfortunately, primary explantation of human tumors for colony formation has met with little success—the major problem being the creation of an environment that gives tumor cells a selective advantage over normal cells (Hamburger and Salmon, 1977b). Two groups of investigators did have some success in obtaining colony growth in a soft agar system with pediatric solid tumors (rhabdomyosarcomas and hepatoblastomas) (McAllister and Reed, 1968; Altman *et al.*, 1975).

The major breakthrough in culturing progenitor cells of human tumors came with the work of Hamburger and Salmon (1977a,b; Hamburger *et al.*, 1978, 1979; Jones *et al.*, 1979; Salmon *et al.*, 1978). They devised a system using soft agar (with a bottom layer containing conditioned media from spleens of BALB/d mice primed with mineral oil) for assay of human myeloma stem cells (Hamburger and Salmon, 1977a,b; Hamburger *et al.*, 1979). Using this method they have been able to grow colonies from 75% of 70 patients with multiple myeloma or related monoclonal disorders (Hamburger and Salmon, 1977a,b). The number of colonies which grew was proportional to the number of cells plated (making a quantitative test of drug sensitivity a possibility). Morphologic, histochemical, and functional criteria (including the presence of intracytoplasmic immunoglobulin) showed the colonies growing in the agar were myeloma cells.

Using the same system Hamburger and Salmon attempted to grow a variety of metastatic cancers with some success including oat cell carcinoma of the lung, non-Hodgkin's lymphoma, adenocarcinoma of the ovary, melanoma, and neuroblastoma (Hamburger and Salmon, 1977b). They have recently extended their observations in ovarian carcinoma with 85% of 31 ovarian cancer biopsy and effusion specimens forming tumor colonies *in vitro* (Hamburger *et al.*, 1978). Morphologic and histochemical criteria confirmed that the colonies consisted of cells with the same characteristics as the original tumor. Results of cytogenetic studies were also consistent with a malignant origin for the tumor colonies.

The human tumor stem cell system has also been more extensively studied in non-Hodgkin's lymphoma. Lymphoid colony growth was obtained in 11 (61%) of 18 bone marrows microscopically involved by tumor and in 3 (50%) of 6 lymph nodes histologically involved by lymphocytic lymphoma. Conversely, colony growth was observed in only a single instance from 49 bone marrows without overt lymphoma and was not observed in cultures of 4 normal lymph nodes, 2 normal spleens, 10 normal bone marrows, and 6 peripheral blood specimens.

The most important clinical development with the *in vitro* stem cell assay came from Salmon and colleagues with their report of using the system to quantitate the differential sensitivity of human tumors to various anticancer agents (Salmon *et al.*, 1978). Using the *in vitro* stem cell assay they performed 32 retrospective or prospective clinical studies in 9 patients with myeloma and 9 with ovarian cancer. These patients were treated with standard anticancer drugs which were also tested *in vitro*. Each tumor was cultured using the stem cell assay technique after incubation of the single cell suspension with various drug concentrations for 1 hour. The number of colonies which eventually grew out on drug-treated specimens were compared to the number of colonies on control plates. The data were expressed as colonies surviving versus drug concentration. In 8 cases of myeloma and in 3 cases of ovarian carcinoma *in vitro* sensitivity (as defined by the area under the drug concentration curve) corresponded with *in vivo* sensitivity whereas in one case of myeloma it did not. *In vitro* resistance correlated with clinical resistance in all 5 comparisons in myeloma and all 15 in ovarian cancer. They concluded that the assay warranted larger scale testing to determine its efficacy for selection of new agents and for individualization of cancer chemotherapy regimens.

Their experience was recently updated (Salmon *et al.*, 1979). There have been 92 *in vitro–in vivo* correlations available for 20 patients with ovarian cancer and 16 patients with multiple myeloma. Sixteen correlations demonstrated sensitivity *in vitro* and *in vivo*, 8 showed sensitivity *in vitro* and resistance *in vivo* (false positive test), 1 was resistant *in vitro* and sensitive *in vivo* (false negative test), and 67 showed both *in vivo* and *in vitro* resistance. Overall then, in myeloma and ovarian cancer the false positive rate for the system is 8 of 92 (9%) and the false negative rate is 1 of 92 (1%). These early correlations are impressive and certainly warrant rapid well-designed follow-up studies.

Over the past year our laboratory has been studying the human tumor stem cell assay system. This research has taken 4 major directions. The following discussion will cover these 4 areas of research, namely.

1. Types of tumors cultured.
2. Confirmatory evidence that tumor *is* growing than fibroblasts or granulocyte–macrophage colonies.
3. Difficulties encountered with the system.
4. Clinical and basic science applications of the human tumor stem cell system.

Our findings are reported in detail elsewhere (Von Hoff and Johnson, 1979; Von Hoff, 1980). Basically, we have shown that a wide variety of tumors can be grown from a number of sources including ascites,

TABLE I

GROWTH OF TUMOR STEM CELL COLONIES FROM VARIOUS HUMAN NEOPLASMS

Type of tumor (source of sample)[a]	Number of patients with + culture/total tested
Ovarian (A,T,P)	27/35
Neuroblastoma (M)	21/26
Melanoma (P,N,T)	10/16
Colorectal (A)	7/10
Breast (A,T,P)	8/12
Lung cancer (T,M,P)	
Oat cell	11/14
Squamous cell	12/13
Adenocarcinoma	6/7
Head and neck	7/16
Testicular (T)	2/4
Multiple myeloma	3/5
Osteogenic sarcoma (T)	3/5
Rhabdomyosarcoma (M,T)	3/6
Islet cell carcinoma (T)	3/3
Endometrial	3/3
Pancreatic carcinoma	4/4
Cervix	3/3
Ewings sarcoma (M)	2/2
Renal	2/3
Thyroid (T)	1/2
Hepatoma	2/2
Prostate	3/5
Wilms	1/2
T-Cell lymphoma (P)	1/1
Parathyroid	1/1
Burkitts lymphoma (T)	0/1
Hodgkin's disease (T)	0/1
CML	0/1
Glioma (T)	0/1
Thymoma	0/1
Undifferentiated sarcoma (P)	0/1
CLL	0/2
Malignant fibrous histiocytoma (T)	0/1
Hairy cell leukemia	0/1
Normal marrow (M)	0/6

[a] A, Ascites; P, pleural fluid; T, solid tumor; M, marrow; N, lymph node. Overall, 146 of the 209 tumors attempted have grown (70%).

pleural effusions, bone marrow, and solid tumor specimens (see Table I).

From the preliminary studies (Von Hoff and Johnson, 1979) there is good evidence that the tumor cells grown in culture are producing the same tumor markers that they are producing in the patient. This information provides additional evidence that the human tumor stem cell culture system reflects the *in vivo* situation. Our laboratory has noted a number of problems with the system: not all tumors will grow in the system; the tumors have a low plating efficiency with 50–100 colonies developing per 500,000 nucleated cells plated; and the technique is time consuming in terms of specimen preparation (6 hours) and colony counting (4–6 hours per drug experiment). Difficulities with the system noted for clinical application include the 2–3 weeks it takes for colonies to develop, and lack of adequate data on which to choose the appropriate incubation time with drug.

Early *in vitro–in vivo* correlations have shown excellent results in the first 151 correlations. Overall, the accuracy for a positive prediction of the assay was 0.70 while the accuracy for a negative prediction of the assay was 0.94 (Von Hoff, 1980).

If the results from Salmon *et al.* (1978) and from our laboratory can be reproduced by other investigators the use of the human tumor stem cell assay system to predict for response of an individual patient's tumor *in vivo* seems promising.

V. Summary

The concept of *in vitro* tests to predict for *in vivo* response to an antitumor agent is not a new idea. There are minimal requirements that these tests must possess in order to be both useful and practical. Each *in vitro* test must deal with a number of general technical problems including selection of the proper culture media, preparation of single cell suspensions, eliminating growth of unwanted cells, and selection of appropriate *in vitro* drug concentrations and exposure times. There are also other, as yet unrecognized factors, to consider.

The specific types of *in vitro* predictive tests that have had *in vitro–in vivo* clinical correlation studies include tests relying on changes in cell morphology, tests relying on measurements of cell viability, *in vitro* tests based on primary site of action, *in vitro* tests measuring inhibition of cellular metabolism, measurements of radioactive precursor incorporation, measurements of labeling index of the tumor, and finally *in vitro* measurement of reproductive capability.

As discussed above, each of the tests has both advantages and disadvantages. At the present time the most attractive *in vitro* system appears to be a human tumor stem cell assay system which purportedly measures the reproductive capability of the tumor. However, other tests might be equally attractive if they had additional clinical correlations performed.

From the information presented in this article it is quite clear that there is room for a great deal of additional work in the field of *in vitro* predictive tests for response to cancer chemotherapy.

References

Abaza, N. A., Leighton, S., and Zajac, B. A. (1978). *Cancer* **42,** 1364–1374.

Adams, R. L. P., Berryman, S., and Thompson, A. (1971). *Biochim. Biophys. Acta* **240,** 455–462.

Akagi, T., and Kimoto, T. (1976). *Gann* **67,** 483–492.

Altman, A. J., Grussi, F. G., Rierden, W. J., and Baehner, R. L. (1975). *Cancer Res.* **35,** 1809.

Beeby, D. I., Fasty, G. C., Gazet, J. C., Grigor, K., and Neville, A. M. (1975). *Br. J. Cancer* **31,** 317–327.

Bender, R. A., Gieger, W. A., Drake, J. C., and Ziegler, J. L. (1976). *Br. J. Cancer* **34,** 484–492.

Berry, R. J., Laing, A. H., and Wells, J. (1975). *Br. J. Cancer* **31,** 218–227.

Bertino, J. R., Huymocl, W. M., and Capizzi, R. (1971). *Natl. Cancer Inst. Monogr.* **34,** 179.

Bevenbaum, M. D., Sheard, C. E., Reittie, J. R., and Bundick, R. V. (1974). *Br. J. Cancer* **30,** 13–32.

Bhuyan, B. K., Loughman, B. E., Fraser, T. J., and Day, K. J. (1976). *Exp. Cell Res.* **92,** 275–280.

Bickiss, J. J., Henderson, I. W. D., and Quastel, J. H. (1966). *Cancer* **19,** 103–113.

Bishun, N. P., Reed, J., and Williams, D. (1977). *Cytobios* **19,** 41–44.

Black, M. M., and Speer, F. D. (1954). *J. Natl. Cancer Inst.* **14,** 1147–1158.

Bloom, B. R., and Bennett, B. (1966). Science **153,** 80–82.

Bogden, A. E., Ward, A., Gulkin, T. A., Esber, H. J., and Kelton, D. E. (1979). *Proc. Am. Assoc. Cancer Res.* **20,** 323.

Bose, B. M., Vanky, F., and Klein, E. (1977). *Int. J. Cancer* **20,** 512–519.

Brittain, M. G., Pretlow, T. P., and Pretlow T. G. (1977). *Cancer* **40,** 2479–2486.

Brown, C. H., and Carbone, P. O. (1971). *J. Natl. Cancer Inst.* **46,** 989.

Bruce, W. R., Meeker, B. E., and Baleriote, F. A. (1966). *J. Natl. Cancer Inst.* **37,** 233.

Burke, R. E., Mira, J. G., Datta, R., Zava, D. T., and McQuire, W. L. (1978). *Cancer Res.* **38,** 2813–2817.

Chang, P., Wiernik, P., and Bachur, N. (1977). *Proc. Am. Assoc. Cancer Res. ASCO* **18,** 352.

Cline, M. (1969). *N. Engl. J. Med.* **280,** 955.

Cline, M., and Rosenbaum, C. (1969). *Blood* **30,** 176–187.

Cobb, L. M., and Mitchley, B. C. V. (1974). *Cancer Chemother. Rep.* **58,** 645–651.

Costachel, O., Fadei, L., and Badea, E. (1969). *Z. Krebsforsch.* **72,** 24–31.

Creasey, W. A., Sartorelli, A. C., and Johns, D. G., eds. (1975). "Handbook of Experimental Pharmacology," Vol. 38, Part 2, pp. 232–256. Springer-Verlay, Berlin and New York.

Crowther, D., Beard, M. E. J., Bateman, C. J. T., and Sewell, R. L. (1975). *Br. J. Cancer* **32,** 456–464.
Dendy, P. O., Bozman, G., and Wheeler, T. K. (1970). *Lancet* **2,** 68–72.
Dendy, P. O., Dawson, M. P. A., Warner, D. M. A., and Honess, D. J. (1976). "Human Tumors in Short-Term Culture" (P. P. Dendy, ed.), pp. 139–149, 24–27. Academic Press, New York.
Dickson, J. A., and Suzge, M. (1976). "Human Tumors in Short-Term Culture" ed. (P. O. Dendy, ed.), pp. 107–138. Academic Press, New York.
DiPaolo, J. A. (1971). *Natl. Cancer Inst. Monogr.* **34,** 240–245.
Durkin, W. J., Ghanta, V. K., Balch, C. M., Davis, D. W., and Hiramoto, R. M. (1978). *Cancer Res.* **39,** 402–407.
Eagle, H., and Foley, G. E. (1956). *Am. J. Med.* **21,** 739–749.
Erickson, L. C., Bradley, M. D., and Kohn, K. W. (1978). *Cancer Res.* **38,** 672–677.
Eskova, A., Fuska, J., Ivanitskaya, L. P., and Makukho, L. V. (1977). *Neoplasma* **24,** 239–242.
Fjelde, A. (1955). *Cancer* **8,** 845–851.
Freshney, R. I. (1972). *Lancet* **II,** 488–489.
Freshney, R. I. (1976). "Human Tumors in Short-Term Culture" (P. O. Dendy, ed.), pp. 150–155. Academic Press, New York.
Giovanella, B. C., Stehlin, J. S., Jr., Williams, L. J., Jr., Lee, S. S., and Shepard, R. C. (1978). *Cancer* **42,** 2269–2281.
Graff, J. P., and Blakley, R. L. (1978). *Cancer Res.* **38,** 3847–3853.
Graham, F. L., and Whitmore, G. F. (1970). *Cancer Res.* **30,** 2627–2635.
Grunwald, H. W., Rosner, F., and Hirshact, Y. (1978). *Am. J. Hematol.* **4,** 35–46.
Ham, R. G. (1974). *J. Natl. Cancer Inst.* **53,** 1459–1463.
Hamburger, A. W., and Salmon, S. E. (1977a). *J. Clin. Invest.* **60,** 846–854.
Hamburger, A. W., and Salmon, S. E. (1977b). *Science* **197,** 461–463.
Hamburger, A. W., Salmon, S. E., Kin, M. B., Trent, J. M., Soehnten, J., Alberts, D. S., and Schmidt, H. J. (1978a). *Cancer Res.* **38,** 3438–3444.
Hamburger, A. W., Kin, M. B., and Salmon, S. E. (1979). *J. Cell Physiol.* **98,** 371–373.
Hart, J. S., George, S. L., Frei, E., II, Bodey, G. P., Nickerson, R. C., and Freireich, E. J. (1977). *Cancer* **39,** 1603–1717.
Hayashi, I., Larner, J., and Sato, G. (1978). *In Vitro* **14,** 23–30.
Hermans, A. F., and Barendsen, G. W. (1969). *Eur. J. Cancer* **5,** 173.
Hewitt, H. B., and Wilson, C. W. (1959). *Br. J. Cancer* **13,** 69.
Hill, R. P., and Bush, R. S. (1969). *Int. J. Radiat. Biol.* **15,** 435.
Hittleman, W. N., and Rao, P. N. (1978). *Cancer Res.* **38,** 416–422.
Ho, D., Whitecar, J., Luce, J. K., and Fuei, E., III (1970). *Cancer Res.* **30,** 466–472.
Hodges, G. M. (1976). "Human Tumors in Short, Term Culture" (P. P. Dendy, ed.), pp. 3–14. Academic Press, New York.
Holmes, H. L., and Little, J. M. (1974). *Lancet* **2,** 985–987.
Hoskiss, J. M., Meynell, G. G., and Sanders, F. K. A. (1956). *Exp. Cell Res.* **11,** 297–305.
Hryniuk, W., and Bertino, J. (1969). *J. Clin. Invest.* **48,** 2140–2155.
Hurley, J., and Yount, L. (1965). *Am. J. Surg.* **109,** 39–42.
Hutchings, S. E., and Sato, G. H. (1978). *Proc. Natl. Acad. Sci. U.S.A.* **75,** 901–904.
Jones, S. E., Hamburger, A. W., Kim, M. B., and Salmon, S. E. (1979). *Blood* **53,** 294–303.
Kann, H. E., Jr. (1978). *Cancer Res.* **38,** 2363–2366.
Kessel, D. (1971). *NCI Monogr.* (34), 138–145.
Kessel, D., and Hall, T. (1969). *Cancer Res.* **29,** 2116–2119.
Kessel, D., Hall, T., and Roberts, D. (1968). *Cancer Res.* **28,** 564–570.

Kessel, D., Hall, T., and Rosenthal, D. (1969). *Cancer Res.* **29,** 459–463.

Kimball, P. M., Brattain, M. G., and Pitts, A. M. (1978). *Br. J. Cancer* **37,** 1015–1918.

Knock, F. E., Galt, R. M., Oester, Y. T., Renaud, O. V., and Sylvester, R. (1971). *Surg. Gynecol. Obstet.* **133,** 458–466.

Knock, F. E., Galt, R. M., Oester, Y. T., and Sylvester, R. (1974). *Oncology* **30,** 1–22.

Kondo, T. (1971). *Natl. Cancer Inst. Monogr.* (34), 251–256.

Kornblitz, P. L., and Szypko, P. E. (1978). *J. Neurosurg.* **48,** 580–586.

Lasfargues, E. Y., and Moore, D. H. (1971). *In Vitro* **7,** 21–25.

Lazons, H., Tegeler, W., Mazzano, H. M., Leroy, J. G., Boone, B. A., and Foley, G. E. (1966). *Cancer Chemother. Rep.* **50,** 543–555.

Leibovitz, A. (1975). "Human Tumor Cells in Vitro" (J. Fogh, ed.), pp. 23–50. Plenum, New York.

Lickiss, J. N., Cane, K. A., and Baikie, A. G. (1974). *Eur. J. Cancer* **10,** 890–814.

Limburg, H., and Heck, U. (1968). *J. Obstet. Gynaecol. Br. Comm.* **75,** 1246–1255.

Lippman, M. E., and Allegra, J. C. (1978). *N. Engl. J. Med.* **299,** 930–933.

Lippman, M. E., Haltemann, R. H., Leventhal, B. G., Perry, S., and Thompson, E. B. (1973). *J. Clin. Invest.* **52,** 1715–1725.

Livingston, R. B. (1979). *Proc. Am. Assoc. Cancer Res. ASCO* **20,** 317.

Livingston, R. B., Sulkes, A., Thirwell, M. P., *et al.* (1977). "Growth Kinetics and Biochemical Regulation of Normal and Malignant Cells" (B. Drewinko and R. M. Humphrey, eds.), pp. 767–785. Williams & Wilkins, Baltimore, Maryland.

Lloyd, H. H., Dulmadge, E. A., and Wilkoff, L. J. (1972). *Cancer Chemother. Rep.* **56,** 585–591.

McAllister, R. M., and Reed, G. (1968). *Pediat. Res.* **2,** 356–360.

McBurney, M., and Whitmore, G. (1975). *Cancer Res.* **35,** 586–590.

McGuire, W. L. (1978). *Semin. Oncol.* **5,** 428–433.

Mather, J., and Sato, G. (1977). "Cell Tissue and Organ Cultures in Neurobiology" (S. Federoff and L. Hertz, eds.), pp. 619–630. Academic Press, New York.

Mattern, J., Jaufmann, M., Wayss, K., and Volm, M. (1976). "Human Tumors in Short-Term Culture" (P. P. Dendy, ed.), pp. 301–310 Academic Press, New York.

Mavligit, G. M., Hersh, E. M., and McBride, C. M. (1973). *J. Natl. Cancer Inst.* **51,** 337–343.

Mavligit, G. M., Barsales, P. B., Gutterman, J. U., Macvay, V., and Hersh, E. M. (1975). *Proc. Soc. Exp. Biol. Med.* **150,** 597–601.

Messner, H., Till, S., and McCullock, E. (1973). *Blood* **42,** 701–710.

Metcalf, D. (1977). Ann. Intern. Med. **7,** 483–494.

Morasca, L. (1976). "Human Tumors in Short-Term Culture" (P. P. Dendy, ed.), pp. 33–35. Academic Press, New York.

Nakata, Y., and Bader, J. P. (1969). *Biochim. Biopyhs. Acta* **190,** 250–256.

Ogawa, M., Bergsagel, D. E., and McCulloch, E. A. (1973). *Blood* **41,** 7.

Park, C. H., Bergsagel, D. E., and McCulloch, E. A. (1971). *J. Natl. Cancer Inst.* **46,** 411.

Pike, B. L., and Robinson, W. A. (1970). *J. Cell. Physiol.* **76,** 77.

Pretlow, T. G., II, Weiss, E. E., and Zettergres, J. G. (1975). *Int. Rev. Exp. Pathol.* **14,** 91–205.

Pretlow, T. G., II, Jones, C. M., and Pretlow, T. P. (1976). *Biophys. Chem.* **5,** 99–106.

Pretlow, G., II, Brattain, M. G., and Kreisberg, J. I. (1977). *Cancer Treat. Rep.* **61,** 157–159.

Raich, P. C. (1978). *Lancet* **1,** 74–76.

Reichard, P., Skold, O., Klein, G., Reversz, L., and Magnusson, P. H. (1962). *Cancer Res.* **22,** 235–243.

Rizzino, A., and Sato, G. (1978). *Proc. Natl. Acad. Sci. U.S.A.* **75,** 1844–1848.
Rockwell, S. (1977). *Lab. Animal Sci.* **27,** 831–851.
Ronai, P. (1969). *Blood* **33,** 408–413.
Roper, P., and Drewinko, B. (1976).*Cancer Res.* **36,** 2182–2188.
Rous, P., and Jones, F. A. (1916). *J. Exp. Med.* **23,** 555.
Saez, R. J., Campbell, R. J., and Laws, E. R. (1977). *J. Neurosurg.* **46,** 320–327.
Salmon, S. E., Hamburger, A. W., Soehnlen, B. S., Durie, B. G. M., Alberts, D. S., and Moon, T. C. (1978). N. Engl. J. Med. **298,** 1321–1327.
Salmon, S. W., Soehnlen, B. J., Durie, B. G. M., Alberts, D. S., Meyskens, F. L., Chen, H. S. G., and Moon, T. E. (1979). *Proc. Am. Assoc. Cancer Res. ASCO* **20,** 340.
Salto, G., and Hayashi, I. (1976). *Arch. Bibl. Med. Exp.* **10,** 120–121.
Scholar, E. M., Brown, P. R., and Parks, R. E., Jr. (1972). *Cancer Res.* **32,** 259–269.
Shackney, S. E., McCormack, G. W., and Cuchural, G. J. (1978). *Ann. Int. Med.* **89,** 107–121.
Sherwin, R. P., and Richters, A. (1975). "Human Tumor Cells in Vitro" ed. (J. Fogl, ed.), pp. 267–297. Plenum, New York.
Shrek, R. (1936). *Am. J. Cancer* **28,** 389–392.
Skoog, L., and Nordeuskjold, B. (1971). *Eur. J. Biochem.* **21,** 279–284.
Sky-Peck, H. (1971). *NCI Monogr.* (34), 197–205.
Smith, I. E., Courtney, V. D., and Gorden, M. Y. (1976). *Br. J. Cancer* **34,** 476–483.
Smyth, J. F., Robins, A. B., and Leese, C. L. (1976). *Eur. J. Cancer* **12,** 567–573.
Speyer, J. L., Collins, T. M., Dedrick, R. L., Brennan, M. F., Londer, H., Devita, V. T., Jr., and Myers, C. E. (1979). *Proc. Am. Assoc. Cancer Res. ASCO* **20,** 352.
Steel, G. G. (1975). "Medical Oncology-Medical Aspects of Malignant Disease" (K. D. Bagshaw, ed.), pp. 49–66. Blackwell, Oxford.
Stewart, C. D., and Burke, P. J. (1971). *Nature (London) New Biol.* **23,** 109–110.
Sulkes, A., Liningston, R., and Taylor, G. (1976). *Proc. Am. Assoc. Cancer Res. ASCO* **17,** 59.
Tannock, I. (1978). *Cancer Treat. Rep.* **62,** 1117–1133.
Taylor, W. G. (1974). *J. Natl. Cancer Inst.* **53,** 1449–1457.
Thirwell, M. P., and Mansell, P. W. A. (1976). *Proc. Am. Assoc. Cancer Res. ASCO* **17,** 307.
Tsukeda, H., Mizuno, S., and Nitta, K. (1978). *Cancer Res.* **38,** 2529–2532.
Tubiana, M., and Malaise, E. (1976). *Cancer Treat. Rep.* **60,** 1887–1895.
Twentyman, P. R. (1977). *Br. J. Cancer* **36,** 642–644.
Twentyman, P. R. (1978). *Cancer Res.* **38,** 2395–2400.
Van Wezel, A. L., Van Hemert, P. A., Parisiur, W., Cucakovich, N. B., and Macmarine, H. G. (1972). *Appl. Microbiol.* **24,** 506–507.
Von Hoff, D. D. (1980). *Proc. Am. Assoc. Cancer Res. ASCO* **21,** 134.
Von Hoff, D. D., and Johnson, G. E. (1979). *Proc. Am. Assoc. Cancer Res. ASCO* **20,** 51.
Waverius, H. M. (1976). "Human Tumors in Short-Term Culture" (P. P. Dendy, ed.), pp. 311–320. Academic Press, New York.
Waymouth, C. (1972). "Growth Nutrition and Metabolism of Cells in Culture" G. H. Rothblat and V. J. Cristofalo, eds.), Vol. 1, pp. 11–47. Academic Press, New York.
Waymouth, C. (1974). *J. Natl. Cancer Inst.* **53,** 1443–1448.
Waymouth, C. (1977). "Cell, Tissue, and Organ Cultures in Neurobiology" (S. Federoff and L. Hertz, eds.), pp. 631–648. Academic Press, New York.
Weisenthal, L. M., and Ruddon, R. W. (1973). *Cancer Res.* **33,** 2923–2935.
Weisenthal, L. M., Von Hoff, D. D., and Lippman, M. E. (1980). *Semin. Oncol.* (in press).
Wheeler, T. L. K., Dendy, P. P., and Dawson, A. (1974). *Oncology* **30,** 362–376.

Wicha, M. S., Liotta, L. A., and Kidwell, W. R. (1979). *Cancer Res.* **29,** 426–435.

Wilcox, W. S., Griswold, D. P., Laster, W. R., Schabel, F. M., and Skipper, H. F. (1965). *Cancer Chemother. Rep.* **47,** 27.

Wilkoff, L. J., Wildox, W. S., Burdeshaw, J. A., Dixon, G. J., and Dulmage, E. A. (1967). *J. Natl. Cancer Inst.* **39,** 965–975.

Wilkoff, L. J., Dulmadge, E. A., and Lloyd, H. H. (1972). *J. Natl. Cancer Inst.* **48,** 685–695.

Williams, G. M., Weisburger, E. K., and Weisburger, J. H. (1971). *Exp. Cell Res.* **69,** 106–112.

Wright, J. C., Cobb., J. P., Gunport, S. L., Safad, D., Walker, D. A., and Golomb, F. M. (1962). *Cancer* **15,** 284–293.

Wolberg, W. H. (1967). *Ann. Surg.* **166,** 609–623.

Wolberg, W. H. (1969). *Cancer Res.* **29,** 2137–2144.

Wolberg, W. H. (1971). *Natl. Cancer Inst. Monogr.* (34), 189–195.

Wolberg, W. H. (1972). *Cancer Res.* **32,** 130–132.

Wolberg, W. H., and Ansfield, F. J. (1971). *Cancer Res.* **31,** 448–450.

Wu, R., and Sato, G. H. (1978). *J. Toxicol. Environ. Health* **4,** 427–448.

Yates, J., and King, R. J. B. (1978). *Cancer Res.* **38,** 4135–4137.

Yuhas, J. M., Toya, R. E., and Paz, N. H. (1974). *J. Natl. Cancer Inst.* **53,** 465–468.

Yuhas, J. M., Tarleten, A. E., and Harman, J. G. (1978). *Cancer Res.* **38,** 3595–3598.

Zittoun, R., Bouchard, M., Facquet-Davis, J., Percie du Sert, M., and Bousser, J. (1975). *Cancer* **35,** 507–513.

Macrophage Activation for Nonspecific Tumor Cytotoxicity

RICHARD M. SCHULTZ

Immunology and Connective Tissue Research
Lilly Research Laboratories
Eli Lilly and Company
Indianapolis, Indiana

MICHAEL A. CHIRIGOS

Laboratory of Chemical Pharmacology
Developmental Therapeutics Program
Division of Cancer Treatment
National Institutes of Health
Bethesda, Maryland

I. Introduction

The significance of the macrophage to host defense against neoplasia has been the subject of numerous reviews (Levy and Wheelock, 1974; Hibbs, 1976a; Siegel, 1976). However, less is known concerning agents

ISBN 0-12-032917-4

that are capable of specifically modifying the functional activity of macrophages. The correlation that has been observed between the ability of immunoadjuvants to enhance host resistance to cancer and their capacity to activate macrophages (Juy and Chedid, 1975; Bruley-Rosset *et al.*, 1976; Morahan and Kaplan, 1976; Schultz *et al.*, 1977c) further emphasizes the need to understand better the mechanisms and agents involved in the pharmacologic control of the macrophage system. Moreover, increasing evidence suggests that the activated macrophage is the major effector of tumor surveillance, rather than the specifically immunologically active lymphocyte. In this article, particular emphasis will be placed on agents that render macrophages nonspecifically, but selectively, tumoricidal, as well as factors that may interfere with their antitumor effector function.

Four major items will be discussed; namely, the agents involved in the nonspecific and specific pathway for induction of activated macrophages along with suggested mechanisms for their activity (Section II), mechanisms by which the activated macrophage kills the susceptible target cell or alters its proliferation (Section III), interfering agents for macrophage function (Section IV), and therapeutic considerations (Section V). It is hoped that this article will reflect the basic information available as well as show the great complexity involved in altering the functional activity of the macrophage system.

A. On the Definition of the Activated State

Of the varied roles played by macrophages, or cells of the mononuclear phagocyte system, perhaps none is more significant to the host's bodily economy than their role in maintaining the purity and "self"-constancy of the internal environment. In addition to their classically described properties of tissue debridement, phagocytosis, and killing of microorganisms, activated macrophages have a surveillance role in differentiating normal from transformed cells and in selectively killing transformed cells by a nonimmunologic contact-mediated event (Alexander and Evans, 1971; Hibbs *et al.*, 1972a,b; Hibbs, 1974a). The rendering of macrophages nonspecifically tumoricidal is defined in this article as macrophage activation. This activation, on the other hand, is often accompanied by a number of other altered properties, including increased phagocytosis and pinocytosis (Nathan *et al.*, 1971; Meade *et al.*, 1974), secretion of substantial quantities of hydrolytic enzymes including acid hydrolases and neutral proteinases (Wahl *et al.*, 1975; Pantalone and Page, 1975, 1977), release of E-type prostaglandins (Kurland and Bockman, 1978; Schultz *et al.*, 1979a), enhanced ability to destroy facultative intracellular parasites (Mackaness, 1964; Fowles *et al.*, 1973), regulation of granulocyte/macrophage stem-cell growth (Ruscetti and Chervenik, 1974; Cline *et al.*, 1974; Ralph *et al.*, 1977), and ability to suppress cell proliferation including lymphocyte mitogenic responses (Keller, 1976b; Kaplan *et al.*, 1977). Since the correlation between these modifications and increased tumoricidal properties is poorly understood, the term "stimulation" is preferred when reference is made to biochemical, functional, or morphologic alterations in the absence of formal proof of increased cytotoxicity for tumor cells. The importance of defining the activated state is underscored by a recent report (Wing *et al.*, 1977) that shows the capacity of macrophages to inhibit the multiplication of intracellular parasites completely dissociated from the capacity to inhibit DNA synthesis of tumor cells. The possibility that various subpopulations of macrophages exist with separate functions has further complicated this issue.

B. Historical Perspective

It has been amply demonstrated that macrophages, once activated either specifically or nonspecifically, have a prominent role in inhibiting or controlling primary and metastatic tumor cell growth. Much of the early basis for our understanding of macrophage activation came from studies on their antimicrobial function. The concept that macrophages need to undergo functional modification in order to express resistance to certain bacterial infections can be traced back to writings of Metchnikoff at the turn of the century (Metchnikoff, 1905). Since the pioneering studies of Lurie (1964) on tuberculosis, the dominant effector role of the macrophage in acquired resistance against facultative intracellular parasites has become increasingly clear. Mackaness (1964) showed that infection of mice with *Mycobacterium bovis* or *Listeria monocytogenes* caused the production of peritoneal macrophages with enhanced ability to kill bacteria *in vitro*. He noted that these macrophages exhibited a greater ability to spread on glass surfaces, were more heavily endowed with mitochondria and lysosomes, and were more phagocytic than their normal counterparts. Although elicitation of these microbicidal effector cells is specific and appears to have a molecular basis via mediators from antigen-stimulated lymphocytes (Simon and Sheagren, 1972; Adams *et al.*, 1973; Fowles *et al.*, 1973), the resultant macrophages show nonspecific resistance against challenge with phylogenetically diverse intracellular organisms including *Salmonella typhimurium, Listeria monocytogenes, Mycobacterium tuberculosis, Pasteurella tularensis, Besnoitia jellisoni,* and *Toxoplasma gondii* (Mackaness, 1969; Ruskin *et al.*, 1969; Simon and Sheagren, 1971).

This resistance to infections caused by unrelated organisms parallels enhanced nonspecific resistance to transplantable and autochthonous tumors (Lunde and Gerlderman, 1971; Hibbs *et al.*, 1972a; Krahenbuhl and Remington, 1974). Jacobsen (1934) may well have been the first to advance the reticuloendothelial theory of malignancy that increased incidence of cancer results from decreased incidence of acute viral or bacterial infections. He concluded (1) that the evidence tends to support the hypothesis that the reticuloendothelial system, when sufficiently activated by infectious processes, may attain the ability to cope with neoplastic disease and (2) that the present (1934) increase in malignant morbidity is due to decreased resistive powers of the reticuloendothelial system occasioned by lessened incidence of infections which had been widely endemic prior to modern health methods.

A number of investigators demonstrated that macrophages isolated from mice chronically infected with a variety of phylogenetically unrelated microorganisms could inhibit the growth of tumor cells *in vitro*. Hibbs and co-workers showed that infection with *Toxoplasma gondii, Besnoitia jellisoni, Listeria monocytogenes,* and *Bacillus Calmette-Guerin* (BCG) induced in mice a population of activated peritoneal macrophages that were tumoricidal *in vitro* (Hibbs *et al.*, 1971, 1972a,b; Hibbs, 1973). Furthermore, Hibbs (1974a) showed that activated, but not normal, macrophages can nonimmunologically destroy, *in vitro,* target cells with tumorigenic potential by a nonphagocytic mechanism requiring direct contact and speculated that the interaction between activated macrophages and target cells is not entirely nonspecific, but is based on a primitive system of nonimmunologic discrimination since normal cells are spared. The observation of selective cytotoxicity of activated macrophages for neoplastic target cells has been confirmed in several laboratories (Alexander and Evans, 1971; Hibbs *et al.*, 1972a; Holtermann *et al.*, 1973; Keller, 1974; Meltzer *et al.*, 1975b; Fidler *et al.*, 1978). Keller (1974) demonstrated that cytocidal killing was achieved not only on tumor cells, but all rapidly replicating cell lines examined, irrespective of whether they were of syngeneic, allogeneic, or xenogeneic origin, or showed normal or neoplastic growth characteristics, were inhibited in their proliferation by activated macrophages. He postulated that inhibition of proliferation could be an important homeostatic regulatory function of the macrophage which would affect every replicating cell. Krahenbuhl and Remington (1974) and Hibbs and associates (1972a) found that nonspecific antitumor cell activity of macrophages obtained from mice chronically infected with intracellular protozoan parasites persisted for more than 6 months while the same activity of macrophages from mice infected with *Listeria monocytogenes* lasted less than 2 weeks.

Hibbs and co-workers (1974b) reported that BCG-activated macrophages are cytotoxic for tumor cells *in vitro* and that the cytotoxicity is mediated by lysosomal enzymes of macrophages origin. The lysosomes of activated macrophages were secreted directly into the cytoplasm of the susceptible target cells, presumably at regions of cell contact and membrane "destabilization." Using cinemicrographic analysis, Meltzer and associates (1976) noted that the translational movement rate of BCG-activated macrophages among neoplastic cells was 4 times greater than that observed among nonneoplastic cells. At 46 hours of *in vitro* culture, at a time when no viable tumor cells remained, the translational movement of BCG-activated macrophages had decreased to that observed in the absence of tumor target cells.

Several studies underline the requirement for a lymphocyte product for expression of nonspecific tumoricidal effect by macrophages. Piessens and his colleagues (1975) demonstrated that macrophages become cytotoxic for syngeneic neoplastic cells after they have been activated *in vitro* by mediator-rich supernatant fluids prepared from lymphocytes sensitized to an antigen unrelated to the target cells. In addition, Churchill and coworkers (1975) showed that macrophages could be activated as suspension cultures with lymphocyte mediators devoid of antigen. Another model for macrophage activation was described by Evans and Alexander (1972). In this model, specific inducing antigen must: (1) interact with sensitized T-derived lymphocytes to produce specific macrophage arming factor (SMAF) and (2) interact with armed (SMAF-bearing) macrophages, to make them nonspecifically tumoricidal.

In contrast to a requirement for lymphocyte-derived products, Alexander and Evans (1971) demonstrated that macrophages were directly transformed into cytotoxic effector cells *in vitro* by endotoxin and polyinosinic–polycytidylic acid [poly(I)·poly(C)]. Similarly, Schultz and co-workers (1977a) provided experimental evidence that pyran copolymer and other polyanionic interferon inducers directly render macrophages tumoricidal. They postulated that interferon was the ultimate inducer of macrophage activation since macrophages exposed to polyanions *in vitro* produce interferon and since chromatography-purified mouse L cell interferon activates macrophages directly.

Finally, a number of conflicting stimuli have been identified that may prevent macrophage-mediated tumor killing in the local environment of the tumor and may be important in the pathogenesis of progressive tumor growth. Although a number of investigators have demonstrated that the ability of immunoadjuvants to enhance host resistance to cancer correlates with their capacity to render macrophages nonspecifically tumoricidal *in vivo* (Juy and Chedid, 1975; Morahan and Kaplan, 1976; Schultz *et al.*, 1977c), much of their clinical usefulness may be compromised by hydrocortisone (Hibbs, 1976b; Schultz *et al.*, 1978e), proteases (Hibbs *et al.*, 1977), high-molecular-weight lipids (Chapman and Hibbs, 1977), and E-type prostaglandins (Schultz *et al.*, 1978d,e). Schultz and associates (1979a) recently suggested that prostaglandins of the E-series liberated from activated macrophages may act locally in negative feedback inhibition to limit tumoricidal activities. In addition, Snyderman and Pike (1976) found an inhibitor of macrophage chemotaxis produced by various transplantable tumors. The same group found that macrophages from animals implanted with syngeneic tumors developed depressed migratory ability *in vivo* and chemotactic responsiveness *in vitro* (Pike and Snyderman, 1976), and that surgical removal of tumors results in a rapid enhancement of monocyte chemotaxis (Snyderman *et al.*, 1975).

II. Pathways for Induction of Activated Macrophages

A large variety of agents have the ability to render macrophages nonspecifically tumoricidal. It is convenient to place these agents in two broad categories of activating mechanisms: those where activation results from the immunologically specific interaction between sensitized lymphocytes and antigen (specific activation) although the expression of the activated state is nonspecific and those where activation does not appear to have an immunological basis (nonspecific activation). Nonspecific activation may reflect direct effects on the macrophage by the agent as well as cytokines released by nonimmune cells (e.g., fibroblast-derived interferon preparations) and lymphokines released by mitogen-stimulated T lymphocytes.

A. Nonspecific Activation

Although considerable historical emphasis has been placed on the requirement for antigen-induced T-lymphocyte products in the activation of macrophages, observations in the athymic *nu/nu* mouse have indicated an alternative mechanism of macrophage activation *in vivo* due to environmental stimuli. Peritoneal macrophages from conventionally housed, but not germ-free housed, *nu/nu* mice were observed to be nonspecifically tumoricidal (Meltzer, 1976), were bactericidal against facultative intracellular bacteria (Cheers and Waller, 1975), and inhibited replication of vaccinia virus (Ramarao *et al.*, 1977) and herpes simplex virus type 2 (Mogensen and Anderson, 1978). Since *nu/nu* mice are resistant to spontaneous tumor development (Rygaard and Paulsen, 1974; Wortis, 1974), these studies suggest that the chronically activated macrophage, in the absence of mature T-derived lymphocytes, may comprise a more effective antitumor surveillance system than the classical T-lymphocyte-dependent mechanism proposed for conventional animals (Burnet, 1970).

1. *Polyanionic Interferon Inducers*

Alexander and Evans (1971) were the first to show that polyanionic substances directly render macrophages nonspecifically cytotoxic for allogeneic and syngeneic tumor cells. They observed that noncytotoxic macrophages, when exposed to minute amounts of the lipid A component of endotoxin, double-stranded RNA, or synthetic poly(I)·poly(C) *in vitro*, inhibit the growth of lymphoma and sarcoma cells. This cytotoxic action of macrophages was not due to secretory products from drug-treated macrophages, but required direct contact between macrophage and target cell. Tumor cells were noted to adhere firmly to activated macrophages. Evans and Alexander (1976) cautioned that "results of experiments in which the toxicity of various compounds toward tumor cells in culture has been tested should be interpreted with caution, particularly if the compounds are known to activate macrophages and if primary cultures of tumor cells were used, since such frequently contain large numbers of macrophages."

Macrophages were similarly activated *in vivo* by an intraperitoneal injection of double-stranded RNA or endotoxin and then washing out the peritoneal macrophages 3–7 days later (Evans, 1974). Maximal activity was not observed until 7 days after injection. Moreover, these agents have been shown to cause complete regressions of some established subcutaneous or intradermal, but not intraperitoneal (ip) tumors when administered either systemically or directly into the tumor (Parr *et al.*, 1973). Maximal therapeutic effect was observed when treatment was started 7 days after lymphoma or fibrosarcoma transplantation. In addition, these polyanionic agents were shown to act prophylactically and protect mice against a subsequent ip tumor challenge.

The kinetics of *in vivo* activation of macrophages by endotoxin and double-stranded RNA are similar to those observed by Kaplan and coworkers (1974) after pyran (a copolymer of divinyl ether and maleic anhydride) administration. They showed that macrophage cytotoxic activity was slightly increased 3 days after ip pyran treatment, was maximal by 5 and 7 days, and had decreased by 11 days after drug administration. Cytotoxicity was largely tumor-selective, although some cytotoxicity for normal mouse embryo cell was detected. Supernatants from pyran-activated macrophages were not cytotoxic for tumor cells. Activated macrophages could be recovered from thymectomized, irradiated, bone marrow-reconstituted mice inoculated with pyran. They suggested that this might explain why pyran protects mice immunosuppressed by adult thymectomy and antilymphocyte serum from polyoma virus oncogenesis and Rauscher virus leukemogenesis (Hirsch *et al.*, 1972).

Several other studies have implicated the nonspecifically activated macrophage in the antitumor activity of pyran. Harmel and Zbar (1975) showed that ip pyran protected mice against intradermal tumor development of a transplantable chemically induced fibrosarcoma and that peritoneal cells from pyran-treated mice suppressed tumor growth in local passive-transfer experiments. Moreover, the antitumor activity of ip pyran therapy against the sc Lewis lung carcinoma (Snodgrass *et al.*, 1975), Madison lung carcinoma (Schultz *et al.*, 1977d), and colon tumor 26 (Schultz *et al.*, 1977c) was associated with an increased mobilization and deposit of morphologically activated macrophages at the tumor site. Necrosis was much more extensive in the lesions of pyran-treated animals, and macrophages were intimately associated wtih necrobiotic tumor cells in each of these studies. Whether this mobilization of macrophages is related to the chemoattractant property of pyran for monocytes (Majeski and Stinnett, 1977) or related to enhancing the immunogenicity of the tumors is yet to be determined.

Schultz and co-workers (1977a,b) further implicated the polyanionic structure of pyran in its ability to render macrophages cytotoxic. They showed that pyran and numerous other polyanions, including dextran sulfate, poly(A)·poly(U), poly(I)·poly(C), and heparin sulfate activated murine peritoneal macrophages *in vitro* to inhibit the growth of MBL-2 leukemia cells. Activation was sharply dose-dependent and required >24 hours after exposure to drug. Single-stranded RNA and the polycation, DEAE-dextran, were without effect on the functional activity of macrophages. Cytotoxicity was again noted to involve increased adherence of tumor cells on macrophage membranes and not soluble factors secreted by activated macrophages into the culture medium. Moreover, the ability of various polyanions to induce cytotoxic macrophages *in vivo* correlated with their ability to enhance host resistance against a transplantable murine lung carcinoma (Schultz *et al.*, 1978b).

Although the exact mechanism by which polyanions render macrophages cytotoxic is presently unknown, at least three distinct possibilities exist. Polyanions may activate macrophages via interferon induction, because macrophage cultures produce interferon after polyanion treatment *in vitro* (Finkelstein *et al.*, 1968; Ibrahim *et al.*, 1976; Neumann and Sorg, 1978) and because antibody-purified fibroblast-derived interferon has been demonstrated to be a potent macrophage activator (Schultz *et al.*, 1977a, 1978a). Moreover, highly specific anti-interferon globulin has been demonstrated to block the ability of type I interferon inducers [e.g., poly(I)·poly(C), pyran copolymer, and LPS] to activate macrophages *in vitro,* indicating that endogenous interferon has to externalize from the producing cell before induction of the tumoricidal state (Schultz and Chirigos, 1979). Alternatively, polyanions may behave as model gene regulators, binding to nuclear histones and releasing template restriction

(Ansevin *et al.*, 1975; Mohr *et al.*, 1978). Results in our laboratory show that ^{14}C-labeled pyran is rapidly taken up by macrophages; much of this activity can be recovered from isolated nuclei extracted from these cells (Papamatheakis *et al.*, 1978). A third possibility is suggested by the ability of polyanions to activate complement by the alternative pathway, resulting in cleavage of C3 into a small fragment, $C3_a$ and a large fragment, $C3_b$. $C3_b$ has been shown to be a naturally occurring stimulator of macrophage function, whereas $C3_a$ is lytic for cells (Ferluga *et al.*, 1978).

2. *Bacterial Components or Products*

Coley, having noted that regressions of some malignant tumors appeared to coincide with the occurrence of erisipelas, began treating cancer patients in 1893 with bacterial culture filtrates (Coley's toxin), which contained endotoxins along with other components, and achieved striking results (for review, see Nauts *et al.*, 1953). As mentioned previously under polyanions, endotoxin renders macrophages nonspecifically tumoricidal (Alexander and Evans, 1971) and has antitumor activity which predominantly affects established tumors (Parr *et al.*, 1973).

Several studies have attempted to characterize the effects of endotoxin on macrophage tumor cell killing. Using pure populations of cloned macrophages as effectors, Weinberg and co-workers (1978) demonstrated that endotoxin can act directly on macrophages in the complete absence of contaminating lymphocytes. The LPS effect on macrophages was reproduced by lipid A. Furthermore, they showed that macrophage differentiation toward the tumoricidal state paralleled the responsiveness of macrophages to endotoxin. While normal macrophages were not rendered tumoricidal even in the presence of 10 μg/ml LPS, peptone-induced macrophages were made cytotoxic by ≥ 500 ng/ml LPS, and nontumoricidal BCG-stimulated macrophages required 0.5 to 1 ng/ml LPS to kill tumor cells. In addition, LPS acted synergistically with lymphokine in activating macrophages. These authors stressed that reagents should be free of LPS contamination before valid interpretations can be made of experiments investigating macrophage tumor cell killing.

Several investigators have made use of the lipid A-nonresponder mouse strain C3H/HeJ to study the effects of endotoxin on macrophage function. Ruco and associates (1978) demonstrated that macrophages from LPS-unresponsive mice, in contrast to LPS-responsive C3H/HeN mice, failed to develop tumoricidal activity after a variety of *in vivo* and *in vitro* activation stimuli and suggested that the gene for control of macrophage cytotoxic capacity is either closely linked or identical to the LPS gene. The C3H/HeJ macrophage appears to have a highly selective defect, since Ruco and Meltzer (1978b) have shown that other macrophage responses (yield, phagocytosis, peroxidase staining in inflammatory exudates induced by BCG, T-cell mitogens, or heterologous serum) in C3H/HeJ and C3H/HeN mice were identical. Similarly, C3H/HeJ macrophages responded normally *in vitro* to chemotactic lymphokine. Possible mechanisms for the potent effect of lipid A on responsive macrophages have previously been discussed in Section II,A,1. Hibbs and co-workers (1977) showed that there was no difference in the amount of lymphokine or endotoxin required to make macrophages tumoricidal in fresh unheated or heat-inactivated (56°C for 30 minutes) guinea pig or mouse serum, suggesting that complement activation was not a critical factor.

Aqueous ether-extracted *Brucella abortus* (Bru-Pel), at doses ≥ 1 ng/ml culture medium, has been shown to render macrophages cytotoxic for leukemia target cells *in vitro* (Schultz *et al.*, 1978c). *Brucella* LPS, in contrast to LPS extracted from *Escherichia coli* and *Salmonella typhimurium,* failed to activate macrophages *in vitro* at all concentrations tested (1 ng–10 μg/ml). Similarly, Bru-Pel, but not *Brucella* LPS, has been shown to be a potent inducer of a "virus-type" interferon (Feingold *et al.*, 1976). The inability of *Brucella* LPS to activate macrophages, in contrast to LPS of *Enterobacteria,* may be explained by differences in the nature and linkages of fatty acids present in its structure (Rietschel *et al.*, 1972). Intraperitoneal treatment of homozygous nude mice with Bru-Pel induced cytotoxic macrophages, further indicating that Bru-Pel activated macrophages through a thymus-independent process (Schultz *et al.*, 1978c). Bru-Pel and *Brucella* LPS were similarly tested in an artificial lung metastasis model. Only Bru-Pel strikingly inhibited tumor nodule formation and was effective when given either 5 days prior to or 1 day after tumor inoculation. Histopathologic studies of the lungs of Bru-Pel-treated mice revealed accumulations of macrophages surrounding the metastatic lung carcinoma foci and arresting their development. The active component(s) of Bru-Pel has not been well defined.

Another bacterial substance that is capable of rendering macrophages nonspecifically cytotoxic is the simple peptidoglycan, a cell wall component of all bacteria. Nauciel and Goguel (1977) showed that peptidoglycan extracted with lysozyme from *Bacillus megaterium* inhibited the growth of a chemically induced fibrosarcoma in syngeneic rats and activated macrophages *in vivo* at a dose of 500 μg/rat. The resultant macrophages exhibited cytotoxicity against all fibrosarcoma lines tested. Evans and Alexander (1976) demonstrated that peptidoglycan at concentrations of a few micrograms per milliliter activated purified cultures of macrophages *in vitro*. One of the possible functions of macrophage lysozyme might consist of an effect arising in the course of its action on bacteria, as some of the bacterial reaction products, such as peptidoglycans from both Gram-positive and Gram-negative bacteria, behave as macrophage-activating agents and immunoadjuvants (Jolles, 1976). In addition, a synthetic analog of water-soluble components of mycobacteria, *N*-acetyl-muramyl-L-alanyl-D-isoglutamine or muramyl dipeptide (MDP), appears to act directly on macrophages to enhance bactericidal (Hadden, 1978) and cytotoxic (Juy and Chedid, 1975) activity.

3. *Virus*

Since purified cultures of resting macrophages are activated by exposure to polyanions and bacterial lipopolysaccharides and secrete substantial levels of interferon (Finkelstein *et al.*, 1968; Ibrahim *et al.*, 1976; Maehara and Ho, 1977; Neumann and Sorg, 1978), Schultz and associates (1977a) tested chromatography-purified Newcastle disease virus (NDV)-induced interferon from mouse L cells and found that this material potently rendered macrophages cytotoxic. The stimulatory factor fell into the present definition of interferon due to its stability at pH 2.0, sensitivity to both heat and trypsin, and species specificity. Human interferon preparations, as compared to mouse, showed a reduction of approximately two logs of activity when tested on mouse macrophages. Although mouse interferon was active at concentrations as low as 1–10 units/ml culture medium, mock interferon preparations lacked activity at all concentrations tested (Schultz and Chirigos, 1978; Schultz *et al.*, 1978a). *In vivo* administered interferon was similarly active at enhancing macrophage cytotoxic function (Schultz *et al.*, 1978a). These authors suggested that the ability of stromal cells to respond to infection and produce soluble mediators (cytokines) which directly enhance macrophage function may form the basis for a primitive form of local tissue immunity. Similarly, Flanagan and co-workers (1973) demonstrated that supernatants derived from virus-infected monkey kidney cells possessed macrophage migration inhibitory (MIF-like) activity.

A number of other investigators have shown that interferon-containing preparations from a variety of sources enhance the phagocytic function of macrophages (Huang *et al.*, 1971; Donahoe and Huang, 1973, 1976; Imanishi *et al.*, 1975), as well as increase the spreading of macrophages on glass surfaces (Rabinovitch *et al.*, 1977). Using recombinant inbred mice that carry either a "high" or a "low" response allele for a gene that controls their interferon levels induced by NDV, Manejias and co-workers (1978) attempted to compare serum interferon titers with phagocytosis of antibody-coated erythrocytes by macrophages. They found that high responders for interferon induction were also found to be high responders for enhancement of phagocytosis by NDV. Conversely, strains that were low responders for interferon induction were similarly found to be low responders for phagocytosis by macrophages. They suggested that their results were compatible with two main possibilities: (1) interferon induced by NDV enhances phagocytosis by macrophages; or (2) a macrophage-activating factor different from interferon is released together with interferon in response to NDV and the activity of this factor correlates with serum interferon titers. Moreover, Schultz and Chirigos (1978) demonstrated the remarkable similarities between the agents that activate macrophages in fibroblast-derived interferon preparations and lymphokine preparations, including conditions for their induction, interferon level required for activation, and physicochemical properties. They suggested that interferon may provide a unifying mechanism for macrophage activation by these diverse preparations.

Other studies have similarly pointed to the ability of viral infection to enhance macrophage activity. Evans (1974) showed that either productive or nonproductive infection of mouse or rat peritoneal macrophages with lactate dehydrogenase-elevating virus rendered the cells cytostatic for SL2 lymphoma and FS4 sarcoma cells. Rodda and White (1976) reported that highly cytotoxic-activated macrophages, not specific for the infecting virus, appeared on day 1, peaked on day 2 to 3, and disappeared within a week after infection of mice with togaviruses. Similarly, Chapes and Tompkins (1978) demonstrated that peritoneal macrophages from hamsters infected with vaccinia virus were nonspecifically cytotoxic for viral-transformed cells as well as neoplastic cells. Peak cytotoxicity occurred 5 days after virus infection. Puccetti and Holden (1979) noted that macrophages with peak cytotoxic activity could be recovered from the peritoneal cavity of mice 14 days after ip inoculation of murine sarcoma virus. In addition, Blanden and Mims (1973) observed that bactericidal macrophages could be obtained from mice 8 days after infection with ectromelia or lymphocytic choriomeningitis viruses.

4. *Mitogen-Stimulated Lymphokine*

Macrophage are activated by soluble mediators released by concanavalin A (Con A)-treated splenocytes *in vitro* (Pfizenmaier *et al.*, 1975; Fidler *et al.,* 1976a, 1978; Schultz and Chirigos, 1978). This factor that renders macrophages cytotoxic is referred to as macrophage-activating factor (MAF) and appears to be analogous to the factor released by sensitized lymphocytes cultured in the presence of specific antigen (see Section II,B). "Active" culture supernatant was produced by mitogen-stimulated T cells, but not mitogen-stimulated B cells (Pfizenmaier *et al.,* 1975). Fidler and co-workers (1976a) demonstrated that rat lymphocytes stimulated with sepharose-bound Con A elaborated a MAF that rendered mouse macrophages cytotoxic against syngeneic and allogeneic tumor cells, but spared normal syngeneic or allogeneic embryo cells. The MAF activity was enhanced after heating at 100°C. Although tumor cells, upon treatment with Con A, display remarkable adhesion to macrophage cell surfaces (Inoue *et al.*, 1972), control experiments excluded the possibility that residual unbound Con A caused the observed macrophage-mediated tumoricidal effects. In a subsequent study, Fidler and associates (1978) showed that transformed cells were killed by these Con A–MAF-activated macrophages regardless of whether or not they express Forssman antigen, display surface changes which permit agglutination by low doses of plant lectins, express SV40 T antigen, have a low saturation density, or exhibit density-dependent inhibition of DNA synthesis. Piessens (1978b) found that following incubation *in vitro* with Con A–MAF, macrophages became capable of binding more tumor cells than nonactivated macrophages. Increased binding occurred rapidly (within 1 hour), did not require the presence of serum in the medium, and was inhibited by treatment with trypsin. Binding by activated macrophages was quantitatively selective for tumor cells and appeared to result from stimulation of a specific macrophage function during the process of activation.

Although levamisole has no direct effect on macrophage function (Schultz *et al.*, 1976; Kelly, 1978), it has been demonstrated to augment the production of MAF by Con A-treated lymphocytes, while having no effect on lymphocyte proliferation (Whitcomb *et al.*, 1976). Levamisole has similarly affected induction of macrophage activation by Q fever rickettsiae and BCG cell walls (Kelly, 1978). This effect varied with the response of the macrophages to the microbial stimulants. In cells that responded poorly to stimulation, levamisole enhanced the response, but levamisole inhibited the response in cells that were highly stimulated by the microbial agents.

We have previously shown that type II IF and the lymphokine that activates macrophages behave alike both in their coordinate production and physicochemical properties (Schultz and Chirigos, 1978). Both type II IF and the concanavalin A-induced MAF elude from Sephadex G-100 with peak activity between 55,000 and 45,000 daltons, and their broad elution profiles suggest that their activity may be due to more than one protein with molecular weights close to one another. Both agents are destroyed with proteolytic enzymes and are labile at pH 2 (Schultz and Chirigos, 1979). However, most activity remained following heating at 56°C for 30 minutes. Their production paralleled each other in spleen cultures, and both have been reported to require macrophage–T lymphocyte collaboration in their production (Epstein, 1976; Rosenstreich *et al.*, 1976). Moreover, it is interesting that concanavalin A-induced MAF, which contains an antigenically unrelated IF (Youngner and Salvin, 1973), was not neutralized by anti-L cell IF globulin (Schultz and Chirigos, 1979).

5. *Others*

Several naturally occurring polysaccharides containing chains of β-(1 → 3)-linked D-glucose residues, such as glucan, scleroglucan, and lentinan, are capable of inducing nonspecific macrophage-mediated cytotoxicity (Mansell *et al.*, 1975; Bomford and Moreno, 1977; Schultz *et al.*, 1977c, 1978f). Of these agents, glucan, part of the outer membrane of *Saccharomyces cerevisiae,* has been studied most extensively. Mansell and DiLuzio (1976) suggested that glucan has distinct advantages over many of the other macrophage-activating agents in being a relatively nontoxic, chemically defined agent without complications due to infection or toxic metabolites. The most effective antitumor therapy with glucan has been intralesional treatment where dissolution of the tumor mass was associated with necrosis of the tumor and a macrophage infiltrate (Mansell *et al.*, 1975). Glucan does not have direct toxicity for tumor cells *in vitro* (Mansell *et al.*, 1975; Schultz *et al.*, 1978f), and Bomford and Moreno (1977) concluded from their investigations into the antitumor effect of glucans and fructosans in an artifical metastasis assay that the activity of these polysaccharides is predominantly nonspecific macrophage-mediated and much weaker than that found with *Corynebacterium parvum*. We observed that glucan renders macrophages both cytostatic and cytocidal for tumor cells in a sharply dose-dependent and thymus-independent manner (Schultz *et al.*, 1977c, 1978f). Glucan also causes a phagocytic hyperfunction and hyperplasia of the macrophage system (DiLuzio *et al.*, 1970).

Although the mechanism of glucan activation of macrophages is unknown, glucan particles, 3 to 4 μm in diameter, are known to be localized within macrophages and possibly exert their stimulatory effect as a result of solubilization (Mansell *et al.*, 1976). Goldberg (1975) has observed that feeding a variety of carbohydrates to mammals causes profound changes in metabolism, including repression of enzyme induction, RNA synthesis, and glucocorticoid activity and a decrease in cyclic AMP levels relative to cyclic GMP. An alternative mechanism for macrophage activation by carbohydrates may be through their ability to stimulate interferon production (Lackovic *et al.*, 1970; Elinov *et al.*, 1972).

Two other biologic agents that induce tumoricidal macrophages include kanamycin, an antibiotic substance produced by *Streptomyces kanamyceticus* and KS-2, a peptide mannan extracted from the culture mycelia of *Lentinus edodes*. Circulating interferon has been reported after treatment of mice with both kanamycin (Ho *et al.*, 1975) and KS-2 (Suzuki *et al.*, 1977). Kanamycin activates macrophage *in vitro* at concentrations as low as 10 μg/ml (R. M. Schultz, unpublished observations), and its inclusion in culture medium as a broad spectrum antibiotic may make valid interpretation of experiments investigating macrophage-mediated tumor cell killing difficult. The antitumor activity of KS-2 has been suggested to result from induction of nonspecifically cytotoxic macrophages (Suzuki *et al.*, 1978).

Ferluga and co-workers (1978) reported that macrophages exposed to the complement cleavage product, $C3_b$, liberated into the medium a soluble cytolytic factor for tumor cells. This factor was pharmacologically indistinguishable from $C3_a$, and cytolytic activity could be neutralized by antiserum directed against $C3_a$. Moreover, they suggested that the ability of various agents (e.g., LPS, dextran sulfate, and zymosan) to activate macrophages may result from their ability to activate the alternative pathway of complement. The large cleavage product of the third component of complement, $C3_b$, activates macrophages to become tumorolytic, while the smaller cleavage product, $C3_a$, is lytic for macrophages as well as various tumor cells, fibroblasts, and mitogen-stimulated lymphocytes (Schorlemmer and Allison, 1976). However, this hypothesis does not appear to account for the selective cytotoxicity of macrophages for transformed cells, nor the cell-to-cell contact mandatory for tumor cell killing which most investigators have observed (see Section III,A).

BM 12.531, a 2-cyansubstituted aziridine, is a synthetic agent capable of activating murine macrophages *in vitro* and *in vivo* (R. M. Schultz, unpublished observation). Peritoneal macrophages were rendered tumoricidal by addition of BM 12.531 to the culture medium at 1–100 μg/ml. Macrophage activation by BM 12.531 was not sharply dose-dependent as that observed by polyanionic interferon inducers. Similarly, peritoneal macrophages harvested 6 days after ip treatment with BM 12.531 at 10 mg/kg were activated to inhibit growth of MBL-2 leukemia cells.

B. Specific Activation

Macrophages may be rendered nonspecifically tumoricidal by the lymphocyte-derived product, macrophage-activating factor (MAF), released by antigen-stimulated T lymphocytes. Active MAF preparations have been obtained from the culture supernatant of: (1) lymphocytes sensitized *in vivo* against intracellular bacterial and protozoan parasites (Meltzer and Bartlett, 1972; Christie and Bomford, 1975; Anderson *et al.*, 1976; Cullen and Ghaffar, 1978; Ruco and Meltzer, 1978a,b) or tumor cells (Fidler, 1975; Fidler *et al.*, 1976b; Kripke *et al.*, 1977) and cultured *in vitro* in the presence of specific antigen; or (2) mixed lymphocyte cultures (Dy *et al.*, 1976; Nabarra *et al.*, 1978). Mitogen-induced MAF has previously been considered in Section II,A,4, since this MAF production does not require a specific recognition of antigen.

Riisgaard and co-workers (1978) have noted a qualitative difference between activating normal macrophages by incubation with sensitized lymphocytes and antigen or with MAF preparations. They noted that in the former system, direct contact between lymphocytes and macrophages was probably necessary and required H-2 compatibility. Furthermore, David and Remold (1976) concluded that activation of macrophages after direct contact with lymphocytes and antigen (in contrast to lymphokine supernatants) required a shorter incubation time and resulted in greater bactericidal activity.

Perhaps the MAF isolated from purified protein derivative of tuberculin (PPD)-stimulated BCG-immune mouse spleen cell culture fluids has been most extensively studied. Ruco and Meltzer (1978a) demonstrated that peritoneal inflammation induced by sterile irritants led to accumulation of macrophages that were more responsive to lymphokines than macrophages from resident cell populations of untreated mice. Tumor cytotoxicity of lymphokine-activated inflammatory macrophages was about 10-fold greater than that by equal numbers of lymphokine-treated resident cells. They suggested that increased lymphokine responsiveness of inflammatory cells was dependent upon influx of young peroxidase-positive mononuclear phagocytes rather than stimulation of resident macrophages. Weinberg and associates (1978) showed that macrophage differentiation toward the tumoricidal state paralleled the responsiveness of macrophages to endotoxin, and that LPS acted synergistically with MAF in activating macrophages. Much of the antitumor activity of BCG appears to be mediated by nonspecifically cytotoxic macrophages (Hanna *et al.*, 1973), and Keller (1977) has presented evidence that antimacrophage agents can abrogate the antitumor effects of *Corynebacterium parvum* and BCG *in vivo*.

The PPD-induced MAF has been characterized as a protein with a molecular weight of 55,000 ± 1600 (Leonard *et al.*, 1978). Since the relative concentration curve of MAF eluted through Sephadex G-100 or G-200 was wider than that of a single protein, MAF activity was suggested to be due to more than one protein with similar molecular weights. This possibility was strengthened by a broad elution range on DEAE-cellulose chromatography from a specific conductance of 3.5 to 8.5 mmho/cm, at pH 7.9. MAF was labile at both pH 4 and 10, and was destroyed by proteolytic enzymes. Eighty percent was destroyed by heating at 56°C for 30 minutes. In affinity chromatography experiments, MAF did not bind to Con A-Sepharose, but it was bound to insolubilized Cibacron-blue and was eluted by an increase in ionic strength.

Churchill and co-workers (1975) have described a system in which normal macrophages were activated as suspension cultures either in mediator-rich supernatants from *o*-chlorobenzoyl-bovine α-globulin-stimulated lymphocytes or in antigen-free sephadex fractions from these supernatants. These activated macrophages killed the syngeneic tumors, Line 1 hepatoma and MCA-25 fibrosarcoma, while under similar conditions, the survival of two normal syngeneic cell types, fibroblasts and kidney cells, was not affected (Piessens *et al.*, 1975).

Fidler and associates (1976b) showed that supernatants of presensitized rat lymphocytes specifically stimulated *in vitro* with several different mouse, dog, and rat tumor cells were capable of rendering normal rat and mouse macrophages nonspecifically cytotoxic *in vitro* to their respective syngeneic tumor cells. The release of MAF by rat lymphocytes sensitized *in vivo* was dependent upon immunologically specific recognition of an antigen *in vitro*. Their data demonstrated that MAF can cross strain and even species specificities. They also suggested that the activation of macrophages *in vivo* is a continuous process of lymphocyte–macrophage interaction, since they could reactivate macrophages by a secondary exposure to MAF. Fidler (1974) demonstrated that the intravenous injection of these specifically activated macrophages may have therapeutic value against pulmonary metastases.

Dy and co-workers (1976), utilizing MAF preparations from mixed lymphocyte cultures, showed that (1) macrophages possess surface structures binding MAF at either 4 or 37°C; (2) these structures are destroyed by pronase; and (3) macrophage activation under the influence of the MAF bound on the cell surface requires an active cellular process inhibited at 4°C and reappearing at 37°C. Lohmann-Matthes (1976) attempted to characterize the MAF derived from spleen cells sensitized against DBA/2 alloantigens and cocultivated with DBA/2 lymphoma cells. This material had a molecular weight of ~30,000 and proved to be stable at −70°C.

Schultz and Chirigos (1978) noted the similarities between MAF and type II (immune) interferon both in their coordinate production and physicochemical characteristics. Both elude from Sephadex G-100 with peak activity between 55,000 and 45,000 daltons, and both are destroyed by proteolytic enzymes and are labile at pH 2. However, most activity remained following heating at 56°C for 30 minutes. Moreover, both MAF and type II interferon have been reported to require macrophage–T lymphocyte collaboration in their production (Babiuk and Rouse, 1976; Epstein, 1976; Rosenstreich *et al.*, 1976). In addition, a highly specific anti-type I interferon globulin preparation that blocks the ability of type I interferon inducers to activate macrophages directly does not neutralize the affect of either MAF or type II interferon on its target cell (Schultz and Chirigos, 1979).

Evans and associates (1973) presented evidence for an alternative mechanism of macrophage activation where macrophages are first armed with a product of immune T cells termed specific macrophage-arming factor (SMAF), and become tumoricidal after exposure to specific antigen. Macrophages armed with a SMAF directed to a transplantable or tumor-specific antigen specifically inhibited the growth of tumor cells bearing this antigen. However, if SMAF-armed macrophages were exposed to the specific antigen *in vitro,* they become capable of inhibiting growth of lymphoma cells in a nonspecific manner.

III. Mechanisms of the Cytotoxic Action of Activated Macrophages

A. Cell-to-Cell Contact

Several investigators have been unable to identify a soluble cytotoxin in the medium bathing activated macrophages and have noted a requirement for direct cell contact for tumor cytotoxicity (Alexander and Evans, 1971; Hibbs *et al.*, 1972a; Schultz *et al.*, 1977a,b). Studies using time-lapse cinemicrography have indicated that the rate of lateral movement of activated, but not normal macrophages is increased after exposure to tumor cells or their soluble by-products as compared to nonneoplastic targets (Meltzer *et al.*, 1975a; Snodgrass *et al.*, 1978) and that intimate contact between target cell and activated macrophage precedes cell killing (Meltzer *et al.*, 1975a; Bucana *et al.*, 1976; Stewart *et al.*, 1976).

Using phase contrast microscopy and lysosomal markers, Hibbs (1974b) presented evidence that the cytotoxic activity of activated macrophages against tumorigenic target cells was mediated by lysosomes of macrophage origin which were secreted directly into the cytoplasm of susceptible target cells. Moreover this reaction could be inhibited by agents which prevent the exocytosis of macrophage lysosomes (hydrocortisone) or which interfere with the action of lysosomal enzymes (trypan blue). Similarly, Bucana and co-workers (1976) presented morphological evidence for the translocation of lysosomal organelles from cytotoxic macrophages into the cytoplasm of tumor target cells and suggested that neoplastic target cell susceptibility may be the result of an active or passive uptake of lysosomes and consequently cytolysis. These results suggest a local membrane fusion or "destabilization" that occurs during direct contact of neoplastic target cells and activated macrophages. In addition, Piessens (1977) demonstrated that increased tumor cell killing by normal macrophages occurs when artificial contacts (presumably via Schiff bases) are established between macrophages and tumor cells.

Preferential tumor cytotoxicity was elegantly shown by Meltzer and associates (1975b), who demonstrated in a mixed neoplastic/nonneoplastic target cell population, BCG-activated macrophages selectively destroyed the neoplastic cells; nonneoplastic cells were not affected as "innocent bystanders." Several other studies have shown that cytotoxicity results from direct cell contact rather than secretion of soluble cytotoxins. Sharma and Piessens (1978a) suggested that cytochalasins, colchicine, and vinblastine inhibit macrophage-mediated cytotoxicity by preventing intimate contact between the effector macrophage and its target. In addition, they (1978b) showed that pretreatment of activated macrophages with trypsin also inhibited tumor cytotoxicity and suggested that protein synthesis may be necessary to maintain an adequate number of "recognition structures" on the macrophage membrane, structures that mediate the initial contact between the activated macrophage and the target tumor.

B. Soluble Factors

Activated macrophages secrete a variety of products, including neutral proteinases, $C3_a$, thymidine, arginase, and E-type prostaglandins, that may adversely affect the growth or viability of cells *in vitro*. However because of the complexity of macrophage culture supernatant in terms of "factors," extreme caution is warranted in the interpretation of data and in making generalizations on the mechanism(s) of action of macrophages on target cells.

Sethi and Brandis (1975) observed that a soluble macrophage product(s) released by nonimmune mouse peritoneal macrophages exposed to endotoxin or from listeria-immune macrophages after incubation with specific antigen mediates cytotoxic activity against malignant cell types and, to a lesser extent, against normal cells. The macrophage product(s) retained cytotoxic activity following storage at −20°C, was stable when heated at 56°C for 30 minutes, and was completely inactivated when exposed at 100°C for 5 minutes. Adams (1978) showed that cell-free supernatants from BCG-activated macrophages selectively lysed murine neoplastic targets and that the factor responsible for cytolytic activity cochromatographed with 1 of 10 peaks of proteolytic activity and was inhibited by bovine pancreatic trypsin inhibitor.

Schorlemmer and associates (1977) have hypothesized that a common factor in macrophage activation is activation of complement by the alternative pathway. This results in cleavage of C3 into a large fragment $C3_b$ and a small fragment $C3_a$. In addition, they presented evidence that attachment of $C3_b$ to the complement receptor on macrophages is a powerful stimulant of these cells, resulting in enzyme secretion (Schorlemmer and Allison, 1976) and acquisition of tumoricidal activity (Ferluga *et al.*, 1978). Although macrophages normally synthesize and release C3 intact, macrophages exposed to $C3_b$, endotoxin from Gram-negative bacteria, or polyanions, cleave the C3 into $C3_a$ and $C3_b$. The latter could produce serial stimulation of macrophages, whereas $C3_a$ is cytotoxic for a variety of normal and malignant cells (Ferluga *et al.*, 1976). However, this mechanism does not appear to account for the selective tumor cytotoxicity observed by many investigators.

Stadecker and co-workers (1977) showed that macrophages secrete thymidine continuously as part of an active synthetic process and suggested that this was due to a macrophage deficiency in thymidine kinase activity. They isolated an inhibitor of EL-4 leukemia DNA synthesis and cell proliferation from macrophage supernatants. Biochemically, the inhibitor appeared to be thymidine, judging from the migration in three different thin-layer systems and on gel filtration. The inhibitor was shown to be synthesized *de novo* by macrophages pulsed with a radiolabeled precursor of thymidine such as [^{14}C]formate. The amount of inhibitor present in tissue culture fluids proved to be sufficient to block the growth of the EL-4 leukemia cell line in a manner that could be prevented with the addition of 2′-deoxycitidine. However, the authors showed that the EL-4 line was exquisitely more sensitive to thymidine blockade than a number of other lines tested.

Currie (1978) suggested that activated macrophages kill tumor cells by releasing arginase. He showed that activation of macrophages by zymosan or LPS induces the production and release of arginase and that the cytotoxic activity of macrophages and of their supernatant media on the target cells is a consequence of arginine deprivation. This cytotoxic effect of mouse macrophage-conditioned media could be prevented by the addition of L-arginine or L-citrulline. Similarly, Kung and associates (1977) presented evidence that arginase may play a role in immunosuppression by activated macrophages. Currie and Basham (1978) demonstrated that complete arginine deprivation in cell culture media produced more rapid cytolysis of malignant cells than normal cells. They suggested that the biological basis for the selective effects of activated macrophages may reside in the L-arginine dependence of the target cells.

IV. Naturally Occurring Inhibitors of Cytotoxic Activity

The cytotoxic action of activated macrophages appears to be regulated by a number of inhibitory molecules in their local environment. Naturally occurring agents, such as a serum component of high molecular weight that is isolated with a low-density lipoprotein (Chapman and Hibbs, 1977), glucocorticoid hormones and their synthetic derivatives (Schultz *et al.*, 1979b), proteinases (Hibbs *et al.*, 1977), and agents leading to intracellular cyclic AMP accumulation (Schultz *et al.*, 1979c), have been shown to suppress macrophage cytotoxicity against tumor cells. Furthermore, Fidler (1977) demonstrated that macrophages from mice receiving hyperchlorinated drinking water have a depressed ability to respond to concanavalin A—MAF *in vitro*. Identification of these inhibitors has raised the possibility that host resistance against cancer may be enhanced by controlling their production and/or release in the microenvironment of the tumor.

A. Agents Which Increase Cellular Cyclic AMP

Agents known to increase intracellular levels of cyclic AMP in a variety of tissues have been shown to suppress several macrophage activities, including depressed monocyte locomotion (Gallin *et al.*, 1978), prevention of MIF-induced inhibition of macrophage migration (Koopman *et al.*, 1973), inhibition of proliferation of committed granulocyte—macrophage progenitor cells (Kurland *et al.*, 1977b), and prevention of interferon-induced macrophage cytotoxic activity (Schultz *et al.*, 1979c). Similarly, Droller and Remington (1975) showed that macrophages activated *in vivo* with the intracellular protozoan, Toxoplasma, had lower levels of adenyl cyclase activity than macrophages from uninfected, control mice. These studies point to a role for cyclic AMP in the negative regulation of macrophage function, although direct evidence for this conclusion awaits corroboration of levels of cyclic AMP in the macrophage with the observed effects of the agents utilized in each of these studies.

Schultz and associates (1978d, 1979a) showed that prostaglandins of the E-series require concentrations of $\geq 10^{-7}$ *M* to suppress tumor killing by interferon-activated macrophages *in vitro*. Inhibition was observed even when prostaglandin E_1 or E_2 was applied after the macrophages had reached full morphologic activation. Similarly, E-type prostaglandins (PGE) have been shown to suppress a number of other macrophage activities *in vitro* (Table I). In addition, Gemsa and co-workers (1978) demonstrated that the process of phagocytosis enhances sensitivity of the macrophage to PGE, along with a subsequent release of PGE, providing a sensitive control mechanism that may regulate macrophage function under physiological conditions. Although fibroblast-derived interferon does not in itself induce prostaglandin release by macrophages (Schultz *et al.*, 1979a), Yaron and associates (1977) showed that fibroblasts treated with interferon or interferon inducers produce E-type prostaglandins, indicating that local fibroblasts could serve a function in limiting interferon-induced macrophage function.

Schultz and co-workers (1979a) showed that ip PGE administration at doses ≥ 5 μg/mouse suppressed macrophage cytotoxic activity *in vivo* and suggested that PGE may play an important role in the pathogenesis of

TABLE I

SUMMARY OF EFFECTS OF PROSTAGLANDINS OF E-SERIES ON MACROPHAGE ACTIVITIES *in Vitro*

Source of cells	Cellular response	Reference
1. Human monocytes	Decreased random locomotion	Gallin *et al.* (1978)
2. Guinea pig peritoneal macrophage	Prevention of lymphokine-induced inhibition of macrophage migration	Koopman *et al.* (1973)
3. Guinea pig peritoneal macrophage	Inhibition of collagenase production	Wahl *et al.* (1977)
4. Mouse bone marrow	Inhibition of proliferation of committed granulocyte–macrophage progenitor cells	Kurland *et al.* (1978)
5. Mouse peritoneal macrophage	Inhibition of release of lysosomal hydrolases	Zurier *et al.* (1971)
6. Mouse peritoneal macrophage	Inhibition of plasminogen activator production	Vassalli *et al.* (1976)
7. Mouse peritoneal macrophage	Inhibition of interferon-induced tumoricidal activity	Schultz *et al.* (1978d, 1979a)

progressive tumor growth. A large number of experimental animal tumors and spontaneous human cancers have been shown to contain and/or produce high levels of PGE (Sykes and Maddox, 1972; Voelkel *et al.*, 1978), suggesting that tumor cells have acquired the capacity to defend themselves against macrophage surveillance (see Section IV,C).

Macrophages appear to synthesize prostaglandins efficiently (Murota *et al.*, 1978; Weidemann *et al.*, 1978; Bonney *et al.*, 1978), and the rate of incorporation of arachidonic acid into prostaglandins can be considerably enhanced during cellular activation (Kurland and Bockman, 1978; Schultz *et al.*, 1979a). Passwell and co-workers (1979) demonstrated increased (PGE) production by human monocytes after membrane receptor activation by Fc fragments of IgG or Con A. However, the contribution of PGE released by macrophages to the diverse functions of this cell remains to be fully elucidated. Although macrophage functions of PGE production and tumoricidal activity completely dissociate (Schultz *et al.*, 1979a; Shaw *et al.*, 1979), the ability of certain activating stimuli (e.g., endotoxic LPS) to induce PGE and interferon release from macrophages may form an intrinsic modulation system of negative and positive feedback control of cell function (Fig. 1). Both prostaglandins and interferons are characterized by a high catabolic rate and short biologic half-life in serum (Pike, 1971; Grossberg, 1972). Therefore, these mediators are mainly active locally, being produced by one cell and exerting their effects on the same cell or

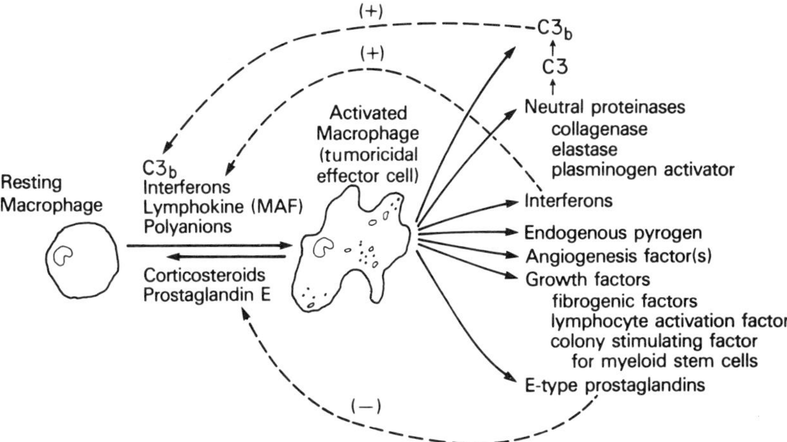

FIG. 1. Monokines released from activated macrophages and feedback mechanisms regulating the activated state. To balance and counteract continuing stimulation of macrophages following enhanced interferon and $C3_b$ production by activated macrophages, increased E-type prostaglandin secretion would serve to limit this positive feedback.

neighboring cells. Furthermore, the PGE-producing macrophage may have an important role as suppressor cell for lymphocyte mitogenic responses (Goodwin *et al.*, 1977).

Since PGE have been demonstrated to activate membrane adenylate cyclase and increase intracellular levels of cyclic AMP in macrophages (Gemsa *et al.*, 1975, 1978), Schultz and co-workers (1979c) tested a number of other agents known to increase cellular cyclic AMP levels. The β-adrenergic agent, isoproterenol, was without effect at all concentrations tested on activated macrophage function. This observation is similar to that of Kurland and associates (1977a), who showed that the proliferation of committed macrophage progenitor cells was not inhibited by β-adrenergic agonists and suggested that these cells lacked adrenergic receptors. In contrast, the inhibitory effect of cholera toxin on macrophage tumoricidal activity was profound, and it occurred at extremely low toxin concentrations (10^{-12} *M*).

B. CORTICOSTEROIDS

Glucocorticoids have been shown to suppress numerous macrophage functions; these include inhibition of plasminogen activator production (Vassalli *et al.*, 1976), inhibition of prostaglandin production (Bray and Gordon, 1976), decreased chemotaxis and random migration (Rinehart *et al.*, 1974), decreased bactericidal and fungicidal activity (Rinehart *et al.*,

1975), and inhibition of nonspecific tumoricidal activity (Hibbs, 1974b). Using established macrophage cell lines, Ralph and co-workers (1978) demonstrated that corticosteroids abrogated newly induced but not constitutive functions of macrophages, including myeloid colony-stimulating activity production, latex phagocytosis, and antibody-dependent lysis of red blood cell and tumor target cells. Furthermore, Werb and co-workers (1978) showed that monocytes and macrophages contain saturable glucocorticoid-binding proteins, with specificity of binding for cortisol, corticosterone, and related synthetic steroids such as dexamethasone, and that they have dissociation constants for binding within physiological ranges. Only glucocorticoids and progesterone competed for binding to the specific receptors.

Using macrophages activated by *Toxoplasma gondii* infection, Hibbs (1974b) demonstrated that their nonspecific tumoricidal activity was mediated by direct contact between the activated macrophage and the tumor target cell. Lysosomes from the activated macrophage were secreted directly into the cytoplasm of the tumor cell, which subsequently lysed. He suggested that hydrocortisone prevented exocytosis of macrophage lysosomal enzymes by stabilization of the macrophage cell membranes and observed that treatment of *T. gondii*-activated macrophages *in vitro* with hydrocortisone abrogated their expression of antitumor activity. Scott (1975) noted that the nonspecific antitumor activity of *Corynebacterium parvum*-activated mouse macrophages *in vitro* was inhibited by their prior treatment with cortisone acetate *in vivo*. Inhibition was marked (60%) 24 hours after cortisone injection and was still significant at 7 days. Dimitriu (1976) showed that corticosteroids do not prevent MAF production by sensitized lymphocytes, but they alter the capacity of normal macrophages to be activated upon exposure to MAF. Schultz and associates (1979b) demonstrated that corticosteroids and their synthetic derivatives administered *in vivo* or *in vitro* suppressed the cytotoxicity of interferon-activated macrophages. This effect of glucocorticosteroids is of particular interest, both because their relative antiinflammatory potencies correlated with their ability to inhibit macrophage function in culture and because this effect occurs at near physiological concentrations. Glucocorticoid activity did not appear to result from inhibition of enzyme release from macrophages, since soluble factors do not appear to be responsible for the cytotoxic effect of interferon-treated macrophages on their target cells (Schultz *et al.*, 1977a). Although the mechanism by which corticosteroids act on inhibiting macrophage cytotoxic activity is unknown, their activity may be mediated by either stabilization of macrophage membranes (Weissman and Thomas, 1963) or stimulation of cyclic AMP (Logsdon *et al.*, 1972).

Stress has previously been shown to impair interferon production (Solomon *et al.*, 1967) and suppress immunologic responsiveness (Amkraut and Solomon, 1975; Monjan and Collector, 1977). In addition, Schultz and co-workers (1979b) noted that acute stress of mice by physical restraint results in a decreased ability of macrophages to be activated by interferon treatment *in vivo* and *in vitro*. They postulated that corticosteroids were at least in part responsible for the inability of macrophages from stressed animals to respond to interferon, since acute stress is known to increase circulating glucocorticoid levels (Solomon *et al.*, 1967; Monjan and Collector, 1977).

C. Lipids and Tumor Products

Hibbs and associates (1977) showed that the tumoricidal potential of activated macrophages is not sharply delineated, but instead controlled by a threshold that is dependent on the net influences of antagonistic environmental chemical signals. An intrinsic macrophage cytotoxic effector system was described which was modulated by serum and other environmental factors that can enhance or suppress tumor killing. Chapman and Hibbs (1977) demonstrated that the tumoricidal capabilities of macrophages can be reversibly inhibited by a lipoprotein of high molecular weight, and that the inhibition appears to be reproduced by enrichment of macrophage plasma membranes with cholesterol. Since macrophages synthesize little or no cholesterol (Werb and Cohn, 1971), macrophage membrane cholesterol is subject to modulation by the microenvironmental determinants of cholesterol flux.

Numerous investigators have presented evidence that tumor products can influence macrophage activities. They may depress chemotactic responses (Snyderman and Pike, 1976; Stevenson and Meltzer, 1976; Snyderman *et al.*, 1978; Kjeldsberg and Pay, 1978; Normann, 1978), inhibit phagocytosis (Gudewicz and Saba, 1977; Ramarao and Tompkins, 1978), decrease expression of Fc receptors (Rhodes *et al.*, 1979), and decrease spreading and attachment to substratum (Cantarow *et al.*, 1978).

Snyderman and Pike (1976) demonstrated that the implantation of syngeneic neoplasms in mice depresses the animal's ability to localize macrophages at inflammatory sites. They identified a low-molecular-weight (6000 to 10,000) factor released by growing tumors that inhibits the accumulation of macrophages *in vivo* and chemotactic responsiveness *in vitro*. They suggested that "neoplastic cells may abrogate immunosurveillance by releasing products that prevent potentially tumoricidal macrophages from accumulating at sites of deveoping malignancies." Stevenson and Meltzer (1976) similarly showed that the *in vitro* chemotactic responses of peritoneal macrophages from mice bearing transplantable syngeneic 3-

methylcholanthrene-induced tumors in their footpads were depressed to about 50% of normal levels. The chemotactic defect to both lymphocyte- and complement-derived stimuli was evident before the appearance of palpable tumor and persisted until the death of the animal by 6–8 weeks. Normann (1978) noted that in DBA/2 mice bearing transplanted, syngeneic P815 mastocytoma, the macrophage accumulation was impaired when the cancer grew intraperitoneally. He determined that $4-16 \times 10^6$ mastocytoma cells were required to inhibit monocyte responsiveness to proteose peptone. Impairment of monocyte inflammation could be passively transferred with ascitic fluid. Normann and co-workers later (1979) found that the tumor-induced antiinflammatory effect directed against macrophages was promptly corrected by tumor excision but recurred with metastasis.

The chemotactic responsiveness of peripheral blood monocytes was also measured in patients with malignant solid tumors (Snyderman *et al.*, 1978; Kjeldsberg and Pay, 1978). Snyderman and co-workers (1978) found that monocyte chemotactic responsiveness was normal in patients with benign breast masses and those previously having breast cancer resected and remaining clinically free of disease. In contrast, monocytes of patients with active breast cancer were depressed in their chemotactic responsiveness, which could be corrected by surgical removal of tumor. Kjeldsberg and Pay (1978) showed that the monocyte chemotaxis was defective in 45% of patients with cancers of the lung and prostate. Serum chemotactic factor inactivator(s) that inhibit chemotaxis of normal monocytes were detected in 90% of the patients.

V. Therapeutic Considerations

Several factors have been identified that affect the tumoricidal activity of activated macrophages (Table II). These factors influence both the macrophage concentration as well as the functional state of macrophages in and around the tumor site. The latter appears to be largely dependent on the balance between opposing chemical signals which determine the extent of macrophage activation in the microenvironment of the tumor. However, the macrophage functional state is also dependent on the degree of maturity of macrophages responding to the tumor and genetic factors which determine the responsiveness to activating stimuli.

A. Macrophage Tumor Content

The macrophage content of tumors appears to be closely associated with therapeutic efficacy of agents that enhance nonspecific host resist-

TABLE II

Some Possible Factors Affecting Macrophage Surveillance in the Microenvironment of the Tumor

Factor	Reference
Density of macrophages within tumor	
1. Macrophage tumor content directly proportional to immunogenicity of tumor	Eccles and Alexander (1974)
2. Certain tumors produce soluble factors that interfere with macrophage chemotaxis	Pike and Snyderman (1976)
Macrophage functional state within tumor	
1. Activation signals need to be present in tumor microenvironment, although activating agents tend to remain in the anatomical compartment into which they were injected	Hibbs (1976b)
2. Newly formed blood-derived monocyte more responsive to activating stimuli than more mature resident macrophage	Ruco and Meltzer (1978a); Poste and Kirsh (1979)
3. Several microenvironmental chemical signals including E-type prostaglandins, corticosteroids, proteinases, and high-density lipoproteins can suppress activated macrophage tumor killing	Schultz *et al.* (1979a,b); Hibbs *et al.* (1977)
4. Genetic factors control macrophage responsiveness to lymphokine and nonimmunologic-derived stimuli that activate macrophages	Boraschi and Meltzer (1979)

ance to neoplasia [e.g., BCG (Hanna *et al.*, 1973), glucan (Mansell *et al.*, 1975), and pyran copolymer (Schultz *et al.*, 1977c,d)]. Evans (1972) described a method whereby the macrophage content of syngeneic mouse and rat fibrosarcomas can be estimated by trypsinization of minced tumor fragments. He demonstrated that necrotic tumors do not show a higher level of macrophages than healthy tumors, suggesting that the ingestion of dead cells itself is not an adequate explanation for the macrophage infiltration. Using a series of six different rat sarcomas grown in normal syngeneic recipients, Eccles and Alexander (1974) showed that the macrophage tumor content is inversely related to the rate of spontaneous metastasis. Similarly, Wood and Gillespie (1975) showed that tumor cell suspensions from murine chemically induced fibrosarcomas depleted of macrophages by adherence to plastic injected into normal syngeneic mice develop an increased potential for metastasis. By contrast, control animals that received tumor cell suspensions containing their normal complement of macrophages invariably developed progressive localized tumors. Russell and McIntosh (1977) demonstrated that macrophages isolated from regressing Moloney sarcomas are more cytotoxic than those recovered from progressing sarcomas. Several other investigators have shown that macrophages harvested directly from tumor tissue are cytotoxic for tumor cells *in vitro* (Evans, 1973; Mantovani, 1978; Stewart and Beetham, 1978). Moreover, Keller (1976a) showed promotion of tumor growth *in vivo* by antimacrophage agents including silica and carrageenan. These studies collectively argue that the tumor-associated macrophage may modulate tumor growth and metastasis.

Since macrophage-mediated tumor destruction results predominantly from a nonphagocytic contact-mediated event (see Section III,A), successful therapy is dependent on achieving adequate cell density at the tumor site. The hypothesis that macrophages enter the tumor as part of a specific reaction of the host directed against tumor-specific antigens is supported by the observations that the macrophage content of tumors is directly related to the immunogenicity of the sarcoma used (Eccles and Alexander, 1974). However, tumors themselves may produce soluble factors that interfere with effective macrophage mobilization (Pike and Snyderman, 1976). The adoptive transfer of macrophages has been shown to be of therapeutic value in a number of studies. Fidler (1974) showed that the intravenous injection of specifically activated macrophages inhibited pulmonary metastasis. Piessens (1978a) showed that macrophages activated *in vitro* with lymphocyte mediators inhibited local tumor growth *in vivo*. Schultz and co-workers (1976) demonstrated that macrophages from tumor allograft-bearing mice were specifically cytotoxic (armed) for the appropriate target cells, and that activating agents acted synergistically to augment specific macrophage cytolysis of tumor cells. Schultz and associates later (1978g) demonstrated that these armed-activated macrophages can eradicate cancer in the syngeneic host. "Cures" required the synergistic interaction between allograft immunity and nonspecific macrophage activation. Neither tumor-immune nor activated macrophages produced long-term survivors. The tumor-suppressive action of armed-activated macrophages required close contact with tumor cells.

B. Macrophage Functional State within Tumor

Many of the current efforts at immunotherapy of neoplasia employ nonspecific agents such as BCG, *Corynebacterium parvum*, glucan, etc., which presumably act in part by induction of nonspecifically tumoricidal macrophages. The greatest clinical success has been achieved when these adjuvants were injected directly into the tumor lesion, allowing for both mobilization of macrophages to the tumor site and subsequent activation in intimate contact with tumor. Similarly, Hibbs (1977b) has shown that the presence of cytotoxic activated macrophages in the tissue tends to be a local phenomenon, confined to the anatomical compartment(s) that contain high levels of inducing antigen. The continuing presence of activated macrophages requires that the specific antigen, e.g., BCG or toxoplasma, which induced the production of cytotoxic macrophages remains in the tissue and provides a continuing stimulus for elaboration of a chemical signal that maintains macrophage activation.

There appears to be a strong need for understanding the immunopharmacology of these nonspecific macrophage stimulants to improve on the clinical effects conferred by empirical therapy of this type. This is especially the case since a number of conflicting stimuli have been demonstrated which abrogate the ability of agents to induce tumoricidal macrophages (see Section IV). Sufficient quantities of these opposing factors in the microenvironment of the tumor may severely compromise adjuvant-induced host resistance against neoplasms. The ability to control local production of agents that negate macrophage chemotaxis and functional activity may allow for improved immunotherapy of cancer.

The maintenance of macrophage tumoricidal activity also appears to require a continuous influx of new peroxidase-positive macrophages from the circulation. Poste and Kirsh (1979) examined the ability of inflammatory tissue macrophages harvested on glass converslips implanted in the sc tissue of C57B1/6 mice to kill tumor cells *in vitro*. Macrophages present on coverslips implanted for less than 4 days were devoid of spontaneous tumoricidal activity but could be rendered cytotoxic for syngeneic and allogeneic tumor cells *in vitro* with lymphokines released by mitogen-stimulated lymphocytes. Inflammatory macrophages on coverslips implanted for 4 to 7 days showed significant spontaneous cytotoxicity for tumor cells *in vitro*, and their tumoricidal activity could be further increased by additional incubation *in vitro* with lymphokines. With progression, the inflammatory macrophages harvested on coverslips implanted for longer than 7 days lacked spontaneous cytotoxic activity and were also resistant to activation by lymphokines *in vitro*. These alterations in tumoricidal activity and responsiveness to lymphokines were accompanied by a marked reduction in the number of peroxidase-positive macrophages within the population. However, macrophages refractory to reactivation by lymphokines in the extracellular environment could be reactivated by treatment *in vitro* with liposomes containing encapsulated lymphokines. Decay of tumoricidal activity and onset of resistance to activation by lymphokines was not peculiar to inflammatory macrophages isolated from sc lesions, since similar results were obtained by Ruco and Meltzer (1978a) in activated peritoneal macrophage populations.

Borashi and Meltzer (1979) attempted to compare 22 different mouse strains for development of activated tumoricidal macrophages following

BCG infection *in vivo* or lymphokine treatment *in vitro*. Peritoneal macrophages from 8 of 22 strains failed to develop tumoricidal capacity by 7 days after intraperitoneal BCG infection. Macrophages from 6 of 6 *in vivo* nonresponder strains failed to develop tumoricidal capacity after *in vitro* treatment with lymphokines. However, the exact mechanisms for genetic control of macrophage responsiveness remain poorly understood. Development of activated tumoricidal macrophages did not correlate with LPS responsiveness among the strains tested. We have recently found that macrophages from LPS-unresponsive C3H/HeJ mice show a depressed ability to be activated by a number of agents *in vivo* when compared to the LPS-responsive strain C3H/HeN (Fig. 2).

A final consideration may be the compatibility of macrophage-activating agents with more traditional treatment modalities for cancer. Cytostatic drugs including cyclophosphamide (Schultz *et al.*, 1978h) and anthracycline antibiotics (Mantovani, 1977) have been shown to interfere with macrophage activation by biologic agents. A better knowledge of the interaction of chemotherapeutic and/or radiation regimens with adjuvants which affect macrophage function may be instrumental to rationalized immunotherapy protocols.

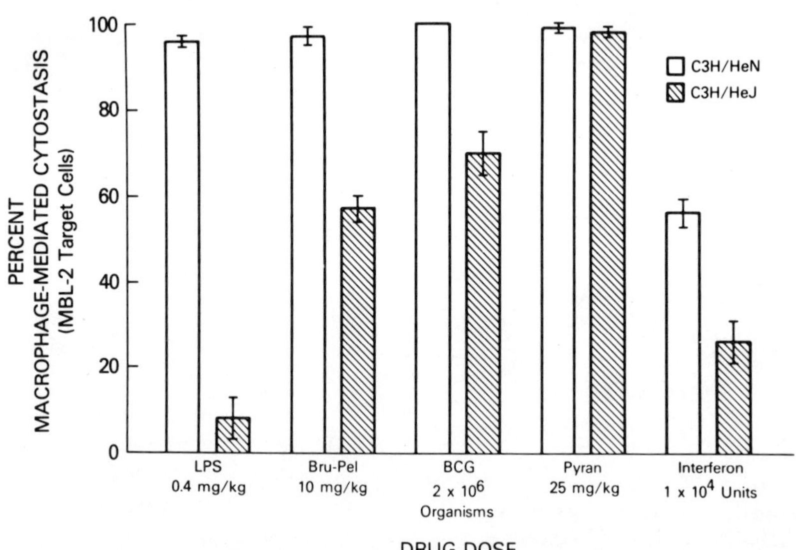

FIG. 2. Comparison of various adjuvants for ability to induce cytotoxic macrophages *in vivo* in C3H/HeN and C3H/HeJ mice. Adjuvants were administered ip at the doses given. Resident peritoneal macrophages were harvested 6 days later and reacted against MBL-2 leukemia target cells. Bars represent mean ± SE obtained from triplicate determinations.

VI. Concluding Remarks

The activated macrophage appears to be ideally suited as a primary antineoplastic surveillance cell. Although the activated macrophage tumoricidal reaction is nonspecific, an elemental sort of discrimination exists in that nonneoplastic target cells are spared. This nonimmunologic recognition of tumor cells appears to involve basic membrane alterations that parallel neoplastic transformation. The activated macrophage tumoricidal reaction may have a primitive phytogenetic origin, since macrophages are activated by cytokines, bacterial products, or polyanions in the complete absence of lymphocytes and immunoglobulins. Macrophages are widely distributed in tissues, and the macrophage plasma membrane is a highly sophisticated sensory organelle capable of detecting subtle changes in its environment.

To date, biochemical marker(s) of the macrophage tumoricidal state have not been convincingly demonstrated. However, measurement of serum lysozyme has been suggested to be a reliable indicator of *in vivo* macrophage function and therapeutic efficacy of immunoadjuvants (Currie, 1976; Schrecker *et al.*, 1979). In addition, Kaplan and Mohanakumar (1977) have presented evidence that a new cell surface antigen present on activated macrophages can differentiate these cells from their normal or stimulated counterparts.

In this article we attempt to summarize what is known about inducers of activated macrophage function. We show that the activated macrophage tumoricidal reaction is not a highly determined event, but rather a relative potential that is regulated by a balance between opposing environmental chemical signals. Thus, tumor cell killing is critically dependent on the local environment in which the macrophages and tumor cells coexist.

References

Adams, D. O. (1978). *J. Reticuloendothel. Soc.* **24,** 21a.

Adams, D. O., Biesecker, J. L., and Koss, L. G. (1973). *J. Reticuloendothel. Soc.* **14,** 550–570.

Alexander, P., and Evans, R. (1971). *Nature (London) New Biol.* **232,** 76–78.

Amkraut, A., and Solomon, G. F. (1975). *Int. J. Psychiat. Med.* **5,** 541–563.

Anderson, S. E., Bautista, S., and Remington, J. S. (1976). *J. Immunol.* **177,** 381–387.

Ansevin, A. T., MacDonald, K. K., Smith, C. E., and Hnilica, L. S. (1975). *J. Biol. Chem.* **250,** 281–289.

Babiuk, L. A., and Rouse, B. T. (1976). *Infect. Immun.* **13,** 1567–1578.

Blanden, R. V., and Mims, C. A. (1973). *AJEBAK* **51,** 393–398.

Bomford, R., and Moreno, C. (1977). *Br. J. Cancer* **36,** 41–48.

Bonney, R. J., Wightman, P. D., Davies, P., Sadowski, S. J., Kueh, F. A., and Humes, J. L. (1978). *Biochem. J.* **176,** 433–442.

Boraschi, D., and Meltzer, M. S. (1979). *Cell. Immunol.* **45,** 188–194.
Bray, M. A., and Gordon, D. (1976). *Br. J. Pharmacol.* **52,** 466P–467P.
Bruley-Rosset, M., Florentin, I., and Mathe, G. (1976). *Agents Action* **6,** 251–255.
Bucana, C., Hoyer, L. C., Hobbs, B., Breesman, S., McDaniel, M., and Hanna, M. G. (1976). *Cancer Res.* **36,** 4444–4458.
Burnet, F. M. (1970). *Prog. Exp. Tumor Res.* **13,** 1–34.
Cantarow, W. D., Cheung, H. T., and Sundharadas, G. (1978). *J. Reticuloendothel. Soc.* **24,** 657–666.
Chapes, S. K., and Tompkins, W. A. F. (1978). *J. Reticuloendothel. Soc.* **24,** 47a.
Chapman, H. A., and Hibbs, J. B. (1977). *Science* **197,** 282–285.
Cheers, C., and Waller, R. (1975). *J. Immunol.* **115,** 844–847.
Christie, G. H., and Bomford, R. (1975). *Cell. Immunol.* **17,** 141–149.
Churchill, W. H., Piessens, W. F., Sulis, C. A., and David, J. R. (1975). *J. Immunol.* **115,** 781–786.
Cline, M. J., Rothman, B., and Golde, D. W. (1974). *J. Cell. Physiol.* **84,** 193–196.
Cullen, R. T., and Ghaffar, A. (1978). *J. Reticuloendothel. Soc.* **24,** 339–349.
Currie, G. A. (1976). *Br. J. Cancer* **33,** 593–599.
Currie, G. A. (1978). *Nature* (*London*) **273,** 758–759.
Currie, C. A., and Basham, C. (1978). *Br. J. Cancer* **38,** 653–659.
David, J. R., and Remold, H. G. (1976). *In* "Immunobiology of the Macrophage" (D. S. Nelson, ed.), pp. 401–426. Academic Press, New York.
DiLuzio, N. R., Pisano, J. C., and Saba, T. M. (1970). *J. Reticuloendothel. Soc.* **7,** 731–742.
Dimitriu, A. (1976). *Cell. Immunol.* **21,** 79–87.
Donahoe, R. M., and Huang, K.-Y. (1973). *Infect. Immun.* **7,** 501–503.
Donahoe, R. M., and Huang, K.-Y. (1976). *Infect. Immun.* **13,** 1250–1257.
Droller, M. J., and Remington, J. S. (1975). *Cell. Immunol.* **19,** 349–355.
Dy, M., Dimitriu, A., Gougerot, M. A., and Hamburger, J. (1976). *J. Reticuloendothel. Soc.* **20,** 93–102.
Eccles, S. A., and Alexander, P. (1974). *Nature* (*London*) **250,** 667–669.
Elinov, H. P., Vitovskaya, G. A., Aksencv, O. A., Ageeva, O. N., and Agmaeva, A. E. (1972). *Biokhimiya* **37,** 590–593.
Epstein, L. B. (1976). *In* "Immunobiology of the Macrophage" (D. S. Nelson, ed.), pp. 201–234. Academic Press, New York.
Evans, R. (1972). *Transplantation* **14,** 468–473.
Evans, R. (1973). *Br. J. Cancer* **28,** Suppl. I, 19–25.
Evans, R. (1974). *In* "Modulation of Host Immune Resistance in the Prevention or Treatment of Induced Neoplasias" (M. A. Chirigos, ed.), pp. 295–301. U.S. Gov. Printing Office, Washington, D.C.
Evans, R., and Alexander, P. (1972). *Nature* (*London*) *New Biol.* **236,** 168–170.
Evans, R., and Alexander, P. (1976). *In* "Immunobiology of the Macrophage" (D. S. Nelson, ed.), pp. 535–576. Academic Press, New York.
Evans, R., Cox, H., and Alexander, P. (1973). *Proc. Soc. Exp. Biol. Med.* **143,** 256–259.
Feingold, D. S., Keleti, G., and Youngner, J. S. (1976). *Infect. Immun.* **13,** 763–767.
Ferluga, J., Schorlemmer, H. U., Baptista,, L. C., and Allison, A. C. (1976). *Br. J. Cancer* **34,** 626–634.
Ferluga, J., Schorlemmer, H. U., Baptista, L. C., and Allison, A. C. (1978). *Clin. Exp. Immunol.* **31,** 512–517.
Fidler, I. J. (1974). *Cancer Res.* **34,** 1074–1077.
Fidler, I. J. (1975). *J. Natl. Cancer Inst.* **55,** 1159–1163.
Fidler, I. J. (1977). *Nature* (*London*) **270,** 735–736.
Fidler, I. J., Darnell, J. H., and Budmen, M. B. (1976a). *Cancer Res.* **36,** 3608–3615.

Fidler, I. J., Darnell, J. H., and Budmen, M. B. (1976b). *J. Immunol.* **177**, 666–673.
Fidler, I. J., Roblin, R. O., and Poste, G. (1978). *Cell. Immunol.* **38**, 131–146.
Finkelstein, M. S., Bausek, G. H., and Merigan, T. C. (1968). *Science* **161**, 465–468.
Flanagan, T. D., Yoshida, T., and Cohen, S. (1973). *Infect. Immun.* **8**, 145–150.
Fowles, R. E., Fajardo, I. M., Leibowitch, J. L., and David, J. R. (1973). *J. Exp. Med.* **138**, 952–964.
Gallin, J. I., Sandler, J. A., Clyman, R. I., Manganiello, V. C., and Vaughan, M. (1978). *J. Immunol.* **120**, 492–496.
Gemsa, D., Steggemann, L., Menzel, J., and Till, G. (1975). *J. Immunol.* **114**, 1422–1424.
Gemsa, D., Seitz, M., Kramer, W., Till, G., and Resch, K. (1978). *J. Immunol.* **120**, 1187–1194.
Goldberg, M. L. (1975). *Life Sci.* **17**, 1747–1754.
Goodwin, J. S., Messner, R. P., Bankhurst, A. D., Peake, G. T., Saiki, J. H., and Williams, R. C. (1977). *N. Engl. J. Med.* **297**, 963–968.
Grossberg, S. E. (1972). *N. Engl. J. Med.* **287**, 13–19.
Gudewicz, P. W., and Saba, T. M. (1977). *Br. J. Cancer* **36**, 670–677.
Hadden, J. W. (1978). *Cancer Treat. Rep.* **62**, 1981–1986.
Hanna, M. G., Snodgrass, M. J., Zbar, B., and Rapp. H. J. (1973). *Natl. Cancer Inst. Monogr.* **39**, 71–84.
Harmel, R. P., and Zbar, B. (1975). *J. Natl. Cancer Inst.* **54**, 989–992.
Hibbs, J. B. (1973). *Science* **180**, 868–870.
Hibbs, J. B. (1974a). *J. Natl. Cancer Inst.* **53**, 1487–1492.
Hibbs, J. B. (1974b). *Science* **184**, 468–471.
Hibbs, J. B. (1976a). *J. Reticuloendothel. Soc.* **20**, 223–231.
Hibbs, J. B. (1976b). *In* "The Macrophage in Neoplasia" (M. A. Fink, ed.), pp. 83–111. Academic Press, New York.
Hibbs, J. B., Lambert, L. H., and Remington, J. S. (1971). *J. Infect. Dis* **124**, 587–592.
Hibbs, J. B., Lambert, L. H., and Remington, J. S. (1972a). *Nature (London) New Biol.* **235**, 48–50.
Hibbs, J. B., Lambert, L. H., and Remington, J. S. (1972b). *Science* **177**, 998–1000.
Hibbs, J. B., Taintor, R. R., Chapman, H. A., and Weinberg, J. B. (1977). *Science* **197**, 279–282.
Hirsch, M. S., Black, P. H., Wood, M. L., and Monaco, A. P. (1972). *J. Immunol.* **108**, 1312–1318.
Ho, M., Armstrong, J. A., and Breinig, M. C. (1975). *Annu. Rev. Microbiol.* **29**, 131–161.
Holtermann, O. A., Klein, E., and Casale, G. P. (1973). *Cell. Immunol.* **9**, 339–352.
Huang, K.-Y., Donahoe, R. M., Gordon, F. B., and Dressler, H. R. (1971). *Infect. Immun.* **4**, 581–588.
Ibrahim, A. L., Zee, Y. C., and Osebold, J. W. (1976). *Proc. Soc. Exp. Biol. Med.* **152**, 483–488.
Imanishi, J., Yokota, Y., Kishida, T., Mukainanka, T., and Matsuo, A. (1975). *Acta Virol.* **19**, 52–58.
Inoue, M., Mori, M., Utsumi, K., and Seno, S. (1972). *Gann* **63**, 795–799.
Jacobsen, C. (1934). *Arch. Dermatol. Syph.* **169**, 562–576.
Jolles, P. (1976). *Biomedicine* **25**, 275–276.
Juy, D., and Chedid, L. (1975). *Proc. Natl. Acad. Sci. U.S.A.* **72**, 4105–4109.
Kaplan, A. M., and Mohanakumar, T. (1977). *J. Exp. Med.* **146**, 1461–1466.
Kaplan, A. M., Morahan, P. S., and Regelson, W. (1974). *J. Natl. Cancer Inst.* **52**, 1919–1921.
Kaplan, A. M., Baird, L. G., and Morahan, P. S. (1977). *In* "Control of Neoplasia by Modulation of the Immune System" (M. A. Chirigos, ed.), pp. 461–474. Raven, New York.

Keller, R. (1974). *Br. J. Cancer* **30,** 401–415.
Keller, R. (1976a). *J. Natl. Cancer Inst.* **57,** 1355–1361.
Keller, R. (1976b). *In* "Immunobiology of the Macrophage" (D. S. Nelson, ed.), pp. 487–508. Academic Press, New York.
Keller, R. (1977). *J. Natl. Cancer Inst.* **59,** 1751–1753.
Kelly, M. T. (1978). *J. Reticuloendothel. Soc.* **24,** 139–145.
Kjeldsberg, C. R., and Pay, G. D. (1978). *Cancer* **41,** 2236–2241.
Koopman, W. J., Gillis, M. H., and David, J. R. (1973). *J. Immunol.* **110,** 1609–1614.
Krahenbuhl, L., and Remington, J. S. (1974). *J. Immunol.* **113,** 507–516.
Kripke, M. L., Budmen, M. B., and Fidler, I. J. (1977). *Cell. Immunol.* **30,** 341–352.
Kung, J. T., Brooks, S. B., Jakway, J. P., Leonard, L. L., and Talmage, D. W. (1977). *J. Exp. Med.* **146,** 665–672.
Kurland J. I., and Bockman, R. (1978). *J. Exp. Med.* **147,** 952–957.
Kurland, J. I., Hadden, J. W., and Moore, M. A. S. (1977a). *Cancer Res.* **37,** 4534–4539.
Kurland, J. I., Kincade, P. W., and Moore, M. A. S. (1977b). *J. Exp. Med.* **146,** 1420–1435.
Kurland, J. I., Bockman, R. S., Broxmeyer, H. E., and Moore, M. A. S. (1978). *Science* **199,** 552–555.
Lackovic, V., Borecky, L., Sike, D., Masler, L., and Bauer, S. (1970). *Proc. Soc. Exp. Biol. Med.* **134,** 874–879.
Leonard, E. J., Ruco, L. P., and Meltzer, M. S. (1978). *Cell. Immunol.* **41,** 347–357.
Levy, M. H., and Wheelock, E. F. (1974). *Adv. Cancer Res.* **20,** 131–163.
Logsdon, P. J., Middleton, E., and Coffey, R. G. (1972). *J. Allergy Clin. Immunol.* **50,** 45–56.
Lohmann-Matthes, M.-L. (1976). *In* "Immunobiology of the Macrophage" (D. S. Nelson, ed.), pp. 463–486. Academic Press, New York.
Lunde, M. N., and Gerlderman, A. H. (1971). *J. Natl. Cancer Inst.* **47,** 485–488.
Lurie, M. B. (1964). *In* "Resistance to Tuberculosis: Experimental Studies in Native and Acquired Defensive Mechanisms." Harvard Univ. Press, Cambridge, Massachusetts.
Mackaness, G. B. (1964). *J. Exp. Med.* **120,** 105–114.
Mackaness, G. B. (1969). *J. Exp. Med.* **129,** 973–992.
Maehara, N., and Ho, M. (1977). *Infect. Immun.* **15,** 78–83.
Majeski, J. A., and Stinnett, J. D. (1977). *J. Natl. Cancer Inst.* **58,** 781–783.
Manejias, R. E., Hamburg, S. I., and Rabinovitch, M. (1978). *Cell. Immunol.* **38,** 209–213.
Mansell, P. W. A., and DiLuzio, N. R. (1976). *In* "The Macrophage in Neoplasia" (M. A. Fink, ed.), pp. 227–243. Academic Press, New York.
Mansell, P. W. A., Ichinose, H., Reed, R. J., Krementz, E. T., McNamee, R., and DiLuzio, N. R. (1975). *J. Natl. Cancer Inst.* **54,** 571–580.
Mansell, P. W. A., DiLuzio, N. R., McNamee, R., Rowden, G., and Proctor, J. W. (1976). *Ann. N. Y. Acad. Sci.* **277,** 20–44.
Mantovani, A. (1977). *Cancer Res.* **37,** 815–820.
Mantovani, A. (1978). *Int. J. Cancer* **22,** 741–746.
Meade, C. J., Lechmann, P. J., and Brenner, S. (1974). *Immunology* **27,** 227–239.
Meltzer, M. S. (1976). *Cell. Immunol.* **22,** 176–181.
Meltzer, M. S., and Bartlett, G. L. (1972). *J. Natl. Cancer Inst.* **49,** 1439–1443.
Meltzer, M. S., Tucker, R. W., and Breuer, A. C. (1975a). *Cell. Immunol.* **17,** 30–42.
Meltzer, M. S., Tucker, R. W., Sanford, K. K., and Leonard, E. J. (1975b). *J. Natl. Cancer Inst.* **54,** 1177–1184.
Meltzer, M. S., Stevenson, M., Tucker, R. W., and Leonard, E. J. (1976). *In* "The Macrophage in Neoplasia" (M. A. Fink, ed.), pp. 211–226. Academic Press, New York.
Metchnikoff, E. (1905). *In* "Immunity in Infection Diseases" (F. G. Binnie, transl.). Cambridge Univ. Press, London and New York.

Mogensen, S. C., and Andersen, H. K. (1978). *Infect. Immun.* **19,** 792–798.
Mohr, S. J., Massicot, J. G., and Chirigos, M. A. (1978). *Cancer Res.* **38,** 1610–1616.
Monjan, A. A., and Collector, M. I. (1977). *Science* **196,** 307–309.
Morahan, P. S., and Kaplan, A. M. (1976). *Int. J. Cancer* **17,** 82–89.
Murota, S., Kawamura, M., and Morita, I. (1978). *Biochim. Biophys. Acta* **528,** 507–511.
Nabarra, B., Cavelier, J. F., Dy, M., and Dimitriu, A. (1978). *J. Reticuloendothel. Soc.* **24,** 489–498.
Nathan, C. F., Karnovsky, M. L., and David, J. R. (1971). *J. Exp. Med.* **133,** 1356–1376.
Nauciel, C., and Goguel, A. F. (1977). *J. Natl. Cancer Inst.* **59,** 1723–1726.
Nauts, H. C., Fowler, G. A., and Bogatko, F. H. (1953). *Acta Med. Scand.* **45,** Suppl., 276.
Neumann, C., and Sorg, C., (1978). *Z. Immunitaetsforsch.* **155,** 48–49.
Normann, S. J. (1978). *J. Natl. Cancer Inst.* **60,** 1091–1096.
Normann, S. J., Schardt, M., and Sorkin, E. (1979). *Int. J. Cancer* **23,** 110–113.
Pantalone, R., and Page, R. C. (1975). *Proc. Natl. Acad. Sci. U.S.A.* **72,** 2091–2094.
Pantalone, R., and Page, R. C. (1977). *J. Reticuloendothel. Soc.* **21,** 343–357.
Papamatheakis, J. D., Schultz, R. M., Chirigos, M. A., and Massicot, J. G. (1978) *Cancer Treat. Rep.* **62,** 1845–1851.
Parr, I., Wheeler, E., and Alexander, P. (1973). *Br. J. Cancer* **27,** 370–389.
Passwell, J. H., Dayer, J.-M., and Merler, E. (1979). *J. Immunol.* **123,** 115–120.
Pfizenmaier, K., Trostmann, H., Rollinghoff, M., and Wagner, H. (1975). *Immunology* **29,** 967–976.
Piessens, W. F. (1977). *J. Immunol.* **119,** 167–172.
Piessens, W. F. (1978a). *Fed. Proc.* **26,** 440A.
Piessens, W. F. (1978b). *Cell. Immunol.* **35,** 303–317.
Piessens, W. F., Churchill, W. H., and David, J. R. (1975). *J. Immunol.* **114,** 293–299.
Pike, J. E. (1971). *Sci. Am.* **225** (Nov.), 84–94.
Pike, M. C., and Snyderman, R. (1976). *J. Immunol.* **117,** 1243–1249.
Poste, G., and Kirsh, R. (1979). (1979). *Cancer Res.* **39,** 2582–2590.
Puccetti, P., and Holden, H. T. (1979). *Int. J. Cancer* **23,** 123–133.
Rabinovitch, M., Manejias, R. E., Russo, M., and Abbey, E. E. (1977). *Cell. Immunol.* **29,** 86–95.
Ralph, P., Broxmeyer, H. E., and Nakoinz, I. (1977). *J. Exp. Med.* **146,** 611–616.
Ralph, P., Ito, M., Broxmeyer, H. E., and Makoinz, I. (1978). *J. Immunol.* **121,** 300–303.
Ramarao, G. V. S. V., and Tompkins, W. A. F. (1978). *J. Reticuloendothel. Soc.* **23,** 373–382.
Ramarao, G., Rawls, W. E., Perey, D. Y. E., and Tompkins, W. A. F. (1977). *J. Reticuloendothel. Soc.* **21,** 13–20.
Rhodes, J., Bishop, M., and Benfield, J. (1979). *Science* **203,** 179–182.
Rietschel, E. T., Gottert, H., Luderitz, O., and Westphal, O. (1972). *Eur. J. Biochem.* **28,** 166–173.
Riisgaard, S., Rhodes, J. M., and Bennedsen, J. (1978). *Scand. J. Immunol.* **7,** 209–213.
Rinehart, J. J., Balcerzak, S. P., Sagone, A. L., and LoBuglio, A. F. (1974). *J. Clin. Invest.* **54,** 1337–1343.
Rinehart, J. J., Sagone, A. L., Balcerzak, S. P., Ackerman, G. A., and LoBuglio, A. F. (1975). *N. Engl. J. Med.* **292,** 236–241.
Rodda, S. J., and White, D. O. (1976). *J. Immunol.* **117,** 2067–2072.
Rosenstreich, D. L., Farrar, J. J., and Dougherty, S. (1976). *J. Immunol.* **116,** 131–139.
Ruco, L. P., and Meltzer, M. S. (1978a). *J. Immunol.* **120,** 1054–1062.
Ruco, L. P., and Meltzer, M. S. (1978b). *Cell. Immunol.* **41,** 35–51.
Ruco, L. P., Meltzer, M. S., and Rosenstreich, D. L. (1978). *J. Immunol.* **121,** 543–548.
Ruscetti, F. W., and Chervenik, P. A. (1974). *J. Lab. Clin. Med.* **83,** 64–72.

Ruskin, J., McIntosh, M., and Remington, J. S. (1969). *J. Immunol.* **103,** 252–259.
Russell, S. W., and McIntosh, A. T. (1977). *Nature (London)* **268,** 69–71.
Rygaard, J., and Paulsen, C. O. (1974). *Acta Pathol. Microbiol. Scand.* **82,** 92–106.
Schorlemmer, H. U., and Allison, A. C. (1976). *Immunology* **31,** 781–788.
Schorlemmer, H. U., Bitter-Suermann, D., and Allison, A. C. (1977). *Immunology* **32,** 929–940.
Schrecker, A. W., Schultz, R. M., and Chirigos, M. A. (1979). *J. Immunopharmacol.* **1,** 219–231.
Schultz, R. M., and Chirigos, M. A. (1978). *Cancer Res.* **38,** 1003–1007.
Schultz, R. M., and Chirigos, M. A. (1979). *Cell. Immunol.* **48,** 52–58.
Schultz, R. M., Papamatheakis, J. D., Stylos, W. A., and Chirigos, M. A. (1976). *Cell. Immunol.* **25,** 309–316.
Schultz, R. M., Papamatheakis, J. D., and Chirigos, M. A. (1977a). *Science* **197,** 674–676.
Schultz, R. M., Papamatheakis, J. D., and Chirigos, M. A. (1977b). *Cell. Immunol.* **29,** 403–409.
Schultz, R. M., Papamatheakis, J. D., Luetzeler, J., and Chirigos, M. A. (1977c). *Cancer Res.* **37,** 3338–3343.
Schultz, R. M., Papamatheakis, J. D., Luetzeler, J., Ruiz, P., and Chirigos, M. A. (1977d). *Cancer Res.* **37,** 358–364.
Schultz, R. M., Chirigos, M. A., and Heine, U. I. (1978a). *Cell. Immunol.* **35,** 84–91.
Schultz, R. M., Papamatheakis, J. D., and Chirigos, M. A. (1978b). *In* "Immune Modulation and Control of Neoplasia by Adjuvant Therapy" (M. A. Chirigos, ed.), pp. 459–467. Raven, New York.
Schultz, R. M., Pavlidis, N. A., and Chirigos, M. A. (1978c). *Cancer Res.* **38,** 3427–3431.
Schultz, R. M., Pavlidis, N. A., Stylos, W. A., and Chirigos, M. A. (1978d). *Science* **202,** 320–321.
Schultz, R. M., Pavlidis, N. A., Stylos, W. A., and Chirigos, M. A. (1978e). *Cancer Treat. Rep.* **62,** 1889–1892.
Schultz, R. M., Papamatheakis, J. D., and Chirigos, M. A. (1978f). *In* "Immune Modulation and Control of Neoplasia by Adjuvant Therapy" (M. A. Chirigos, ed.), pp. 241–248. Raven, New York.
Schultz, R. M., Chirigos, M. A., and Papamatheakis, J. D. (1978g). *Cancer Immunol. Immunother.* **3,** 183–187.
Schultz, R. M., Pavlidis, N. A., Chirigos, M. A., and Weiss, J. F. (1978h). *Cell. Immunol.* **38,** 302–309.
Schultz, R. M., Stoychkov, J. N., Pavlidis, N., Chirigos, M. A., and Olkowski, Z. L. (1979a). *J. Reticuloendothel. Soc.* **26,** 93–102.
Schultz, R. M., Chirigos, M. A., Stoychkov, J. N., and Pavlidis, N. A. (1979b). *J. Reticuloendothel. Soc.* **26,** 83–92.
Schultz, R. M., Pavlidis, N. A., Stoychkov, J. N., and Chirigos, M. A. (1979c). *Cell. Immunol.* **42,** 71–78.
Scott, M. T. (1975). *J. Natl. Cancer Inst.* **54,** 789–792.
Sethi, K. K., and Brandis, H. (1975). *J. Natl. Cancer Inst.* **55,** 393–395.
Sharma, S. D., and Piessens, W. F. (1978a). *Cell. Immunol.* **38,** 276–285.
Sharma, S. D., and Piessens, W. F. (1978b). *Cell. Immunol.* **38,** 264–275.
Shaw, J. O., Russell, S. W., Printz, M. P., and Skidzel, R. A. (1979). *J. Immunol.* **123,** 50–54.
Siegel, B. V. (1976). *J. Reticuloendothel. Soc.* **20,** 219–222.
Simon, H. B., and Sheagren, J. N. (1971). *J. Exp. Med.* **133,** 1377–1389.
Simon, H. B., and Sheagren, J. N. (1972). *Cell. Immunol.* **4,** 163–174.

Snodgrass, M. J., Morahan, P. S., and Kaplan, A. M. (1975). *J. Natl. Cancer Inst.* **55,** 455–462.
Snodgrass, M. J., Harris, T. M., and Kaplan, A. M. (1978). *Cancer Res.* **38,** 2925–2929.
Snyderman, R., and Pike, M. C. (1976). *Science* **192,** 370–372.
Snyderman, R., Pike, M. C., Meadows, L., Hemstreet, G., and Wells, S. (1975). *Clin. Res.* **23,** 297A.
Snyderman, R., Meadows, L., Holder, W., and Wells, S. (1978). *J. Natl. Cancer Inst.* **60,** 737–740.
Solomon, G. F., Merigan, T. C., and Levine, S. (1967). *Proc. Soc. Exp. Biol. Med.* **126,** 74–79.
Stadecker, M. J., Calderon, J., Karnovsky, M. L., and Unanue, E. R. (1977). *J. Immunol.* **119,** 1738–1743.
Stevenson, M. M., and Meltzer, M. S. (1976). *J. Natl. Cancer Inst.* **57,** 847–852.
Stewart, C. C., and Beetham, K. L. (1978). *Int. J. Cancer* **22,** 152–159.
Stewart, C. C., Adles, C., and Hibbs, J. B. (1976). *In* "The Reticuloendothelial System in Health and Disease: Immunologic and Pathologic Aspects" (H. Friedman, M. R. Escobar, and S. M. Reichard, eds.), pp. 423–433. Plenum, New York.
Suzuki, F., Ishida, N., Maeda, H., and Fujii, T. (1977). *Proc. Annu. Meet. Jap. Cancer Assoc., 36th* (Abstr. 79).
Suzuki, C., Suzuki, F., Umenai, T., Ishida, N., Maeda, H., Takiguchi, S., Kobayashi, S., and Fujii, T. (1978). *Jap. J. Bacteriol* **33,** 78–83.
Sykes, J. A., and Maddox, I. S. (1972). *Nature (London) New Biol.* **237,** 59–61.
Vassalli, J., Hamilton, J., and Reich, E. (1976). *Cell.* **8,** 271–281.
Voelkel, E. F., Levine, L., Alper, C. A., and Tashjian, A. H. (1978). *J. Exp. Med.* **147,** 1078–1088.
Wahl, L. M., Wahl, S. M., Mergenhagen, S. E., and Martin, G. R. (1975). *Science* **187,** 261–262.
Wahl, L. M., Olsen, C. E., Sandberg, A. L., and Mergenhagen, S. E. (1977). *Proc. Natl. Acad. Sci U.S.A.* **74,** 4955–4958.
Weidemann, M. J., Peskar, B. A., Wrogemann, K., Rietschel, E. T., Staudinger, H., and Fischer, H. (1978). *FEBS Lett.* **89,** 136–140.
Weinberg, J. B., Chapman, H. A., and Hibbs, J. B. (1978). *J. Immunol.* **121,** 72–80.
Weissman, G., and Thomas, L. (1963). *J. Clin. Invest.* **42,** 661–669.
Werb, Z., and Cohn, Z. (1971). *J. Exp. Med.* **134,** 1545–1552.
Werb, Z., Foley, R., and Munck, A. (1978). *J. Exp. Med.* **147,** 1684–1694.
Whitcomb, M. E., Merluzzi, V. J., and Cooperband, S. R. (1976). *Cell. Immunol.* **21,** 272–277.
Wing, E. J., Gardner, I. D., Ryning, F. W., and Remington, J. S. (1977). *Nature (London)* **268,** 642–644.
Wood, G. W., and Gillespie, G. Y. (1975). *Int. J. Cancer* **16,** 1022–1029.
Wortis, H. H. (1974). *Contemp. Top. Immunol.* **3,** 243–262.
Yaron, M., Yaron, I., Gurari-Rotman, D., Revel, M., Lindner, H. R., and Zor, U. (1977). *Nature (London)* **267,** 457–459.
Youngner, J. S., and Salvin, S. B. (1973). *J. Immunol.* **111,** 1914–1922.
Zurier, R. B., Dukor, P., and Weissman, G. (1971). *Clin. Res.* **19,** 453–457.

ADVANCES IN PHARMACOLOGY AND CHEMOTHERAPY, VOL. 17

Prenatal and Neonatal Toxicology and Pathology of Heavy Metals

LOUIS W. CHANG AND PAUL R. WADE

Department of Pathology
University of Arkansas for Medical Sciences
Little Rock, Arkansas

JOEL G. POUNDS

Department of Health and Human Services
Food and Drug Administration
National Center for Toxicological Research
Jefferson, Arkansas

KENNETH R. REUHL

Division of Biological Sciences
National Research Council of Canada
Ottawa, Canada

I. General Concept on Teratogenesis

The general toxic potential of many heavy metals, such as mercury, cadmium, lead, copper, arsenic, zinc, silver, gold, and molybdenum, is

ISBN 0-12-032917-4

well recognized. Mammalian embryos are found to be extremely susceptible to the influence of chemical compounds including heavy metals. Many metallic salts are found to induce abnormal development and malformations of embryos. These elements are recognized as teratogenic metals.

The vulnerability of the embryo toward teratogenesis varies with the teratogen involved and the different stages of the embryonic development. Teratogenic effects are usually more severe during the critical organogensis and histogenesis periods than in the fetal or maturation periods.

Chemical agents which have similar structures or molecular size as the essential nutrients cross the placental barrier readily. Such chemical agents include many of the heavy metals and trace elements. Maternal homeostasis and detoxification potential influences the level of toxic metals that may reach the placental membrane. Thus it is very difficult to establish the precise level of teratogen reaching the fetus. The embryocidal and teratogenic effects may overlap at a given dose level. Therefore, it is difficult to establish a clear-cut dose–effect situation.

Among the trace metals, many are known to be teratogenic: lithium (Li), molybdenum (Mo), zinc (Zn), cadium (Cd), mercury (Hg), lead (Pb), aresenic (As), aluminum (Al), indium (In), thallium (Tl), tellurium (Te), and selenium (Se). In the present article, only those metals, Hg, Cd, and Pb, which have the greatest health hazard will be presented. Because the established information on the toxic effects of each metal varies in the literature, different emphasis will be put on each of these toxic metals in the present article.

II. Toxic Effects of Mercury on Development

A. Introduction

Methylmercury is a widespread and highly toxic environmental pollutant. Although this compound has been recognized as a potential health hazard to laboratory and industrial workers for many years (Hunter *et al.*, 1940; Hunter and Russell, 1954), it was not until the disasterous outbreak of poisoning in Minamata Bay, Japan, during the 1950s that scientists first recognized the potential danger of the organomercurial as an environmental toxicant (Kurland *et al.*; 1960; Takeuchi, 1968; Chang, 1977).

Toxic exposure to methylmercury results primarily in neurological damage, characterized chiefly by ataxia, sensory disturbances, and changes in mental state (Takeuchi, 1968). An unexpected and alarming finding of the Minamata Bay episode was the indication that the fetus has a high vulnerability toward methylmercury toxicity. The congenitally affected children displayed a progressive neurologic disturbance resembling cerebral palsy but manifested other neurologic problems as well. In Japan, of the first 120 patients with confirmed methylmercury poisoning, 19 were infants showing symptoms of "fetal Minamata disease." By 1976, 40 cases of fetal Minamata disease had been positively identified in the Minamata area (Harada, 1976).

B. Human Studies

1. *Clinical Findings*

Studies of infants prenatally exposed to methylmercury have confirmed that the developing human nervous system is highly sensitive to the deleterious effects of this toxicant (Takeuchi, 1968; Takeuchi *et al.*, 1977; Matsumoto *et al.*, 1964; Harada, 1976, 1977). The signs and symptoms resulting from "fetal Minamata disease" have been well documented (Takeuchi, 1968; Snyder, 1971; Amin-Zaki *et al.*, 1974a; Harada, 1976, 1977; Koos and Longo, 1976; Choi *et al.*, 1978). The type and severity of the nervous system injury is variable, depending upon the duration and intensity of exposure and the gestational stage during which the exposure occurred (Takeuchi *et al.*, 1977). In addition, therapeutic efforts to reduce maternal mercury levels (Bakir *et al.*, 1973) and interactions with naturally occurring mercury antagonists such as selenium or vitamin E may moderate the toxicity of the compound (Evans *et al.*, 1977). The expression of fetal injury varies widely between individuals, ranging from barely detectible mental and/or physical deficits to complete physical incapacitation and profound mental retardation (Harada, 1976, 1977). The number of children who may be suffering from mild neurological damage following fetal exposure has not been determined (Takeuchi *et al.*, 1977).

The available clinical data concerning methylmercury intoxication *in utero* have been mainly derived from two large outbreaks of human poisoning: one in Minamata Bay and Niigata, Japan, during the 1950s and early 1960s; and the other in Iraq during the winter of 1971–1972 (Takeuchi, 1968; Tsubaki and Irukayama, 1977; Bakir *et al.*, 1973; WHO Bullentin, 1976).

In both symptomatic and asymptomatic females, child delivery was usually uneventful. Although gross abnormalities of the skull and teeth were reported in some fetal Minamata victims (Murakami, 1972), none were noted in the 6 cases reported from Iraq (Amin-Zaki *et al.*, 1974a,b). This difference may be attributed to the difference in duration of exposure to the toxin. The first signs of neurologic injury in the Minamata cases began to appear in infants weeks to months after birth (Harada, 1976,

TABLE I

PREVALENCE OF SYMPTOMS IN 22 CASES OF PRENATAL METHYLMERCURY INTOXICATION IN MINAMATA[a,b]

Symptoms	Prevalence (%)
Mental disturbance	100
Ataxia	100
Impairment of gait	100
Disturbance in speech	100
Disturbance in chewing and swallowing	100
Brisk and increased tendon reflex	82
Pathological reflexes	54
Involuntary movement	73
Salivation	77
Forced laughing	27

[a] From Reuhl and Chang (1979).

[b] Visual fields and hearing not examined (Harada, 1968).

1977). Lethargy, delayed movement, failure to follow visual stimuli, uncoordinated sucking or swallowing, and convulsions were frequent signs. As the victims grew older, additional indications of neurologic injury were noted. Primitive reflexes were late in disappearing. A marked impairment of coordination was a consistent finding throughout infancy and childhood. Both spastic and flaccid paralysis were noted among the patients. General developmental mileposts, such as grasping, crawling, standing, and walking, were usually delayed or, in some cases, never achieved. Excessive salivation and forced laughter were frequently seen. Blindness was present in 5 of 15 patients in the Iraqi series, and in the single case reported by Snyder (1971). Blindness was not observed among the 40 congenital Minamata cases when initially studied, but constriction of visual fields was noted when the patients were tested several years later (Harada, 1976). Hearing defects and speech disorders are also frequently observed abnormalities. The prevalence of the major signs and symptoms in 22 cases studied by Harada (1968) is seen in Table I.

Although motor defects, chiefly ataxia, predominated in the early course of the poisoning, mental disturbances were present and became more obvious as the infants matured. Mental changes were identified in 100% of the Japanese fetal Minamata disease patients (Harada, 1976), and, although the final studies are not yet available, it is highly likely that mental deficits will also be observed in the Iraqi patients. The severity of the mental damage varied. The first signs of mental involvement were frequently decreased alertness and changes in emotional state. In the most severely affected cases, the child was profoundly retarded. All of the 23 patients discussed by Harada (1977) had an I.Q. of 75 or less, and 8 were idiotic.

2. *Placental and Mammary Transfer*

Methylmercury readily crosses the placental barrier and accumulates in the developing fetus. With time, levels of methylmercury in the fetal system may exceed those of the mother. Analysis of blood taken from maternal–infant pairs exposed to methylmercury revealed a 28% greater concentration of methylmercury in the infant's blood (Tejning, 1968). Elevated ratios of umbilical cord blood and maternal blood-mercury levels have been confirmed in normal obstetrical patients with low level mercury exposure (Fujita and Takabatake, 1977; Suzuki *et al.*, 1971; Pitkin *et al.*, 1976). The mechanisms accounting for the high level of methylmercury accumulation in the fetal blood are not clear. Studies by White and Rothstein (1973) detected no major differences in mercury binding or release between adult or fetal erythrocytes, indicating that differences between adult and fetal hemoglobin do not account for the disparity in mercury levels. The elevated infant–maternal blood-mercury ratio may be maintained for a considerable time postpartum (Amin-Zaki *et al.*, 1974a,b). Nursing may contribute to maintaining high blood-mercury levels in the infant (Pitkin *et al.*, 1976; Fujita and Takabatake, 1977). A recent report indicates that lactation decreases the blood clearance time of methylmercury (Greenwood *et al.*, 1978). The halftime clearance in blood of human males and nonlactating females is approximately 75 days, while it is only 42 days in lactating females. This finding has been confirmed in mice, where lactation decreases the blood half-time from 9.3 days in nonlactating females to 5.6 days in those nursing. While exact reasons for the increased blood clearance are unclear, three postulates have been presented to account for the phenomenon. First, it is possible that excretion via lactation results in a rapid decrease in blood-mercury burden. However, calculations indicate that loss of methylmercury via milk accounts for only 3% of the reduction in body burden. This loss in milk cannot account for the change in blood-mercury half-life. A second possibility is that increased food intake by lactating females could enhance biliary excretion. A final postulate is that an altered hormonal status of the lactating female may influence the rate of methylmercury removal from the blood.

3. *Neuropathology of Human Fetal Minamata Disease*

The literature contains few detailed descriptions of the neuropathology resulting from *in utero* methylmercury poisoning. To date, only four autopsy examinations have been fully reported; two originating in the Minamata Bay area (Matsumoto *et al.*, 1964), and two from Iraq (Choi *et al.*, 1978). Examination of peripheral nerve biopsy material has also been reported (Takeuchi, 1977).

The neuropathologic findings in the Japanese and Iraqi cases are considered separately to permit closer comparison of the salient features of the chronic and acute forms of fetal methylmercury intoxication.

a. Japanese Cases. Grossly, the brains were small and symmetrically atrophic. Brain weights were reduced one-half to one-third when compared to age-matched controls. Cerebral convolutions were narrowed, and cerebellar hemispheres and vermis showed evidence of atrophy. Coronal sections of the brains revealed reduction in the size of the corpus callosum and generalized thinning of the cortex. Cerebral white matter appeared poorly developed, and the basal ganglia were small.

Microscopically, multiple sections revealed that toxic injury was widely spread throughout the brain. This is in marked contrast to the infantile and adult forms, which show considerable anatomic selectivity (Hunter and Russell, 1954; Takeuchi, 1968). Disruption of the cerebral and cerebellar cytoarchitecture was striking. Columnar groups of neurons were observed in the temporal lobes bilaterally. Resting matrix cells lined the periventricular region, and atypical neurons, described as hypoplastic and dysplastic, were identified in the cortex. Neuronal loss, involving primarily the granule and small pyramidal cells, was seen throughout the cerebrum. Proliferation of glial cells, especially microglia, was observed in areas of diffuse neuronal loss. Although no active demyelination was noted, the white matter was poorly myelinated, and neurons were observed in the cerebral medulla. Such characteristic microscopic findings are seen only in the prenatal methylmercury poisoning and serve to differentiate the fetal from the infantile form of the disease.

The cerebellar hemispheres and vermis were atrophic, with a thinning of both the granular and molecular layers. Granule cell loss was most pronounced in the depths of the sulci, particularly in the culmen and declive of Monticulus, but was not as severe as that seen in cases of adult methylmercury poisoning. Occasional Purkinje cells demonstrated dendritic swelling and infrequently degeneration. Basket cells and parallel fibers were also damaged. As in the cerebrum, the cerebellar white matter was poorly developed but without active demyelination. The spinal cords were unremarkable except for poor myelination of pyramidal and corticospinal tracts.

Changes in components of the peripheral nervous system (PNS), such as the dorsal root ganglia and nerve fibers, are important in the overall pathology of methylmercury poisoning in the adult (Takeuchi, 1968;

Miyakawa *et al.*, 1976; Eto and Takeuchi, 1977). Little is known about the influence of congenital methylmercury exposure on the PNS. Recently, Takeuchi *et al.* (1977) reported light and electron microscopic findings in sural nerve material taken from three patients with documented congenital methylmercury poisoning. Major findings consisted of extensive loss of myelinated fibers and incomplete myelination of remaining axons. Occasionally, the myelin sheaths were markedly distended, apparently as a result of abnormal remyelination. Small groups of nerve fibers were found to be devoid of myelin sheaths. A proliferation of Schwann cells and a marked increase of collagen within the nerve bundle was also observed.

b. Iraqi Cases. The brains of both infants were described as small. The frontal lobes were shorter than normal, with atypical gyral patterns. Multiple small, narrow gyri were seen in the parietal, temporal, and occipital lobes. Cut sections revealed a heterotopic area of gray matter in the white matter of the occipital lobe of one brain. The white matter of both cerebrum and cerebellum appeared slightly less in volume. The corpus callosum and basal ganglia were grossly normal.

Microscopically, both brains were characterized by a marked disruption of the cytoarchitecture. Many nests of heterotopic neurons were seen in the white matter of the cerebrum and cerebellum. The normal pattern of neurons were seen in the white matter of the cerebrum and cerebellum. The normal pattern of neurons in the cerebral cortex was disrupted by irregular aggregates or vertical columns of neurons. In other areas the cortical layers were described as having an "undulating" pattern, and in these areas the overlying gyri had not developed. Large numbers of plump, gemistocytic astrocytes were noted in the white matter of both cerebrum and cerebellum. No reactive proliferation of microglia was observed. The cerebellum also contained multiple heterotopic neurons in the white matter. These neurons appeared to be both granule and Purkinje cells. Unlike the Japanese cases, there was no neuronal necrosis in either cerebellum or cerebrum.

Both Japanese and Iraqi cases are characterized by a reduction of brain size and major disturbances in the cellular architecture. The resting matrix cells were reported in the Japanese cases, and the multiple nests of heterotopic neurons indicate that interference with normal neuronal migration underlies methylmercury's effect on the developing nervous system. These changes in cytoarchitecture appear to be permanent, as they were seen in the 2- and 6-year-old Japanese cases. It is highly likely that these migration defects would disrupt the synaptic circuitry in the brain. Defective synaptic communication could underlie some of the behavioral or electrophysiological defects reported in these victims. The differences in the morphologic appearance between the Japanese and Iraqi reports may rest largely in the length of postnatal survival. The Iraqi cases, with a short survival period, represent a more "pure" form of the fetal disease, essentially uncomplicated by postnatal toxic damage. The relatively long survival of the Japanese cases permitted full manifestation of the effects of toxic injury which is reflected in the small brain weight and extensive loss of neurons. The chronicity of the exposure may also influence the neuropathological findings.

C. Animal Studies

Animal models of transplacental methylmercury intoxication have contributed to our understanding of the mercury–fetal interaction. Most of the experimental work can be divided into four general areas: maternal–fetal exchange of methylmercury (or exchange via maternal milk after birth), teratology/pathology, behavior, and biochemistry. These are discussed separately.

1. *Placental and Mammary Transfer*

The mammalian placenta protects the developing fetus from external influences by enveloping it in a stable physical environment and by regulating transport of materials from the mother to the fetus. In general, the placenta is quite efficient at excluding detrimental substances from entering the fetal blood stream while permitting the passage of essential nutrients and trace metals. Methylmercury, however, is capable of passing through the "placental barrier" of mammals and injuring the developing organism. Pharmacokinetic and tissue distribution studies have documented tranplacental tissue passage of methylmercury in mice (Suzuki *et al.*, 1967; Childs, 1973; Olson and Massaro, 1977a), rats (Yang *et al.*, 1972; Casterline and Williams, 1972; Null *et al.*, 1973; Mansour *et al.*, 1973, 1974; Yamaguchi and Nunotani, 1974; Garcia *et al.*, 1974a; King *et al.*, 1976), hamsters (Gale and Hanlow, 1976), guinea pigs (Kelman and Sasser, 1977), and rhesus monkeys (Reynolds and Pitkin, 1975). Inorganic and aryl mercurials may also cross the placenta, but do so to a much smaller extent (Mansour *et al.*, 1973, 1974; Garret *et al.*, 1972; Suzuki *et al.*, 1967).

The amount of methylmercury which accumulates in the fetus is a function of the administered dose, the period of gestation at which it is given, and the time interval between the dose administration and sample analysis. Following a single administration of methylmercury, the fetal-mercury burden continues to increase for several days before reaching a peak. Elimination of methylmercury from the fetus occurs primarily through exchange with the maternal circulation and the rate of excretion varies significantly between species. Studies of tissue and blood levels of maternal and fetal animals following both single and multiple methylmercury administrations have revealed that the fetus may carry a heavier tissue concentration than the maternal animal.

Garcia *et al.* (1974a) found 27% more radiolabeled methylmercury in the blood of newborn rats than in maternal blood following oral administration of methylmercury on gestational day 16. Other studies, however, have shown that the ratio of fetal to maternal blood mercury remains less than one throughout gestation (Mansour *et al.*, 1974; Wannag, 1976; Casterline and Williams, 1972). Differences in results probably reflect different species and variations in administered dose or sample times.

As in the adult form of Minamata disease, the kidney, liver, and brain are preferential sites of deposition for methylmercury. Concentrations in the fetal brains are frequently higher than those in the maternal brains. Methylmercury appears in the brain of the fetus as early as 10 minutes following intravenous administration (Reynolds and Pitkin, 1975), but it frequently takes several days for the peak concentrations to be achieved (Yang *et al.*, 1972). Increasing brain-mercury levels are a result of continuing deposition from blood-bound mercury and from a redistribution of methylmercury from other organs. Levels of mercury in the fetus as well as the rate of accumulation have been related to the amount of mercury given.

The relative amount of mercury in the brain, however, may not follow the whole body relationship. Null and co-workers (1973) compared the levels of methylmercury in the brains of the fetus and their mothers as well as in the nonpregnant female rats exposed to equal levels of mercury. The concentration of mercury in the fetal brain was found to be at least twice that of their mothers. It has been calculated that if fetal brain mercury is corrected for the mercury bound to blood cells within the cerebral vasculature, the ratio of fetal to maternal brain mercury concentration is even higher (Wannag, 1976).

Work from several laboratories has shown that the placenta may alter the rate and amount of methylmercury transfer between mother and fetus (Reynolds and Pitkin, 1975; Garcia *et al.*, 1974a,b). Evidence indicates that the rate of mercury transfer is much greater in the direction from the mother toward the fetus than in the reverse direction (Reynolds and Pitkin, 1975). Such phenomenon may contribute to the "trapping" of mercury in the fetal tissue.

Transfer of methylmercury from the lactating mother to her offspring has been documented both in humans and in experimental animals (Amin-Zaki *et al.*, 1974b; Greenwood *et al.*, 1978; Pitkin *et al.*, 1976; Fujita and Takabatake, 1977; Garcia *et al.*, 1974a; Yang *et al.*, 1973; Mansour *et al.*,

1973). Neurological lesions characteristic of methylmercury poisoning have been observed in animals which were exposed to mercury only via mother's milk (Deshimaru, 1969). However, the extent to which methylmercury in mother's milk contributes to the injury observed in the infant is still unknown. Yang *et al*. (1973) calculated that it would require feeding a lactating female rat approximately 17 to 25 mg of methylmercury before neurological problems in the pups could be induced. Such calculations are based on the assumption that 1% of the dose fed to the lactating mother will pass to the offspring during a 21-day weaning period. This postulation correlates well with the findings of Deshimaru (1969), who found neurological lesions in newborns which were nursed by mothers treated with 14–16 mg of methylmercury over a period of 18 days.

Garcia *et al*. (1974b) investigated the stability of methylmercury in the milk of rats and discovered that the covalent bond of methylmercury may be broken in the fat and casein fractions of the milk. This indicates that both organic and inorganic mercury are present in maternal milk. Since organic and inorganic mercury are transferred to the pup through milk with about the same efficiency (Mansour *et al*., 1973), the potential contribution of inorganic mercury to the overall toxicity on the suckling infants must also be borne in mind.

2. *Teratology and Pathology of Experimental Fetal Minamata Disease*

The effects of *in utero* methylmercury exposure have been studied with various animal models. The compound is embryolethal in most species examined to date. The sensitivity of both the mother and the fetus to the toxic effect of methylmercury is influenced by many factors, particularily the species and strain of the experimental animal studied (Spyker *et al*., 1972; Su and Okita, 1976b), the duration of exposure during pregnancy (Harris *et al*., 1972), the amount of mercury administered to the pregnant animal (Spyker, 1972; Harris *et al*., 1972), and the route of exposure (Lown *et al*., 1977). Variations in the experimental design of studies already in the literature frequently makes direct comparison or correlation of existing data difficult.

Intrauterine death is a frequent result of congenital organomercurial intoxication, and is usually manifested by fetal reabsorption or stillbirth. When given during developmentally sensitive periods, particularly during the days of rapid organogenesis, relatively low levels of methylmercury can produce a high fetal mortality. Harris *et al*. (1972), using golden hamsters, reported that a single intraperitoneal (ip) injection of 8 mg/kg methylmercury on the eighth gestational day resulted in a 42% incidence of fetal death and a 36% incidence of grossly malformed pups. The same dose administered on day 4 of gestation resulted in only 5% mortality and 8% malformations, while administration on day 10 caused 30% intrauterine death but no gross malformations. Increased fetal vulnerability during the period of organogenesis has been reported by other workers (Spyker *et al.*, 1972).

Strains within a species frequently show a marked variation in susceptibility to methylmercury. Spyker and Smithberg (1972) compared the incidence of intrauterine death in two strains of mice (129 Sv/Sl and A/J) and found that a single ip administration of 8 mg/kg to pregnant 129 Sv/Sl mice between fetal days 9 and 13 resulted in over 80% of the fetal implants being resorbed. The same dose produced significantly lower lethality (less than 40% of the implants were resorbed) in the A/J strain. However, approximately 72% of the A/J offspring were malformed. In addition, a significant difference in maternal sensitivity to methylmercury was observed. Thirty-one percent of the pregnant females of the 129 Sv/Sl strain died when treated on days 9, 10, or 11, while only 11% of the pregnant A/J females died. Su and Okita (1976b) also found a marked difference in methylmercury sensitivity among C57BL, CD, and 129 Sv/Sl strains of mice treated subcutaneously (sc) with several doses of methylmercury on day 10 of gestation.

Congenital malformations are another frequent manifestation of methylmercury's impact on developing organisms. The most common malformations produced in experimental animals have been cleft palate (Spyker and Smithberg, 1972; Su and Okita, 1976b), limb defects (Harris *et al.*, 1972), and brain and facial malformations (Spyker and Smithberg, 1972; Gilani, 1975). Under some experimental conditions methylmercury may be an extremely potent teratogen. A 97% incidence of cleft palate was observed in 129 Sv/Sl mouse fetuses following six consecutive injections of 5 mg methylmercury/kg on days 7–12 (Su and Okita, 1976b). Other workers have also reported high incidence of cleft palates in their experimental animals following methylmercury exposure (Spyker and Smithberg, 1972; Harris *et al.*, 1972; Olson and Massaro, 1977b). While the precise mechanism by which methylmercury induces a cleft palate is unknown, it has been suggested that the inhibitory effect on protein synthesis may disrupt the regulatory processes controlling closure of the palate (Olson and Massaro, 1977b). Morphological changes have also been detected in the fetal liver (Ware *et al.*, 1974) and kidney (Chang and Sprecher, 1976a,b).

The neuropathological lesions resulting from experimental fetal methylmercury poisoning were initially reported in the Japanese literature (Moriyama, 1967; Tatetsu *et al.*, 1968), and are summarized in a comprehensive review by Murakami (1972). The most severe methylmercury-induced congenital abnormalities are exencephaly and encephalocele

(Spyker and Smithberg, 1972; Gilani, 1975). Hydrocephalus has also been observed by several authors (Harris *et al.*, 1972; Murakami, 1972). The type or cause of the hydrocephalus was not described.

Light microscopic studies of the CNS of congenitally treated animals have revealed a variety of pathologic findings. Loss of neurons and cytoarchitectural changes have been reported in the cerebrums of rat pups exposed to 5 mg/kg methylmercury on gestational days 0–12 (Murakami, 1972). Cystic changes and small hemorrhages in the cortex and white matter were reported by Tatetsu *et al.* (1968) following exposure to 1 mg/kg throughout gestation. Unspecified white matter destruction was seen in the temporal lobes of rats receiving 7.5 mg/kg on days 7–14 (Fuyuta *et al.*, 1978). In the cerebellum, the lesions involved primarily the granule cell layers. Delayed migration of the external granular cell layer was observed in mice following exposure to 1 mg/kg on gestational days 6–17 (Khera and Tabacova, 1973). Alterations of cerebral and cerebellar architecture, with hypoplastic and atrophic neurons and incomplete granular cell layer formation, have been reported in cats following chronic methylmercury poisoning during gestation (Harada, 1977; Khera, 1973). If the kitten survived, marked ataxia usually appeared. Atopic neurons, dendritic swelling of the Purkinje cells, and degeneration of the granule cells were also observed in our laboratory.

Recently, Chang *et al.* (1977a,b) reported ultrastructural evidence of cellular damage in the brains of mice and rats prenatally exposed to low doses of methylmercury during gestation. In the cerebellum, both Purkinje and granular cell neurons contained abnormal accumulations of lysosomes. Disorientation and shortening of the rough endoplasmic reticulum was seen in Purkinje cells. Occasional neurites contained dilated saccules resembling smooth endoplasmic reticulum, and segmentally incomplete myelination of axons was frequently encountered. Large cytosegresomes, floccular degeneration, and neuronal necrosis were common. Follow-up studies indicate that such toxic changes may persist into adult life. Abnormalities of myelin formation, with accumulation of large myelin ovoids, and degenerating axons, could still be demonstrated in the cerebellum of adult rats and hamsters a year after a single prenatal administration of methylmercury (Chang, unpublished observations).

3. *Behavioral Studies*

Behavioral studies of offspring from mercury-treated animals have shown promise in detecting subtle nervous system damage before any classical neurological symptoms appear, or when exposure levels fall below those capable of inducing symptoms (Spyker, 1975). It has been reported that a single, low dose of methylmercury to pregnant animals could result in behaviorally abnormal offspring (Spyker *et al.*, 1972). Su and Okita (1976a) exposed mice to various amounts of methylmercury on gestational day 10 and performed behavioral studies on postnatal days 24, 44, and 64. Open-field tests revealed abnormalities manifested by prolonged center-square latency, decreased ambulatory and exploratory activity, lower frequency of grooming and urination, and increased backing movements when compared to the controls. Depression of spontaneous locomotor activity was also observed in the pups, but was found to increase toward normal levels with time. The treated offspring were also found to be abnormally sensitive to the induction of convulsions by flurothyl.

Hughes and Annau (1976) conducted extensive tests on the offspring of mice treated with either 1, 2, 3, 5, or 10 mg/kg methylmercury on day 8 of gestation. Little difference was found between the experimental animals and the controls when tested for motor skills. However, definite differences from controls were detected in passive avoidance task and in the number of consecutive avoidances in the shuttle box, indicating that the deficit was one of learning rather than of motor impairment. Unlike Spyker *et al.* (1972) and Su and Okita (1976a), the authors noted no differences in the results of open-field tests. Differences in strain or experimental procedure may account for this discrepancy.

Musch *et al.* (1978) used operant conditioning procedures to tests rats which had been exposed to 0.05 or 2.0 mg/kg of methylmercury on days 6, 7, 8, and 9 of gestation. The authors used an operant conditioning schedule referred to as "Differential Reinforcement of High Rates" (DRH). Test results showed that significant differences between experimental and control groups appeared with increasing demand on performance. The reduction of successful performance was dose related and reflected a decreased learning rate among the treated animals.

Since methylmercury has been reported to be excreted in mother's milk and to cause neurologic and behavioral changes in suckling rat pups (Deshimaru, 1969), it is of some importance to attempt to differentiate the effects of congenital exposure from those of exposure during infancy. Brown *et al.* (1972) tested water escape T-maze performance in mice. The initial tests demonstrated deficits in all of the treated groups, i.e., those exposed to mercury prenatally, postnatally through milk, and both pre- and postnatally. Testing a week later revealed that only the pups treated prenatally and those treated both prenatally and postnatally showed persistent learning defects. This indicates that there may be a qualitative difference in sensitivity to methylmercury between prenatal and postnatal exposure, and that the fetal brain is more sensitive than the neonatal brain. Similar findings were reported by Zenick *et al.* (1973).

Recent electrophysiological, biochemical, and ultrastructural studies have begun to elucidate some of the possible underlying mechanisms which could contribute to behavioral alterations. Dyer *et al.* (1978) reported alterations in cortically recorded visual evoked potentials in 60-day-old rats treated with 5.0 mg methylmercury/kg on day 7 of gestation. The treated animals demonstrated elevated P1-N1 and P2-N2 amplitudes (measurements of retinal-striate system activity), and shortened P2 and N2 latencies. It was hypothesized that the shortened P2 and N2 latencies might result from damage to small neurons whose axons have slow conduction velocities. Such speculation correlates with the findings of Chang and co-workers (1977a,b) demonstrating defects of myelination and degenerative changes in small neurons and their processes following *in utero* methylmercury treatment of mice and hamsters.

4. *Biochemical Studies*

Although there have been numerous studies of biochemical alterations in the nervous system of adult animals following methylmercury intoxication (Omata *et al.*, 1978; Farris and Smith, 1975; Brubaker *et al.*, 1973; Verity *et al.*, 1977; Cavanagh and Chen, 1971; Yoshino *et al.*, 1966; Chang *et al.*, 1972a,b, 1973), only a few investigations have been performed to analyze neurochemical changes of congenital methylmercury poisoning.

Much of the evidence for a direct biochemical effect comes from enzyme histochemical studies. Using cerebellum of mouse pups treated with 1.0 mg/kg/day during gestational days 6–17, Khera and Nera (1971) observed an inhibition of DPN diaphorase, succinic dehydrogenase, cytochrome oxidase, and ATPase on day 1 of postnatal life. However, only cytochrome oxidase was still decreased when the animals were examined on day 7. A subsequent study confirmed the depression of DPN diaphorase, succinic dehydrogenase, and cytochrome oxidase when the animals were examined on the second postnatal day. There was no difference in enzyme activity observed between control and experimental animals examined after day 14, indicating that the depression of the enzyme activity was only transient. The activities of choline acetyltransferase, cholinesterase, and acetylcholinesterase were not significantly altered following *in utero* administration of 8 or 10 mg/kg to mice or hamsters (Spyker *et al.*, 1972).

Alterations in lipid metabolism following prenatal methylmercury administration have recently been reported (Menon *et al.*, 1978). Inhibition of the incorporation of the label from (DL)-3-OH[3-^{14}C]butyrate into the total extractable brain lipid was observed in brain slices from prenatally treated rats during the period of active myelination. Further studies revealed a reduction of incorporation of 3-OH-butyrate into cholesterol, free fatty acids, phosphatidylcholine, and phosphatidylserine on day 14, while incorporation of the label into sphingomyelin was greatly increased at this time. By day 21, all parameters of incorporation returned to control levels. Data indicate inhibition of the steps between the uptake of 3-OH-butyrate and its conversion to lipids. In addition, it was thought that there was a further defect either in the conversion of cystidine diphosphate choline to phosphatidylcholine or a defect in myelination. Abnormal myelin profiles have been observed in peripheral nerves of humans (Takeuchi *et al.*, 1978) and rodent cerebellum (Chang, unpublished data) following *in utero* methylmercury exposure. It has not been determined if an abnormal process of myelination or chemically defective myelin underlies this defect.

Exposure to methylmercury during early postnatal life produces lasting biochemical changes in the brains of developing animals. Taylor and DiStefano (1976) investigated the influence of methylmercury on biogenic amines in neonatal rat pups. A dose of 5 mg/kg ip on days 5, 6, and 7 postpartum resulted in a decrease in serotonin, 5-hydroxyindoleacetic acid, and norepinephrine when measured on day 8. From day 8 to day 15, levels of biogenic amines steadily increased and surpassed control levels. After day 15, brain catecholamine levels varied widely and showed no consistent trends. Serotonin (5-hydroxytryptamine) levels, however, remained elevated until the experiment was terminated on day 60. Both tryptophan hydroxylase activity and serotonin turnover were reduced on day 8, and monoamine oxidase, which degrades both serotonin and catecholamines, was decreased by 15% on day 15 and 17% on day 27. Levels of both tryptophan hydroxylase, the rate-limiting enzyme in this pathway, and the amino acid tryptophan, a substrate for the enzyme, were significantly reduced. The significance of these findings is not fully understood. It is possible that alterations in biogenic amines may induce behavioral changes in young methylmercury-intoxicated animals, or may cause morphologic damage to neural elements, but such speculations are unconfirmed. Further, it is yet unknown whether *in utero* exposure to organomercurials will yield similar findings.

Studies utilizing whole fetuses have revealed significant decreases in total fetal protein and DNA content following administration of methylmercury. Olson and Massaro (1977b) reported that injection of 5 mg/kg on day 12 of gestation was followed by a maximal reduction of fetal protein levels 48 hours after mercury administration, while fetal DNA levels were maximally decreased 72 hours postinjection. Protein levels returned to normal about 24 hours before the DNA levels, suggesting that altered protein synthesis could result in a decreased rate of cell growth and an increased cell cycle time by reducing DNA levels. Such a mechanism might explain the retarded growth in mercury-treated animals and may underly the developmental malformations reported, as well as the delayed limb regeneration seen in mercury-treated amphibians (Chang *et al.*, 1976). A reduction in protein synthesis has also been reported in adult animals treated with methylmercury (Omata *et al.*, 1978; Syversen, 1977; Farris and Smith, 1975; Cavanagh and Chen, 1971; Yoshino *et al.*, 1966). Other workers have observed an induction of protein synthesis in brains of adult male rats treated with methylmercury hydroxide (Brubaker *et al.*, 1973). The difference between the findings of Brubaker and co-workers and those of other workers may be due to either the cell population studied or procedural differences (Chang, 1977).

The transport of amino acids across the placenta of mercury-treated animals has also been studied (Olson and Massaro, 1977b). A reduction in the levels of alanine, valine, methionine, leucine, and isoleucine was found in the fetus 12 hours after methylmercury (5 mg/kg) was given to the mother on the twelfth day of gestation. Reduced placental transport of certain amino acids was also noted at this time. Such reduction of placental transport may explain the reduced fetal amino acid levels and the decreased protein synthesis in the fetus.

Damage to other organ systems may also contribute to the development of neuropathologic lesions. Snell *et al.* (1977) investigated alterations in carbohydrate metabolism in the offspring of rats treated with a subcutaneous injection either 4 or 8 mg/kg methylmercury on gestational day 9. Animals were sacrificed either 2 days before term, shortly after birth, or on postnatal day 6. Biochemical analysis of the fetal rats showed decreased plasma glucose and liver glycogen concentrations as well as decreased hepatic glucose 6-phosphatase (G-6-P) activity when compared with controls. In neonatal pups, impaired glycogen mobilization was observed within the first few hours of life, and was associated with a severe protracted hypoglycemia. It was suggested that the hypoglycemia resulted from either (1) a lowered hepatic G-6-P activity in fetal animals limiting the production of free glucose from glycogen-derived glucose phosphate, or (2) defective glycogen mobilization at birth. These factors are not mutually exclusive and may be operating simultaneously. On postnatal day 6, the animals showed elevated levels of hepatic glycogen and decreased body weight. The extent to which the protracted hypoglycemia at birth contributes to CNS dysfunction or injury is unclear. The CNS is highly sensitive to alterations in glucose concentrations and it is conceivable that hypoglycemia occurring at a highly sensitive period of brain development could contribute to the observed clinical and behavioral alterations (Snell *et al.*, 1977).

Fetal hepatic mitochondria have been shown to be sensitive to methylmercury exposure. Fowler and Woods (1977) exposed female rats to drinking water containing 0, 3, 5, or 10 ppm methylmercury for 4 weeks prior to mating. Following successful impregnation, the animals were continued on the mercury dose until sacrificed on gestational day 19. A significant reduction of amino acid uptake was found in the mercury-exposed pups. A decrease in the structural proteins made within the mitochondria was also noted. Enzyme studies confirmed that the mitochondrial alterations were localized to the membranes. Monoamine oxidase, cytochrome oxidase, and ALA-synthetase were all reduced in a dose-related fashion. Malate dehydrogenase, a mitochondrial matrix enzyme, showed no alteration in activity at any of the dose levels examined. In addition, respiratory control was lost in animals exposed to 3 ppm mercury and state 3 respiration was completely suppressed in animals treated with 5–10 ppm mercury (Fowler and Woods, 1977). Similar mitochondrial changes may also occur in the nervous system of the fetus. Alterations of mitochondrial enzymes have been observed in brains of adult animals (Yoshino *et al.*, 1966). These findings support the morphological observations of Chang and Hartmann (1972) who, by means of electron microscopic histochemical techniques, demonstrated the close association of mercury with the mitochondrial membranes. Morphometric analysis also revealed a reduction in volume density of the hepatic mitochondria (Fowler and Woods, 1977).

The effects of fetal exposure to methylmercury on biochemical systems may not appear until later in the animal's life. Robbins *et al.* (1978) observed a decrease in the hepatic cytochrome P-450-dependent systems of methylmercury-treated male rats studied after 26 weeks of life; changes were not observed in earlier life. It is interesting to note that while a significant reduction in cytochrome P-450, NADPH–cytochrome c reductase, ethylmorphine *N*-demethylase, and benzoapyrene hydroxylase was observed in male rats, these enzyme levels remained normal in the female animals. This finding indicates a sex-related difference in toxicity. Confirmation of this work in other species is still unavailable.

III. Toxic Effects of Cadmium on Development

A. Introduction

Cadmium should be considered as an important health hazard because (1) it is used in various industrial processes and products which drastically increases its presence or contamination in the environment; (2) it has an exceptionally long biological half-life in the human system (about 30 years) (Kjellstrom *et al.*, 1971); (3) it produces very specific pathological effects in various systems in adult animals (Parizek, 1957; Mennear, 1979; Chang *et al.*, 1980); and (4) it produces teratologic changes and deaths in fetuses (Parizek, 1964; Rohrer *et al.*, 1979) and placental necrosis, especially in the pars fetalis, in pregnant mothers. Such pathological changes are clinically and morphologically similar to those of toxemia of pregnancy in humans (Parizek, 1965).

In the present article, the impact of cadmium on pregnancy and fetal development will be presented.

B. Human Studies

Cadmium can be detected in both human placental and fetal tissues. It was found that the cadmium content in human tissues varies with geographic regions (Thuerauf *et al.*, 1975). There was a significant increase in placental cadmium in individuals residing in industrialized areas compared to those living in rural areas. By studying still borns, Bryce-Smith *et al.* (1977) demonstrated that significantly (10-fold) higher cadmium levels were found in the fetal skeletal tissues than those reported in normally aborted human fetuses (Chaube, 1973). Although these authors suggested that the high cadmium levels in these stillborns might be related to the intrauterine death of these fetuses, such speculation still needs to be proved.

By means of atomic absorption analysis, Baglan *et al.* (1974) demonstrated that the elemental levels of cadmium in the placenta reflected the blood concentration of cadmium in the infant and mother. Another study by Baumslag *et al.* (1974) suggested that cadmium levels in neonatal hair may give an indication of the maternal body burden of this particular metal.

C. Placental Transfer of Cadmium

1. *Human Studies*

Until the last decade it was thought that the placenta provided complete protection for the human fetus against cadmium accumulation (Schroeder and Balassa, 1961). Later studies have shown that cadmium can cross the placental barrier and reach the human fetus (Flick *et al.*, 1971; Scanlon, 1972).

Recent studies on placental transfer of cadmium in humans revealed that: (1) the placenta is an important (but incomplete) barrier in protecting the fetus from cadmium accumulation (Lauwerys *et al.*, 1978); (2) there is a correlation of maternal blood, placenta, and fetal blood cadmium concentrations (Lauwerys et al., 1978; Roels *et al.*, 1978); (3) mothers who smoke have a higher blood cadmium content with an increased cadmium accumulation in the placenta as compared to nonsmoking mothers (Buchet *et al.*, 1978; Roels *et al.*, 1978); and (4) the placenta concentrates approximately 10-fold more cadmium than the maternal blood.

Although it is known that the placenta does not act as a complete barrier in preventing cadmium from reaching the human fetus, it should be stressed that no baseline data exist for the threshold of cadmium toxicity in human fetuses.

2. *Animal Studies*

Several important parameters related to the placental trasfer of cadmium in laboratory animals should be considered: (1) species of animal (and in some cases the strain of a particular species), (2) the route of maternal exposure to cadmium, (3) the gestational age of the offspring at the time of exposure, (4) the amount of cadmium given to the pregnant animals.

A variety of animal spécies including mice (Berlin and Ulberg, 1963; Wolkowski, 1974), hamsters (Ferm *et al.*, 1969), guinea pigs (Kelman and Walter, 1977), and rats (Rohrer *et al.*, 1978, 1979; Ahokas and Dilts, 1979; Sonawane *et al.*, 1975) have been used for investigation. Berlin and Ullberg (1963), using autoradiography, showed an uptake of cadmium in mice placenta after intravenous injection of labeled cadmium (^{109}Cd). No cadmium accumulation in the fetuses was observed. Because of the extreme concentration difference between the mother and the fetus (Sonawane *et al.*, 1975) it was suggested that whole-body autoradiography may not be sensitive enough to detect the extremely small amounts of cadmium in fetal tissues (Wolkowski, 1974).

Later studies with mice which were injected (iv) with ^{109}Cd on the twentieth day of gestation (just befor birth) showed that cadmium could cross the placenta and reach the fetus. Neonatal mice showed a cadmium content of approximately 0.09% of the maternal dose as determined by whole-body scintillation counting (Tanaka *et al.*, 1972).

Differences in placental transfer of cadmium has been demonstrated between strains of mice (Wolkowski, 1974). In both a "Cd-susceptible" (B10) and a "Cd-resistant" (NAW) strain, cadmium was shown to cross the placenta and localize in embryos as early as 30 minutes after subcutaneous injection. However, a significant difference in cadmium content was found in the cadmium-binding protein (MW 10,000) of the embryonic cytosol between the two strains of mice. While the "Cd-susceptible" mice showed a higher cadmium content in the embryonic cytosol protein, the "Cd-resistant" mice showed more cadmium binding to a higher molecular weight protein (MW about 19,000) in the placenta. It was postulated that the "Cd-resistant" mice are able to "trap" the cadmium at the placental level by means of a higher molecular weight Cd-binding protein and reduce the fetal exposure to this toxic metal.

Placental transfer of cadmium has also been demonstrated in neonatal hamsters with ^{109}Cd administered on the eighth day of gestation (Ferm *et al.*, 1969). A 60-fold decrease in embryo-cadmium content was detected between day 9 and day 12 of gestation. It was postulated that the developing yolk sac might be actively removing some of the cadmium from the fetus. This postulation, however, needs to be confirmed by future experimentation. The "protective" function of the yolk sac was not observed in mice where the yolk sac ceases to exist in late gestational stage resulting an increased fetal mortality (Chernoff, 1973; Wolkowski, 1974).

It was found that the fetal and neonatal gut and liver concentrate a significant amount of cadmium as a result of *in utero* exposure to cadmium in early gestational period (Lucis *et al.*, 1972). Sonawane *et al.* (1975) showed that cadmium may cross the placenta at any time of the pregnancy. The placental and fetal cadmium concentrations also increase with the dose of exposure and with the gestational stage of the animals (Sonawane *et al.*, 1975). Ahokas and Dilts (1979) also demonstrated that only a small amount of cadmium reached the embryo prior to the formation of a functional placenta. After establishment of the placenta, large accumulation of cadmium was detected in the placenta with comparatively little cadmium transferred to the fetus. However, the placental cadmium transfer increased with the dose of exposure (Ahokas and Dilts, 1979).

In an attempt to determine the extent of placental barrier to cadmium transfer, Kelman and Walter (1977) measured the blood cadmium concentrations on either side of perfused guinea pig placentas. They found that cadmium was cleared very rapidly from the maternal blood, and that this clearance was linearly related to perfusion rate. It was suggested that the low transference of cadmium from the mother to the fetus is influenced by factors such as maternal metallothionein function or the maternal plasma cadmium levels and may not be related to the effectiveness of the placental barrier.

Recent studies indicate that a cadmium-binding protein (CBP) found in the maternal system or in the placenta may play an important role in the fetotoxicity induced by cadmium. The synthesis of this CBP is believed to be zinc dependent. Investigation by Parizek *et al.* (1968) demonstrated that zinc-deficient rats displayed greater fetotoxicity upon exposure to cadmium. However, no significant difference in fetal cadmium content was observed between control or zinc-deficient animals (Rohrer *et al.*, 1978). Thus the CBP may exert its protective effect on the fetus by complexing with the cadmium at the maternal or placental level without reducing the placental cadmium transfer or the fetal cadmium content. The precise protective mechanism, however, still needs to be elucidated.

D. Mammary Transport of Cadmium

Mammary transport of cadmium to the newborn is still an area of research that needs more investigation. Tanaka and co-workers have shown that approximately 60% of radiolabeled cadmium reached the newborn mice via the mother's milk when the mother was injected (iv) with cadmium 24–36 hours before parturition (Tanaka *et al.*, 1972). It was demonstrated that the cadmium burden in neonates dropped from 0.09% (at birth) to 0.05% (at weaning) of the maternal dose when prenatally exposed animals were nursed by control females. On the other hand, control neonates (without previous cadmium exposure) accumulated 0.05% of the maternal dose within 24 hours when nursed by cadmium-treated females. These animals accumulated a maximum of 0.3% of the maternal dose after 14 days of nursing. Their body burden of cadmium, however, gradually declined to a level of 0.08% of the maternal dose after weaning.

It has been shown with rats that ^{109}Cd when administered to females on the day of parturition can be detected at low levels in the colostrum. The amount of cadmium remains at a fairly constant, low level throughout the period of nursing (Lucis *et al.*, 1972). Most of the cadmium detected in the offspring of these rats is concentrated in the intestines with only very slight amounts in the liver. It is interesting to note that in rats most of the ^{109}Cd is transmitted by mother's milk within 2 days after birth. The mammary tissue was found to contain comparatively high levels of ^{109}Cd at the initial period of lactation. This high level of cadmium persisted in mammary tissue well after lactation had ceased. Cadmium in the mammary tissue was found to bind to a protein of a molecular weight much higher than the Cd-binding protein found in other organs. Such Cd-binding protein was believed to reduce the toxic potential of cadmium and provide some protective measure for the neonates (Lucis *et al.*, 1971).

E. Pathological Effects of Cadmium on the Placenta

Using pregnant albino rats, Parizek (1964) first reported that a single subcutaneous injection of 0.04 m*M* (4.5 mg) $CdCl_2$/kg body weight given to the animal on gestational day 17 to 21 resulted in degenerative changes of the placenta (pars fetalis) and hemorrhage within 24 hours of administration. Despite the removal of fetuses from the womb prior to cadmium injection, the placenta remaining *in situ* still exhibited vascular degeneration upon cadmium administration.

Chiquoine (1965) performed a subsequent experiment with mice to examine the sensitivity of the placenta to cadmium toxicity in relationship to the time of pregnancy. Animals were injected (sc) with 6.7 mg $CdCl_2$/kg body weight between gestational day 6 and 17. It was found that injection of cadmium on days 1 to 5 of pregnancy resulted in normal fetuses at parturition. Gross signs of placental and decidual necrosis and hemorrhage were observed in animals injected with the same dose of cadmium after the thirteenth day of pregnancy. Hemorrhage within the uterus and embryonic death were found in these animals. Between day 6 and 12 of pregnancy, similar alteration of the uterine vascular system and microscopic changes in the embryos showing varying degrees of autolysis and degeneration were observed. It was concluded that a single injection of cadmium chloride given to pregnant mice on any day from the sixth to the seventeenth of pregnancy results in intrauterine death of the embryos and localized necrosis of the placenta or adjacent decidual tissue. Despite the acute and rapid placental necrosis and fetal death, no irrevocable harm was reported in the maternal animals.

Webb (1970) also reported consistent placental necrosis and intrauterine embryonic death in rats which were injected (sc) with 2.5 mg $CdCl_2$/kg body weight on day 11, 15, 17, and 18 of pregnancy. Preinjection of cadmium prior to mating produced only very minimal effect on the pregnancy. It was concluded that preexisting stores of cadmium, accumulated before pregnancy, are not mobilized by the maternal animal to produce any significant damage to the developing fetus.

F. Teratogenic Effects of Cadmium

1. *Gross Changes in the Fetuses*

Laboratory findings by Parizek (1965) indicated that pregnant animals were more sensitive to the toxic effects of cadmium than nonpregnant ones. When pregnant rats were injected with the same dose of cadmium (2.4 mg/kg) after the sixteenth day of pregnancy as that given to non pregnant females, the pregnant animals experienced a 76% mortality rate while no deaths occurred in the nonpregnant animals. Furthermore, it was demonstrated by Schroeder *et al.* (1971) that doses of cadmium nonlethal to nongravid rats significantly increased the mortality rate of gravid animals. Continuous ingestation of sublethal doses of cadmium over a long period of time by male or female animals was sufficient to cause a complete breeding failure in mice.

A number of studies have demonstrated that cadmium interferes with prenatal mammalian development and may cause a wide range of malformations (Ferm and Carpenter, 1968; Mulvihill *et al.*, 1970; Ferm, 1971; Chernoff, 1973; Barr, 1973). Despite various factors such as strain of animals, route of administration, dose of cadmium given, and period of gestation that may influence the teratogenic effects of cadmium, facial malformations seem to be a consistant and prominent finding in cadmium-induced teratology.

Mulvihill *et al.* (1970) investigated the facial malformation in hamster fetuses induced by intravenous administration of cadmium sulfate (0.44 mg/kg) on day 8 of pregnancy. Delayed ossification of the palatine shelves as well as the absence or bifurcation of the cartilaginous nasal system was found in the 14-day fetuses. Other skeletal defects (ribs, limbs, and skull) were also observed in rat and mice embryos after cadmium exposure (Barr, 1972, 1973; Ferm, 1971; Gale and Ferm, 1974). Besides skeletal abnormalies, Barr (1972) reported a markedly attenuated abdominal musculature, undescended testicles, and deformities of eyes and ears of rat fetuses exposed to 1–2 mg/kg of cadmium on day 9–11 of gestation.

2. *Factors Which Influence Cadmium-Induced Teratology*

The teratogenetic effect of cadmium apparantly is sensitive to species of animal studied, route of exposure, dose of exposure, and time of exposure. In mice, orally administered cadmium salts produce embryo mortality, fetal malformation, and runting of development (Schroeder and Mitchener, 1971). Intravenous cadmium sulfate in hamsters produces mainly facial malformation (Mulvihill *et al.*, 1970) while other forms of abnormality were reported in rats (Barr, 1972). Thus the interpretation as well as conclusions drawn from teratological studies should be made with caution.

a. Species and Strain Differences. Cadmium seemingly presents a different teratological picture in hamsters, rats, and mice (Ferm and Carpenter, 1968; Mulvihill *et al.*, 1970; Barr, 1972, 1973; Schroeder and Mitchener, 1971). Barr (1973) further documents that even within the same species and strain, sensitivity to cadmium-induced teratology may be varied even in different stocks of the same strain of animals. By using two stocks of Wistar rats (obtained from two commerical sources), Barr reported that one stock (S) had a much higher fetal mortality than the other stock (C). Malformation of the face, which is characteristic of cadmium teratogenesis in hamsters, was totally absent in rats from either stock. However, offspring from both stocks of rats showed high incidences of anophthalmia, microphthalmia, and hydrocephaly. Thinning (attenuation) of the abdominal wall was observed in both stocks of animals. The deficiency of the abdominal wall in the C stock was significantly associated with persistence of the left umbilical artery, ear dysplasia, undescended testes, and renal agenesis. However, none of these associations were significant in the offspring of the S stock. Anal atresia was found in 21% of the fetuses in the S stock exposed to cadmium on the tenth gestational day. Such abnormaly was not observed in the C stock animals similarly exposed to cadmium. Furthermore, forelimb malformation was observed almost exclusively in the left forelimb following day 10 cadmium exposure in the S stock. Total absence or severe hypoplasia of the postaxial portion of the paw was observed in 25% of the fetuses. Female fetuses seemed to be more affected than the males. No forelimb defects were found in the C stock animals treated on day 9 or day 10.

The important work by Barr (1973) strikes a note of caution that the susceptibility of animals to cadmium toxicity is extremely variable. Variations within the same species and strain may occur. Any comparison of experiments and interpretation of teratological findings should be conducted with extreme caution.

b. Influence by Dosage of Cadmium and Route of Exposure. Sonawane *et al.* (1975) by means of radioactive-labeled cadmium studied the placental transfer of cadmium in rats. Higher percentages of administered cadmium were found in the fetuses with increasing dose. When a pregnant rat was injected with low, medium, and high doses of cadmium at day 12 of gestation, fetuses accumulated 0.0001, 0.003, and 0.009% of the injected dose, respectively, representing an approximately 90-fold increase in the percentage of cadmium uptake by the fetuses when high dose condition was compared with that of low dose.

A dose-related fetal mortality response was found when cadmium was administered on days 14–17 of gestation. A 4.4% mortality rate at 4.0 mg/kg increased to a 51.6% rate with 12.0 mg/kg dose (Chernoff, 1973).

Since the route of administration such as oral, intravenous injection, intraperitoneal injection, and subcutaneous injection dictates how rapidly the cadmium ion will be absorbed into the maternal blood and transferred to the fetal system, the fact that the route of cadmium administration plays an important role in influencing the teratological effects is expected. Barr (1973) demonstrated with Wistar rats that fetal malformation could be produced by cadmium when given intraperitoneally, no teratological effect was observed when the same dose of cadmium was administered by means of subcutaneous injection. Both oral and intravenous administration of cadmium have also been shown to be effectively teratogenic (Ferm and Carpenter, 1968; Rohrer, *et al.*, 1979).

c. Influence of Gestational Age. Dencker (1975) studied the fetal uptake of cadmium in various gestational stages and reported that cadmium accumulated in the primitive gut of the embryo (hamster and mouse) when cadmium was administered (iv) on day 8 of gestation. No cadmium was detected in the embryos if injected on or after the ninth day (hamster) or eleventh day (mouse) of gestation. It was postulated that cadmium was able to pass from the yolk sac cavity into the primitive gut before the closure of the vitelline duct but not later. Sonawane *et al.* (1975), however, demonstrated that in the rats there was a significant gestational age relationship with cadmium transfer. Higher percentages of administered cadmium was found in the fetus with increasing gestational age.

In support to Dencker's (1975) study and in contrast to the report by Sonawane *et al.* (1975), Ahokas and Dilts (1979) reported their findings in rats exposed to labeled cadmium chloride on various gestational periods. It was found that embryo levels of cadmium were highest prior to formation of the functional placenta. After placental formation, there was a reduction in fetal cadmium uptake, while the placental accumulation of cadmium increased with gestational age. The authors interpreted these findings as the embryo accumulates the greatest percentage of ingested cadmium between implantation and placentation, the early period of organogenesis, and the placenta offered protection to the fetus by trapping the cadmium during the last trimester of the pregnancy.

Chernoff (1973) demonstrated that higher mortality rate was found in rat embryo when the pregnant animals were injected with cadmium at a later gestational period. Such fetal mortality, however, may be related to placental damage rather than direct fetal destruction as suggested by the findings of Ahokas and Dilts (1979). Experiments by Ferm (1971) and Gale and Ferm (1974) also indicated that teratological malformation varied with different gestational exposure.

IV. Toxic Effects of Lead on Development

A. Introduction

The adverse effects of lead in the biological systems have been well documented (National Academy of Sciences, 1972; Goyer and Rhyne, 1973; Waldron and Stofen, 1974; Griffin and Knelson, 1975; Nordberg, 1976; Environmental Protection Agency, 1977; Nriagu, 1978; National Research Council of Canada, 1978). The organ systems which are considered to be the "target systems" of lead intoxication are the nervous system (Blackman, 1937; Popoff *et al.*, 1963; Greengard *et al.*, 1965; Pentschew, 1965; Krigman and Hogan, 1974; Clasen *et al.*, 1974), the renal system (Lilis *et al.*, 1969; Cramer *et al.*, 1974; Wedeen *et al.*, 1975), and the hematopoietic system (Waldron, 1964; Hernberg *et al.*, 1967, 1970; Paglia *et al.*, 1975). Although these three organ systems have historically been associated with lead poisoning, ample experimental or clinical data suggest that lead may exert a deleterious influence on the endocrine system (Wright *et al.*, 1975; Sandstead *et al.*, 1970), the immune system (Koller and Kovacic, 1974; Wilde *et al.*, 1974; Muller *et al.*, 1977; Faith *et al.*, 1979), the cardiovascular system (Sharrett and Feinleib, 1975; Stofen, 1974), and the reproductive system (Stowe and Goyer, 1971; Hilderbrand *et al.*, 1973; Varma *et al.*, 1974; Lancranjan *et al.*, 1975).

The U.S. Environmental Protection Agency has estimated that approximately 900,000 newborn children are at risk of lead intoxication from lead absorption via their mothers (EPA, 1977). The National Bureau of Standards (1976) has recently estimated that over 600,000 children have blood lead levels equal to or greater than 40 μg/dl. These findings are clearly a cause for concern in view of the incidious nature of lead, and many diverse manifestations of perinatal lead intoxication.

As with many environmental toxicants, the developing organism is very sensitive to lead poisoning (Lin-Fu, 1973; Jugo, 1977). The effects of lead on human development due to both childhood and occupational exposure have been extensively reviewed (Rosen and Sorell, 1978; Posner *et al.*, 1978; David *et al.*, 1979; Center for Disease Control, 1978; Gordon *et al.*, 1979; Timpo *et al.*, 1979; Angle and McIntire, 1979).

There is an extensive body of literature in the area of the toxic effects of lead on development. In the present article, we will present a basic current concept in lead poisoning to include only the transplacental toxicity and the teratogenicity of lead compounds.

B. Placental Transfer of Lead

The harmful effects of lead on the fertility and reproduction of humans as a result of occupational exposure have long been recognized (Lane, 1949). It is found that lead crosses the placenta readily producing an increase in blood lead levels in the fetus. The fetal blood lead levels correlate closely with that in the maternal blood (Clark, 1977; Roels *et al.*, 1978; Buchet *et al.*, 1978; Lauwerys *et al.*, 1978; Hubermont *et al.*, 1978). Although overt congenital lead intoxication was an infrequent finding (Angle and McIntire, 1964; Palmisano *et al.*, 1963; Ryu *et al.*, 1978; Timpo *et al.*, 1979), spontaneous abortion and fetal death as a result of lead exposure has been reported (Rom, 1976).

Kostial and Momcilovic (1974) injected tracer doses of ^{203}Pb and ^{47}Ca into pregnant rats and noted that the placental transport of ^{47}Ca was eight times greater than that of ^{203}Pb. These investigators postulated that either lead was transported by passive transfer or the rodent placenta acted as a partial barrier to the placental movement of lead. However, other investigators (McClain and Becker, 1975) reported detectable quantities of ^{210}Pb in the rat fetus only 2 minutes following intravenous injection of the tracer to the maternal system. Of the intravenously administered ^{210}Pb, 0.7% was found in the fetus when the tracer was given on the eleventh day of gestational age. This deposition of lead increased to 3.4% when the administration was given on day 20 (Green and Gruner, 1974). In a similar study, Carpenter (1974), using both scintillation and autoradiographic techniques, demonstrated the rapid transfer of ^{210}Pb across the rodent placenta. McClain and Siekierka (1975a,b) infused radiolabeled lead nitrate and ^{210}Pb-chelating compounds into rats on day 18 of pregnancy at a rate of 0.5 mg/kg/min. It was found that the Pb-chelated compounds (lead-EDTA, Pb-nitrolotriacetate, and Pb-penicillamine) are transferred across the placenta more readily than Pb^{2+} ions alone. However, the potential fetotoxicity of these lead-chelate complexes is less than that with free lead ions. It is postulated that the lead chelates are less tissue bound and are more rapidly cleared from the maternal blood.

The effects of lead inhalation with or without the presence of carbon monoxide on pregnant and nonpregnant rats were investigated by Prigge *et al.* (1977). It was found that although the lead storage capacity in the adult liver was lowered by the presence of 500 ppm carbon monoxide, the blood lead concentration of these animals was increased. Moreover, the lead level in the fetus was also increased with carbon monoxide inhalation. Such increased fetal lead levels might be related to the higher maternal blood lead level under the influence of carbon monoxide. In a study with pregnant and nonpregnant animals, Buchet *et al.* (1977) demonstrated that pregnancy remobilized lead stores in the female producing increased lead levels in the blood and soft tissues of both the mother and the neonates. Such lead redistribution was found to be associated with an increase in free tissue protoporphyrins (FTP) in the maternal liver, heart, and brain as well as in the neonatal liver.

C. Mammary Transfer of Lead

The use of the lactating dam as a vehicle for delivery of lead to neonatal rats and mice has been employed by many investigators (Pentschew and Garro, 1966; Michaelson and Sauerhoff, 1974). By such approach, most investigators failed to estimate the lead intake by the pups via the milk (Silbergeld and Goldberg, 1973; Brown, 1975; Maker *et al.*, 1975). By means of a radioactive tracer technique, Kostial and Momcilovic (1974) demonstrated that 10.1–14.2% of ^{203}Pb injected into female rats was transferred to the suckling pups via lactation, while transplacental transfer amounted to only 3%. There is some evidence indicating that the intestinal absorption of lead is also greatly enhanced by milk (Kello and Kostial, 1973). In view of this information, it is clear that mammary transfer may pose as a significant source of lead to the newborns.

D Teratogenic Effects of Lead

1. *Human Studies*

While it is certain that lead crosses human and animal placentas, the importance of lead as a human teratogen remains debatable. However, spontaneous abortion in human patients as a result of high lead exposure has been reported (Taussig, 1936; Wilson, 1966). Boulos (1976) reported that the incidence of miscarriage was three times higher in women who were occupationally exposed to lead than in the control population. Similar observations were also reported by Fahim *et al.* (1976). Early membrane ruptures were increased from 0.41 to 17% and the incidences of preterm delivery also increased from 3 to 13%.

2. *Animals Studies*

a. Rat. Rats are found to be relatively refractory to lead-induced teratologic changes. McClain and Becker (1975) reported that a single intravenous injection of lead nitrate (50–70 mg/kg during days 8–17 of gestation) crossed the placenta readily, but teratologic changes (urorectocaudal malformations) were observed only when the injections were administered on day 9 of pregnancy. Moreover, it was found that embryo- and fetotoxicity were most prominent when lead was administered on days 10–15. After day 16, the fetotoxic effects of lead were minimal. This study demonstrated the importance of gestational stage in the susceptibility of lead-induced fetotoxicity.

Kennedy *et al.* (1975) compared the teratogenic potentials of lead acetate (0 to 714 mg/kg) and tetraethyllead (TEL)(0–10 mg/kg) in the CD-1 mice and the COBS rats. The animals were exposed to these compounds for 10 days during the period of rapid organogenesis (days 5–15 for mice and days 6–16 for rats). Although fetal resorption and general retardation of development were observed, neither of these lead compounds caused gross congenital malformations.

Multigeneration studies involving rats fed with 250 ppm (Kimmel *et al.*, 1979) and 1000 ppm (Jessup, 1967) of lead also failed to demonstrate any detectable malformation in these generations. A recent study by Granahan and Huber (1979), however, successfully induced a variety of malformations in rat neonates by feeding the pregnant animals with a diet containing 1000 ppm of lead throughout pregnancy. McClain and Siekierka (1975a,b) evaluated the teratogenic and embryotoxic potential of lead nitrate and lead-chelator complexes (Pb-edetic acid, Pb-nitrolotriacetic acid, Pb-imidodiacetic acid, and Pb-penicillamine). It was reported that in the rat, lead-chelates were less teratogenic than free lead ions. This study implies that chelation may help to reduce the toxicity and teratogenicity of lead.

b. Mouse. Jacquet *et al.* (1975a,b) showed that a dietary intake of 0.25 to 0.5% lead acetate by female mice reduced the incidence of pregnancy and increased the frequency of spontaneous abortion. Subsequent studies by Jacquet (1976, 1977) and Jacquet *et al.* (1977) demonstrated that the failure of fetal implanation may be related to a deficiency of progesterone in the maternal plasma. These authors suggested that lead may depress the progesterone activity in the pregnant female and precipitate the instability of pregnancy. Wide and Nilsson (1977) examined the effect of lead chloride on embryonic development in the NMRI mouse. Three developmental stages were examined: the attachment of the blastocyst, the invasion of the trophoblast, and the formation of the primitive streak. It was found that the stage of trophoblast invasion was most susceptible to lead.

c. Hamster. Early work on lead-induced teratogenesis in the hamster was done using a noninbred strain. Lead salts were found to be very fetotoxic producing high incidence of tail bud abnormalities in the fetuses (Ferm and Carpenter, 1967; Ferm and Ferm, 1971). Detailed morphological investigation of these lead-induced tail lesions revealed that local edema, blisters, and hematomas played an important role in the pathogenesis of these malformations (Carpenter and Ferm, 1977). In a recent study Gale (1978) examined the teratologic response of five inbred and one noninbred strains of hamster to the toxicity of lead nitrate. It was concluded that four strains (three of the inbred and one noninbred strain) were susceptible to lead toxicity showing fetal resorptions, tailbud malformations, hydrocephalus, and skeletal defects. Two of the inbred strains, however, were relatively refractory to these effects. It was postulated that the yolk sac placenta played a role in regulating the amount of lead transfer from the maternal to the fetal system, and the amount of lead reaching the fetus would influence the outcome of fetotoxicity and malformation. The resistant strains apparently had a smaller placental transport of lead preventing a large amount of lead from reaching the developing fetus.

d. Other Animal Models. Lead has also been shown to be teratogenic in other animal species. Kruckenberg *et al.* (1976) reported that intravenous administration of lead acetate into pregnant prairie voles (*Microtus ochrogaster*) caused exencephaly and spina bifida at a dose level of 32 mg/kg. No teratogenic response was noted at dose levels of 8 or 16 mg/kg. Total fetal resorption was observed at dose level of 64 mg/kg.

Holcombe *et al.* (1976) exposed three generations of brook trout to lead (0.9–474 ng/liter of water) and reported severe spinal deformities (scoliosis) in second and third generations of the fish when the lead concentration was greater than 119 ng Pb/liter of water.

The ability of lead salts to interfere with morphogenesis and development of the chick embryo has long been recognized (Hammett and Wallace, 1928; Catizone and Gray, 1941). Gilani (1975) further demonstrated the teratogenic effects of lead by injecting 5–80 mg of lead salt into chick eggs. Even at the lowest dose level (5 mg Pb/egg), reduction of body size

(10%), deformation of neck (10%), and malformation of limbs (5%) and beak (5%) were observed. At dose level of 30 mg/Pb/egg or more, exocephalus, hydrocephalus, and microthalmia were observed. Similar observation was reported by Hirano and Kochen (1973). Such changes were believed to be related to an alteration in the cerebral vasculature of the chick embryo (Roy *et al.*, 1974). The incidence of lead-induced malformations in chicks embryos was found to be reduced by the addition of ascorbic acid (King and Liu, 1975). It is believed that ascorbic acid may act as a chelating agent binding to the lead ions thus reducing its toxic potential.

The teratogenicity of lead was, however, not observed in larger animal species such as rabbit (Jessup, 1967), cows (Shupe *et al.*, 1967), and sheep (James *et al.*, 1966; Sharma and Buck, 1976).

E. Behavioral Effects of Lead Poisoning

Behavioral toxicology in lead poisoning represents a very important aspect of the toxic impact of this metal. Because of the large body of literature and complexity involved with this area of research, it will be difficult to condense the information into any reasonable length in this portion of the article. The authors, therefore, feel that it is more beneficial for the readers to seek specific reviews in this area of toxicology (Repko and Corum, 1979; Jason and Kellogg, 1980).

V. Concluding Remarks

It can be stated that mercury, cadmium, and lead all have deleterious impacts on the development of the fetus; however, the specific fetotoxicity and teratogenicity of each of these metals differ. It is difficult to make any definitive conclusion or to extrapolate the animal findings to human situations. Many of the problems are associated with the differences in animal species used in the studies, the dose levels used, the chronicity of the intoxications, the gestational stages explored, and the lack of interdisciplinary (biochemical, morphological, physiological, and functional) correlations. Thus a direct comparison of the findings is almost impossible.

The phenomena of metal–metal interaction and metal–element interaction within maternal and fetal systems make the overall understanding of metal toxicology that much more complex. There is no doubt that metal-induced teratology represents one of the most important areas in toxicology. More investigation is needed to elucidate further the many intriguing but still unanswered questions related to metal-induced developmental abnormalies.

Acknowledgments

The authors wish to thank Ms. Cindy Flippo for her able assistance in the preparation of the manuscript. We also acknowledge the courtesy of Pathotox Publishers, Inc. for permission of reusing portions of the article which we have published in *Neurotoxicology*.

References

Ahokas, R. A., and Dilts, P. V. (1979). *Am. J. Obstet. Gynecol.* **135** (2), 219–222.

Amin-Zaki, L., Elhassani, S., Majeed, M. A., Clarkson, T. W., and Greenwood, M. (1974a). *Pediatrics* **54,** 587–595.

Amin-Zaki, L., Elhassani, S., Majeed, M. A., Clarkson, T. W., Doherty, R. A., and Greenwood, M. R. (1974b). *J. Pediatr.* **85,** 81–84.

Amin-Zaki, L., Majeed, M. A., Clarkson, T. W., and Greenwood, M. R. (1978). *Br. Med. J.* **1,** 613–616.

Angle, C. R., and McIntire, M. S. (1979). *Am. J. Dis. Child.* **108,** 436–445.

Baglan, R., Brill, A., Schulert, S., Wilson, D., Larsen, K., Dyer, N., Mansour, M., Schaffner, W., Hoffman, L., and Davis, J. (1974). *Environ. Res.* **8,** 64–70.

Bakir, F., Damluji, S. F., AminZaki, L., Murtadha, M., Khalidi, A., Al-Rawi, N.Y., Tikriti, S., Dhahir, H. I., Clarkson, T. W., Smith, J. C., and Doherty, R. A. (1973) *Science* **181,** 230–241.

Barr, M., Jr. (1972). *J. Pediatr.* **81,** 182.

Barr, M., Jr. (1973). *Teratology* **7,** 237–242.

Baumslag, N., Yeager, D., Levin, L., and Petering, H. (1974). *Arch. Environ. Health* **29,** 186

Berlin, M., and Ullberg, S. (1963). *Arch. Environ. Health* **7,** 72–79.

Blackman, S. S. (1937). *Bull. Johns Hopkins Hosp.* **61,** 1–61.

Boulos, B. M. (1976). "Special Problems of Lead in Women Workers," pp. 39–49. HEW Publ. NIDSH NO. 134.

Brown, D. R. (1975). *Toxicol. Appl. Pharmacol.* **32,** 628–637.

Brown, R. V., Zenick, H., Cox, V., Jr., and Fahim, M. S. (1972). *Fed. Proc.* **31,** 1907–1972.

Brubaker, P. E., Klein, R., Herman, S. P., Lucier, G. W., Alexander, L. T., and Long, M. D. (1973). *Exp. Mol. Pathol.* **18,** 253–280.

Bryce-Smith, D., Despande, R., Hughes, J., and Waldron, H. (1977). *Lancet* **1,** 1159.

Buchet, J. P., Lauwerys, R., Roels, H., and Hubermont, G. (1977). *Int. Arch. Occup. Environ. Health* **40,** 33–36.

Buchet, J. P., Roels, H., Hubermont, G., and Lauwerys, R. (1978). *Environ. Res.* **15** (3), 494–503.

Carpenter, S. J. (1974). *Environ. Health Persp.* **7,** 129–137.

Carpenter, S. J., and Ferm, V. H. (1977). *Lab. Invest.* **37,** 369–385.

Casterline, J. L., Jr., and Williams, C. H. (1972). *Bull. Environ. Contam. Toxicol.* **7,** 292–295.

Catizone, O., and Grey, P. (1941). *J. Exp. Zool.* **87,** 71–82.

Cavanagh, J. B., and Chen, F. C. K. (1971). *Acta Neuropathol.* **19,** 216–224.

Center for Disease Control (1978). "Preventing Lead Poisoning in Children, A Statement by the CDC," pp. 40–45. HEW, Washington, D. C.
Chang, L. W. (1977). *Environ. Res.* **14,** 329–379.
Chang, L. W., and Hartmann, H. A. (1972). *Exp. Neurol.* **35,** 122–137.
Chang, L. W., and Sprecher, J. A. (1976a). *Environ. Res.* **11,** 392–406.
Chang, L. W., and Sprecher, J. A. (1976b). *Environ. Res.* **12,** 218–223.
Chang, L. W., Mak, L. L., and Martin, A. H. (1976). *Environ. Res.* **11,** 305–309, 1976.
Chang, L. W., Desnoyers, P. A., and Hartmann, H. A. (1972a). *J. Neuropathol. Exp. Neurol.* **31,** 489–501.
Chang, L. W., Martin, A. H., and Hartmann, H. A. (1972b). *Exp. Neurol.* **37,** 62–67.
Chang, L. W., Desnoyers, P. A., and Hartmann, H. A. (1973). *Acta Neuropathol.* **23,** 77–83.
Chang, L. W., Reuhl, K. R., and Spyker, J. M. (1977a). *Environ. Res.* **13,** 171–185.
Chang, L. W., Reuhl, K. R., and Lee, G. W. (1977b). *Environ. Res.* **14,** 414–423.
Chang, L. W., Reuhl, K. R., and Wade, P. R. (1980). *In* "The Biogeochemistry of Cadmium in the Environment" (J. O. Nriagu, ed.), Wiley, New York (in press).
Chaube, S. (1973). *Arch. Environ. Health* **26,** 237–240.
Chernoff, N. (1973). *Teratology* **8,** 29–32.
Childs, E. A. (1973). *Arch. Environ. Health* **27,** 50–52.
Chiquoine, A. D. (1965). *J. Reprod. Fertil.* **10,** 263–265.
Choi, B. H., Lapham, L. W., Amin-Zaki, L., and Saleem, T. (1978). *J. Neuropathol. Exp. Neurol.* **37,** 719–733.
Clark, A. R. (1977). *Postgrad. Med. J.* **53,** 574–678.
Clasen, R. A., Hartmann, J. F., Starr, A. J., Oogen, P. S., Pandolfi, S., Laing, I., Becker, R., and Hass, G. M. (1974). *Am. J. Pathol.* **74,** 215–240.
Cramer, K., Goyer, R. A., Jogenburg, R., and Wilson, M. H. (1974). *Br. J. Ind. Med.* **31,** 113–127.
Criffin, and Nelson, J. H. K. (1975). *In* "Lead: Environmental Quality and Safety," Suppl. Vol. II, pp. 299–330. Academic Press, New York.
David, O. J., Clark, J., and Hoffman, S. (1979). *Arch. Environ. Health* **76,** 106–112.
Dencker, L. (1975). *J. Reprod. Fertil.* **44,** 461–471.
Deshimaru, M. (1969). *Seishin Shinkeigaku Zasshi* **71,** 506.
Donaldson, W. E. (1976). *Poultry Sci.* **55,** 2280–2284.
Dyer, R. S., Eccles, C. U., and Annau, Z. (1978). *Pharm. Biochem. Behav.* **8,** 137–141.
Environmental Protection Agency (1977). "Air Quality Criteria for Lead." Publ. No. EPA-600/8-77-017. Washington, D. C.
Eto, K., and Takeuchi, T. (1977). *Virchows Arch. B Cell Pathol.* **23,** 109–128.
Evans, H., Garman, R., and Weiss, B. (1977). *Toxicol. Appl. Pharmacol.* **41,** 15–33.
Fahim, M. S., Fahim, Z., and Hall, D. G. (1976). *Res. Commun. Chem. Pathol. Pharmacol.* **13,** 309–331.
Faith, R. E., Luster, M. I., and Kimmel, C. A. (1979). *Clin. Exp. Immunol.* **35,** 413–420.
Farris, F. F., and Smith, J. C. (1975). *Bull. Environ. Contam. Toxicol.* **13,** 451–455.
Ferm, V. (1971). *Biol. Neonate* **19,** 101–107.
Ferm, V. H., and Carpenter, S. J. (1967). *J. Exp. Mol. Pathol.* **7,** 208–213.
Ferm, V., and Carpenter, S. (1968). *Lab. Invest.* **18,** 429–432.
Ferm, V. H., and Ferm, D. W. (1971). *Life Sci.* **10,** 35–39.
Ferm, V. H., Hanlon, D. P., and Urban, J. (1969). *J. Embryol. Exp. Morphol.* **22,** 107–113.
Flick, D. F., Kraybill, H. F., and Dimitroff, J. M. (1971). *Environ. Res.* **4,** 71–85.
Fowler, B. A., and Woods, J. S. (1977). *Lab. Invest.* **36,** 122–130.

Fujita, M., and Takabatake, E. (1977). *Bull. Environ. Contam. Toxicol.* **18,** 205–209.
Fuyuta, M., Fujimoto, T., and Hirata, S. (1978). *Teratology* **18,** 353–366.
Gale, T. F. (1978). *Environ. Res.* **17,** 325–333.
Gale, T., and Ferm, V. (1974). *Biol. Neonate* **23,** 149–160.
Gale, T. F., and Hanlow, D. P. (1976). *Environ. Res.* **12,** 26–31.
Garcia, J. D., Yang, M. G., Wang, H. C., and Belo, P. S. (1974a). *Proc. Soc. Exp. Biol. Med.* **147,** 224–231.
Garcia, J. D., Yang, M. G., Belo, P. S., and Wang, J. H. C. (1974b). *Proc. Soc. Exp. Biol. Med.* **146,** 190–193.
Garrett, N. E., Garrett, R. J., and Archdeacon, J. W. (1972). *Toxicol. Appl. Pharmacol.* **22,** 649–654.
Gilani, S. H. (1975). *Pathol. Microbiol.* **42,** 188–195.
Gordon, M. C., Brown, S., Khosloa, V. N., and Hansen, L. S. (1979). *Oral Surg.* **47,** 500–512.
Goyer, R. A., and Rhyne, B. C. (1973). *Int. Rev. Exp. Pathol.* **12,** 1–77.
Granahan, P., and Huber, A. M. (1979). *Fed. Proc.* **37,** 895.
Green, M., and Gruener, N. (1974). *Res. Comm. Chem. Pathol. Pharmacol.* **8,** 735–738.
Greengard, J., Adams, B., and Berman, E. (1965). *J. Pediatr.* **66,** 707–711.
Greenwood, M. R., Clarkson, T. W., Doherty, R. A., Gates, A. H., Amin-Zaki, L., Elhassani, S., and Majeed, M. A. (1978). *Environ. Res.* **16,** 48–54.
Griffin, T. B., and Knelson, J. H. (1975). "Environmental Quality and Safety: Lead." Academic Press, New York.
Hammett, F. S., and Wallace, V. L. (1928). *J. Exp. Med.* **48,** 659–665.
Harada, Y. (1976). *Bull. Inst. Constitut. Med.* **25,** 1–60.
Harada, Y. (1977). *In* "Minamata Disease-Methylmercury poisoning in Minamata and Niigata, Japan" (T. Tsubaki and K. Irukayama, eds.). Elsevier, Amsterdam.
Harada, Y. (1968). *In* "Minamata Disease" (M. Kutsuna, ed.). Kumamoto Univ., Japan.
Harris, S. B., Wilson, J. G., and Printz, R. H. (1972). *Teratology* **6,** 139–142.
Hernberg, S., Nurminen, M., and Hasan, J. (1967). *Environ. Res.* **1,** 247–261.
Hernberg, S. J., Nikkanen, G., Mellen, G., and Lilius, H. (1970). *Arch. Environ. Health* **21,** 141–145.
Hilderbrand, D. C., Der, R., Griffin, W. T., and Fahim, M. S. (1973). *Am. J. Obstet. Gynecol.* **115,** 1058–1065.
Hirano, A., and Kochen, J. (1973). *Lab. Invest.* **29,** 659–668.
Holcombe, G. W., Benoit, D. A., Leonard, E. N., and McKim, J. M. (1976). *J. Fish. Res. Board Can.* **33,** 1731–1741.
Hubermont, G., Buchet, J. P., Roels, H., and Lauwerys, R. (1978). *Int. Arch. Occup. Environ. Health* **41,** 117–124.
Hughes, J. A., and Annau, Z. (1976). *Pharm. Biochem. Behav.* **4,** 385–391.
Hunter, D., and Russell, D. (1954). *J. Neurol. Neurosurg. Psychiat.* **17,** 235–241.
Hunter, D., Bomford, R., and Russell, D. (1940). *Q. J. Med.* **9,** 193–213.
Jacquet, P. (1977). *Arch. Pathol. Lab. Med.* **101,** 461–463.
Jacquet, P. (1976). *Soc. Biol. Fil.* **170,** 1319–1322.
Jacquet, P., Leonard, A., and Gerber, G. B. (1975a). *Toxicology* **6,** 129–132.
Jacquet, P., Leonard, A., and Gerber, G. B. (1975b). *Experientia* **31,** 1312–1313.
Jacquet, P., Gerber, G. B., and Maes, J. (1977). *Bull. Environ. Contam. Toxicol.* **18,** 271–277.
Jason, K. M., and Kellogg, C. K. (1980). *In* "Lead Toxicity" (R. L. Singhal and J. A. Thomas, eds.), pp. 241–271. Urban and Schwarzenberg, Baltimore, Maryland.

James, L. F., Lazar, V. A., and Binns, W. (1966). *Am. J. Vet. Res.* **27,** 132–135.
Jessup, D. C. (1967). "Lead Acetate. Teratology Study in Rabbits." U.S. National Technical Information Service Rep. Pb-201. Washington, D.C.
Jugo, S. (1977). *Environ. Res.* **13,** 36–46.
Kello, D., and Kostial, K. (1973). *Environ. Res.* **6,** 355–360.
Kelman, B. J., and Sasser, L. B. (1977). *Toxicol. Appl. Pharmacol.* **39,** 119–127.
Kelman, B. J., and Walter, B. K. (1977). *Proc. Soc. Exp. Biol. Med.* **156,** 68–71.
Kennedy, G. L., Arnold, D. W., and Calandra, J. C. (1975). *Food Cosmet. Toxicol.* **13,** 629–632.
Khera, K. S. (1973). *Teratology* **8,** 293–304.
Khera, K. S., and Nera, E. A. (1971). *Teratology* **14,** 233.
Khera, K. S., and Tabacova, S. A. (1973). *Food Cosmet. Toxicol.* **11,** 245–254.
Kimmel, C. A., Grant, L. D., West, G. L., Martinez-Vargas, C. M., McConnell, E. G., Fowler, B. A., Woods, J. S., and Howard, J. L. (1979). *In* "Department of Energy Symposium Series No. 47: Developmental Toxicity of Energy Related Pollutants," pp. 396–409. D.O.E., Washington, D.C.
King, D. W., and Liu, J. (1975). *Fed. Proc.* **34,** 1049.
King, R. B., Robkin, M. A., and Shepard, T. H. (1976). *Teratology* **13,** 275–280.
Kjellstrom, T., Friberg, L., Nordberg, G., and Piscator, M. (1971). *In* "Cadmium in the Environment" (L. Friberg, M. Piscator, and G. Nordberg, eds.), pp. 140–152. CRC Press, Cleveland, Ohio.
Koller, L. D., and Kovacic, S. A. (1974). *Toxicol. Appl. Pharmacol.* **29,** 139.
Koos, B. J., and Longo, L. D. (1976). *Am. J. Obstet. Gynecol.* **126,** 390–409.
Kostial, K., and Momcilovic, B. (1974). *Arch. Environ. Health* **29,** 28–30.
Krigman, M. R., and Hogan, E. L. (1974). *Environ. Health Persp.* **7,** 187–199.
Kruckenberg, S. M., Dennis, S. M., Leipold, H. W., Oehme, F. W., and Cook, J. E. (1976). *Vet. Toxicol.* **18,** 58–60.
Kurland, L. T., Faro, S., and Siedler, H. (1960). *World Neurol.* **1,** 370–395.
Lancranjan, I., Popescu, H. I., Gacaescu, O., Klepsch, I., and Serbanescu, M. (1975). *Arch. Environ. Health* **30,** 395–401.
Lane, R. E. (1949). *Br. J. Ind. Med.* **6,** 125–129.
Lauwerys, R., Buchet, J. P., Roels, H., and Hubermont, G. (1978). *Environ. Res.* **15** (2), 278–289.
Lilis, R., Gavrilesu, N., Nestorescu, B., Durimtiuand, C., and Roventa, A. (1969). *Br. J. Ind. Med.* **25,** 196–202.
Lin-Fu, J. S. (1973). *N. Engl. J. Med.* **289,** 129–1233.
Lown, B. A., Morganti, J. B., Stineman, C. H., and Massaro, E. J. (1977). *Gen. Pharm.* **8,** 97–101.
Lucis, O. J., Lucis, R., and Shaikh, Z. A. (1971). *Proc. Can. Fed. Biol. Soc.* **14,** 52.
Lucis, O. J., Lucis, R., and Shaikh, Z. A. (1972). *Arch. Environ. Health* **25,** 14–22.
McClain, R. M., and Becker, B. A. (1975). *Toxicol. Appl. Pharmacol.* **31,** 72–82.
McClain, R. M., and Siekierka, J. J. (1975a). *Toxicol. Appl. Pharmacol.* **31,** 443–451.
McClain, R. M., and Siekierka, J. J. (1975b). *Toxicol. Appl. Pharmacol.* **31,** 343–442.
Maker, H. S., Lehrer, G. M., and Silides, D. J. (1975). *Environ. Res.* **10,** 76–91.
Mansour, M. M., Dyer, N. C., Hoffman, L. H., Schulert, A. R., and Brill, A. B. (1973). *Environ. Res.* **6,** 479–484.
Mansour, M. M., Syer, N. C., Hoffman, L. H., Davies, J., and Brill, A. B. (1974). *Am. J. Obstet.* **119,** 557–562.
Matsumoto, H., Koya, G., and Takeuchi, T. (1964). *J. Neuropathol. Exp. Neurol.* **24,** 563–574.

Mennear, J. H. (1969). "Cadmium Toxicity," Dekker, New York.
Menon, N., Lopez, R. R., and Kark, R. A. P. (1978). 8th Annual Meeting of Soc. Neuroscience, A1020.
Michaelson, I. A., and Sauerhoff, M. W. (1974). *Toxicol. Appl. Pharmacol.* **28,** 88–96.
Miyakawa, T., Murayama, E., Sumiyoshi, S., Deshimaru, M., Fujimoto, T., Hattori, E., and Shikai, I., (1976). *Acta Neuropathol.* **35,** 131–138.
Moriyama, H. (1967). *J. Kumamoto Med. Soc.* **41,** 506.
Muller, S., Gilbert, K. E., Krause, C., Gross, U., L'Age, J., and Diamantstein, T. (1977). *Experientia* **35,** 667–668.
Mulvihill, J., Gamm, S., and Ferm, V. (1970). *J. Embryol. Exp. Morphol.* **24,** 393–403.
Murakami, U. (1972). *Adv. Exp. Med. Biol.* **27,** 301–336.
Musch, H. R., Bornhausen, M., Kriegel, H., and Greim, H. (1978). *Arch. Toxicol.* **40,** 103–108.
National Academy of Sciences (1972). "Lead: Airborne lead in Perspective," pp. 330–381. National Academy of Science Publication, New York.
National Bureau of Standards (1976). "Survey Manual for Estimating the Incidence of lead Paint in Housing." NBS Technical Note 921. Washington, D.C.
National Research Council of Canada (1978). "Effects of lead in the Environment." NRCC No. 16736, 779.
Nordberg, G. F. (1976). "Effects and Dose-response Relationships of Toxic Metals." Elsevier, Amsterdam.
Nriagu, J. O. (1978). "The Biogeochemistry of Lead in the Environment. Parts A and B." Elsevier/North-Holland, Amsterdam.
Null, D. H., Gartside, P. S., and Wei, E. (1973). *Life Sci.* **12,** 65–72.
Olson, F. C., and Massaro, E. J. (1977a). *Toxicol. Appl. Pharmacol.* **39,** 263–273.
Olson, F. C., and Massaro, E. J. (1977b). *Teratology* **16,** 187–194.
Omata, S., Sakimura, K., Tsubaki, H., and Sugano, H. (1978). *Toxicol. Appl. Pharmacol.* **44,** 367–378.
Paglia, D. E., Valentine, W. H., and Dahlgnen, J. G. (1975). *J. Clin. Invest.* **56,** 1164–1169.
Palmisano, P. A., Sneed, R. C., and Cassady, G. (1963). *J. Pediatr.* **75,** 869–873.
Parizek, J. (1957). *J. Endocrinol.* **15,** 56–63.
Parizek, J. (1964). *J. Reprod. Fertil.* **7,** 263–265.
Parizek, J. (1965). *J. Reprod. Fertil.* **9,** 111–112.
Parizek, J., Ostadalova, I., Benes, I., and Babicky, A. (1968). *J. Reprod. Fertil.* **16,** 507–509.
Pentschew, A. (1965). *Acta Neuropathol.* **5,** 133–160.
Pentschew, A., and Garro, F. (1966). *Acta Neuropathol.* **6,** 266–278.
Pitkin, R. M., Bahns, J. A., Filer, L. J., Jr., and Reynolds, W. A. (1976). *Proc. Soc. Exp. Biol. Med.* **151,** 565–567.
Popoff, N., Weinberg, S., and Feignin, I. (1963). *Neurology* **13,** 101–112.
Posner, H. S., Damstra, T., and Nriagu, J. O. (1978). *In* "The Biogeochemistry of Lead in the environment" (J. O. Nriagu, ed.), Part B, pp. 173–224. Elsevier/North-Holland, Amsterdam.
Prigge, E., Baumert, H. P., Hochainer, D., and Oberdoerster, G. (1977). *Prev. Med.* **165,** 283–293.
Repko, J. D., and Corum, C. R. (1979). "Critical Review and Evaluation of the Neurological and Behavioral Sequelae of Inorganic Lead Absorption." CRC Crit. Rev. Toxicol.
Reuhl, K. R., and Chang, L. W. (1979). *Neurotoxicology* **1,** 21–55.
Reynolds, W. A., and Pitkin, R. M. (1975). *Proc. Soc. Exp. Med.* **148,** 523–526.
Robbins, M. S., Hughes, J. A., Sparber, S. B., and Mannering, G. J. (1978). *Life Sci.* **22,** 287–294.

Roels, H., Hubermont, G., Buchet, J. P., and Lauwerys, R. (1978). *Environ. Res.* **16,** (1–3), 236–247.

Rohrer, S. R., Shaw, S. M., and Van Sickle, D. C. (1969). *In* "Cadmium Toxicity" (J. H. Mennear, ed.), pp. 159–171. Dekker, New York.

Rohrer, S. R., Shaw, S. M., Born, G. S., and Vetter, R. J. (1978). *Bull. Environ. Contam. Toxicol.* **19,** 556–563.

Rohrer, S. R., Shaw, S. M., and Lamar, C. H. (1979). *Bull. Environ. Contam. Toxicol.* **23,** 25–29.

Rom, W. N. (1976). *Mt. Sinai J. Med.* **43,** 542–560.

Rosen, J. F., and Sorell, M. (1978). In "The Biogeochemistry of Lead in the Environment" (J. O. Nriagu, ed.), Part B, pp. 151–172. Elsevier/North-Holland, Amsterdam.

Roy, S., Hirano, A., Kochen, J. A., and Zimmerman, H. M. (1974). *Acta Neuropathol.* **30,** 287–294.

Ryu, E. J., Ziegler, E. E., and Fomon, S. J. (1978). *J. Pediatr.* **93,** 476.

Sandstead, H. H., Michelakis, A. M., and Temple, T. E. (1970). *Arch Environ. Health* **20,** 356–363.

Scanlon, J. (1972). *Clin. Pediatr.* **11** (3), 135–141.

Schroeder, H. A., and Balassa, J. J. (1961). *J. Chron. Dis.* **14,** 236–258.

Schroeder, H., Mitchner, M., and Brattleboro, V. (1971). *Arch. Environ. Health* **23,** 102–106.

Sharma, R. M., and Buck, W. B. (1976). *Vet. Toxicol.* **18,** 186–188.

Sharrett, A. R., and Feinleib, M. (1975). *Prev. Med.* **4,** 20–36.

Shupe, J. L., Binns, W., James, L. F., and Keeler, R. F. (1967). *J. Am. Vet. Med. Assc.* **151,** 198–203.

Silbergeld, E. K., and Goldberg, A. M. (1973). *Life Sci.* **13,** 1275–1283.

Snell, K., Ashby, S. L., and Barton, S. J. (1977). *Toxicology* **8,** 277–283.

Snyder, R. D. (1971). *N. Engl. J. Med.* **284,** 1014–1016.

Sonawane, B. R., Nordberg, M., Nordberg, G. F., and Lucier, G. W. (1975). *Environ. Health Persp.* **12,** 97–102.

Spyker, J. M. (1975). *Fed. Proc.* **34,** 1835–1844.

Spyker, J. M., and Smithberg, M. (1972). *Teratology* **5,** 181–190.

Spyker, J. M., Sparber, S. B., and Goldberg, A. M. (1972). *Science* **177,** 621–623.

Stofen, D. (1974). *J. Mol. Cell. Cardiol.* **6,** 285–290.

Stowe, H. D., and Goyer, R. A. (1971). *Fertil. Steril.* **22,** 755–760.

Su, M., and Okita, G. T. (1976a). *Toxicol. Appl. Pharmacol.* **38,** 195–205.

Su, M., and Okita, G. T. (1976b). *Toxicol. Appl. Pharmacol.* **38,** 207–216.

Suzuki, T., Matsumoto, N., Miyama, T., and Katsunuma, H. (1967). *Ind. Health* **5,** 149–155.

Suzuki, T., Miyama, T., and Katsunuma, H. (1971). *Bull. Environ. Contam. Toxicol.* **5,** 502–508.

Syversen, T. L. M. (1977). *Neuropathol. Appl. Neurobiol.* **3,** 225–236.

Takeuchi, T. (1968). "Minamata Disease." Kumamoto Univ., Japan.

Takeuchi, T. (1977). *Pediatrician* **6,** 69–87.

Takeuchi, T., D'Itri, A. M., Fischer, P. V., Annett, C. S., and Okabe, M. (1977). *Environ. Res.* **13,** 215–228.

Tanaka, M., Matsusaka, N., Yuyama, A., and Kobayashi, H. (1972). *Radioisotopes* **21,** (1), 34–36.

Tatetsu, S., Takagi, M., and Miyakawa, T. (1968). *Psychiat. Neurol. (Jpn)* **70,** 162.

Taussig, F. J. (1936). "Abortion, Spontaneous and Induced." Kimpton, London.

Taylor, L. L., and DiStefano, V. (1976). *Toxicol. Appl. Pharmacol.* **38,** 489–497.

Tejning, S. (1968). Report No. 680529. University Clinic, Lund, Sweden.

Thuerauf, J., Schaller, K., Engelhardt, E., and Gossler, K. (1975). *Int. Arch. Occup. Health* **36,** 19–27.

Timpo, A. E., Amin, J. S., Casalino, M. B., and Yuceoglu, A. M. (1979). *J. Pediatr.* **94,** 765–767.

Tsubaki, T., and Irukayama, T. (1977). "Minamata Disease-Methylmercury Poisoning in Minamata and Niigata, Japan" Elsevier, Amsterdam.

Varma, M. M., Joshi, S. R., and Adeyemi, A. O. (1974). *Experientia* **30,** 486–487.

Verity, M. A., Brown, W. J., Cheung, M., and Czer, G. (1977). *J. Neurochem.* **29,** 673–679.

Waldron, H. A. (1964). *J. Clin. Pathol.* **17,** 405–406.

Waldron, H. A., and Stofen, D. (1974). "Subclinical Lead Poisoning." Academic Press, New York.

Wannag, A. (1976). *Acta Pharmacol. Toxicol.* **38,** 289–298.

Ware, R. A., Chang, L. W., and Burkholder, P. M. (1974). *Nature (London)* **251,** 236–237.

Webb, M. (1970). *J. Reprod. Fertil.* **30,** 99–103.

Wedeen, R. P., Maesaka, J. K., Weiner, B., Lipat, G. A., Lyons, M. M., Vitale, L. F., and Joselow, M. M. (1975). *Am. J. Med.* **59,** 630–641.

White, J. F., and Rothstein, A. (1973). *Toxicol. Appl. Pharmacol.* **26,** 370–384.

Wide, M., and Nilsson, O. (1977). *Teratology* **16,** 273–276.

Wilde, K., Chan, Y., and Joseph, J. M. (1974). *Am. Soc. Microbiol.* **74,** 134–135.

Wilson, J. T. (1966). *Scott. Med. J.* **11,** 73–82.

Wolkowski, R. M. (1974). *Teratology* **10,** 243–262.

World Health Organization (1976). "Conference on Intoxication due to Alkylmercury-treated Seed." Suppl. to Vol. 53. WHO. Geneva.

Wright, G. L., Lessler, M. A., and Iams, S. G. (1975). *Ohio J. Sci.* **75,** 155–161.

Yamaguchi, S., and Nunotani, H. (1974). *Environ. Physiol. Biochem.* **4,** 7–15.

Yang, M. G., Krawford, K. S., Garcia, J. D., Wang, J. H., and Lei, K. Y. (1972). *Proc. Soc. Exp. Med. Biol.* **141,** 1004–1007.

Yang, M. G., Wang, J. H., Garcia, J. D., Post, E., and Lei, K. Y. (1973). *Proc. Soc. Exp. Biol. Med.* **142,** 723–726.

Yoshino, Y., Mozai, T., and Nakao, K. (1966). *J. Neurochem.* **13,** 1223–1231.

Zenick, H., Wright, D. C., and Brown, R. V. (1973). *Fed. Proc.* **32,** 3563.

ADVANCES IN PHARMACOLOGY AND CHEMOTHERAPY, VOL. 17

Salicylates: Molecular Mechanism of Therapeutic Action

DAVID C. ATKINSON[1]

Pharmacology Section, Toxicology Department
Corporate Research Division, Miles Laboratories, Inc.
Elkhart, Indiana

HARRY O. J. COLLIER

Research Department
Miles Laboratories, Ltd.
Stoke Poges, Slough, England

[1] Formerly of the Department of Pharmacology, Reckitt & Colman Pharmaceutical Division, Dansom Lane, Hull HU8 7DS, England.

ISBN 0-12-032917-4

I. General Aspects

A. Assumptions, Questions, and Answers

A wit once defined a drug as any substance that, given to an animal, produces a scientific paper. This definition contains much truth. We consider a drug to be a substance that is used because of its particular effects on living material, namely, its pharmacological effects. We assume that these effects are due to the drug's interaction with one, or more than one, physiological process at a molecular level, in other words, with a natural biochemical process.

We assume also that salicylates resemble many drugs in that they interact with a biochemical process, by binding with a specifically sensitive site (recognition site, active site) on a macromolecule (receptor, enzyme, etc.) that reacts to the bound molecule. For example, if the macromolecule is a receptor for an endogenous messenger substance (hormone, transmitter, mediator, modulator), binding of an endogenous molecule with its recognition site would lead to transmission of a message. Again, if the macromolecule is an enzyme, binding of a substrate molecule with its active site would lead to transformation of the substrate.

This step is particularly vulnerable to drugs, which often act by binding with a receptor intended for a natural substance, because they possess structural features resembling those of the natural substance. As a result of binding, the drug can either activate or inactivate a macromolecule. Thus, muscarine binds with a site on a macromolecule that naturally binds acetylcholine, and, in so doing, activates that macromolecule; whereas atropine binds with this site in a way that inactivates it. If we assume that salicylates have such a molecular mechanism of action, our ultimate task would be to identify the site or sites at which salicylates bind and the results of such binding. As a beginning, however, it would suffice to identify the biochemical process or processes whose inhibition or stimulation by aspirin or sodium salicylate leads to the therapeutic actions of these drugs.

Again, we assume that we are concerned with some of the more potent pharmacological effects of salicylates, namely, those for which they are used. We assume, furthermore, that these effects result from the interactions with biochemical processes that occur when a relatively low concentration of the drug is present at its site of action, because these will happen when other interactions do not. This means, in the terms discussed above, that binding sites with a high affinity for the drug will be those involved in its main therapeutic actions or side-effects. Finally, we assume that the main therapeutic forms in which salicylates are used—aspirin and sodium salicylate—act on the same biochemical process(es), although each may act in its own right and possess different degrees of activity.

Having assumed that salicylates act by affecting a natural biochemical process, through binding with a site on a macromolecule that conducts some part of this process, we discuss the method of identifying this molecular event. We then consider a series of questions concerning the nature of salicylate action, the answers to which lead toward the identification of the critical event. Next, we try, in Section II of this article, to identify the critical action of salicylates and to see how this explains their pharmacological effects. Finally, we consider what insights into the biochemistry and physiology of the body are given by this analysis of the mechanism of action of salicylates.

The answers to these questions have been or are being produced by the theoretical and experimental work of many independent, yet interconnected groups of research workers. The answers produced in this way are never complete, nor do they command total agreement, but rather a consensus of opinion. These answers always lead to fresh questions. Our aim in this article cannot therefore be more than to scan the mechanism of action of the salicylates, while the general understanding of this mechanism is increasing; to take, as it were, a cross-section of this growing branch of knowledge, without stopping its growth.

B. Identifying the Mechanism of Action of a Drug

As we have seen, the molecular mechanism of action of a drug usually involves its binding with a site on a macromolecule that normally takes part in an endogenous biochemical process. To identify this process, it is necessary to study effects of the drug *in vitro,* usually both in isolated organs or tissues and in preparations of cells or homogenates of cells. Findings *in vitro* must then be matched with pharmacological effects *in vivo*. The main criteria of a good match are as follows:

1. The effect of the drug *in vitro* should be such that it would give rise to the pharmacological properties *in vivo*. For example, if the drug is supposed to act by reducing the concentration of an endogenous messenger substance, the substance should itself produce the effect that the drug counteracts.
2. The concentration of drug required to give the effect *in vitro* should correspond with that in the responding tissue *in vivo*.
3. The time-courses of effects of the drug *in vitro* and *in vivo* should likewise correspond, after taking into account factors peculiar to the situation *in vivo*.

4. Drugs having a similar spectrum of activity *in vivo* should show the corresponding effect *in vitro,* and drugs not having that spectrum should not.

5. In a group of like-acting drugs, relative potencies *in vitro* and *in vivo* should correspond, all other factors (biodistribution and metabolism) being taken into account.

6. If the effect of the drug *in vitro* is to inhibit a biosynthetic process, then the drug should lower the concentration of the active product of that process and that product should antagonize the drug *in vivo*.

7. Antagonists of the effect of the drug *in vitro* should also antagonize its pharmacological action *in vivo* and vice versa.

8. If the drug is the active member of a pair of enantiomers, the same relative activity should be observable *in vitro* and *in vivo*.

9. Divergencies from any of these criteria should be readily explicable.

In any investigation of the mechanism of action of a drug, the limitations of *in vitro* methods of assessment and the inherent pitfalls of extrapolation to the *in vivo* situation must not be underestimated. Detailed knowledge concerning the pharmacokinetic properties and biotransformation of the drug in the species in which it exerts its therapeutic actions is needed before such extrapolations can be valid. This is particularly important in the case of the salicylates, since they are extensively bound to plasma albumin and since aspirin is quickly converted to the salicylate ion *in vivo*.

The capacity of a drug to bind with macromolecules relates also to its duration of action. If a drug acts by binding with a receptor, its duration of action may be expected to depend on how long it remains bound. This, in turn, will depend, on the one hand, on the nature of the binding and, on the other hand, on the forces tending to remove the drug from the binding site and from the body fluid bathing the site. If a drug binds firmly to a site at which it is not readily destroyed, or if binding produces a prolonged or irreversible inactivation of the receptor, the drug's action may last long after it has disappeared from the body fluids.

C. Character of Therapeutic Actions of Salicylates

At first sight, the antipyretic, analgesic, and antiinflammatory effects, for which aspirin is so widely taken, appear diverse and unconnected. An underlying connection exists, however, in that all these effects can be characterized as "antidefensive," since fever, pain, and inflammation are natural defensive mechanisms (Collier, 1963, 1969a). Not only the main therapeutic actions of salicylates, but other actions also can be regarded as "antidefensive." Thus, aspirin inhibits contraction of the smooth muscle of the airways, which may be regarded as a defensive response to irritants (Collier, 1968). Likewise, aspirin inhibits secretion of gastric mucus (Menguy and Masters, 1965), which may also be deemed defensive. Again, aspirin blocks the rise in free fatty acids of the blood provoked by cold or fasting, which Bizzi *et al.* (1965) regard as a response to emergency.

A drug that is "antidefensive" might be expected to act only when a defensive process is in operation. In other words, an antidefensive drug should restrain pathological rather than physiological processes. This is at least partly true of aspirin. For example, it lowers body temperature raised in response to infection, but not normal body temperature in man. In acting only in a situation that requires it, aspirin might be described as having a "servo" property.

If defensive reactions are designed to protect the body against threatening influences or invasive parasites, it might seem wrong to inhibit them. There are situations, however, where inhibition of defensive reactions can be therapeutic (Collier, 1974b). Such situations may be of two types. First, where the reaction would be useful if it were limited, but has become excessive in degree or duration, as can occur with itch, pain, cough, inflammation, diarrhea, vomiting, and fever. Second, where the defensive reaction is misguided, as in allergy, rheumatic fever, or autoimmune disease. In either situation, a defensive reaction can itself be fatal, although more usually it is distressing rather than dangerous. Salicylates do not necessarily inhibit all these defensive reactions; they undoubtedly inhibit some of them. The commonness with which aspirin is used bears witness to its effectiveness against these reactions, to the distress that they produce, and to the need that human beings feel to restrain the body from overreacting to produce "too much of a good thing."

D. Bioactive Chemical Forms

1. *Sodium Salicylate*

In considering the mechanism of action of sodium salicylate and aspirin, we need to know whether the activity *in vivo* is due to the drug molecule itself or to a metabolite. It has been believed, at least since Dreser (1899), that the salicylate ion is itself active, but this view has been challenged by several investigators. One reason for this challenge is the discrepancy between the potency of sodium salicylate as an inhibitor of prostaglandin biosynthesis *in vitro* and its potency as an antiinflammatory agent *in vivo*. This point will be discussed in Section II,D.

A second reason for this challenge is the activity of some metabolites of salicylates, such as gentisic and γ-resorcylic acids. Lim (1966) reviewed this question, however, and concluded that at least the analgesic activity of the salicylate ion does not depend on any of its metabolites.

A third reason arises from the suggestion that the salicylate ion could form a more active chelate with ions of heavy metals present in the tissues (Chenoweth, 1956; Sorenson, 1974a,b, 1976a,b). In particular, Sorenson has shown that copper chelates of various antiinflammatory agents are more active than their respective ligands in experimental models of inflammation. Bonta (1969) has found, however, that copper-containing compounds having antiinflammatory activity also caused marked irritation at the site of injection, whereas those without such activity were not irritant. This provides the alternative explanation that the greater activity of copper chelates is due to counterirritation. This alternative is supported by Rainsford and Whitehouse (1976), who showed that, when both drugs were administered parenterally, copper salicylate was more irritant as well as being more active than was sodium salicylate against carrageenin edema of rat paw. They further showed that, by mouth, copper aspirinate was no more active against paw edema than was aspirin. These findings have been essentially confirmed in other laboratories (Williams *et al.*, 1976; D. C. Atkinson, unpublished observations; Lewis, 1978). The reduced oral potency of copper aspirinate could be due to the fact that oral administration less readily produces counterirritant effects than does parenteral (Benitz and Hall, 1963); but, as Rainford and Whitehouse (1976) suggested, it could alternatively result from dissociation of the chelate at gastric pH. Disproof of Sorenson's hypothesis therefore remains incomplete; but nonetheless the hypothesis seems unlikely to be true.

2. *Aspirin*

Does aspirin act in its own right, as the acetylsalicylate ion; does it act as the salicylate ion to which it is in time converted in the body; or does it act in both forms? Dreser (1899) showed that aspirin was converted to the salicylate ion *in vivo* and he believed that the latter was the active form. His belief was challenged more than 40 years later by Lester *et al.* (1946), who observed that the analgesic action of aspirin in man could be correlated with the presence in the blood plasma of the acetylsalicylate, rather than the salicylate ion.

By now, there is good evidence to support the view expressed by Lester and co-workers in 1946, particularly where aspirin is more active than sodium salicylate. Much of this evidence has been reviewed (Collier, 1969a), with the conclusion that aspirin is effective in its own right, at least in certain actions, notably as an analgesic. This conclusion is supported by the finding of Vane (1971) that aspirin is considerably more active than sodium salicylate in inhibiting prostaglandin synthesis by guinea pig lung homogenate.

The higher activity of aspirin, compared with sodium salicylate, might be accounted for by (1) the reactivity of the acetyl group (Pinckard *et al.*, 1968), (2) the lower plasma protein binding capacity (Lester *et al.*, 1946), or (3) some other factor.

It would also be expected that the salicylate ion into which aspirin is converted would contribute to the overall activity of aspirin. This is probably true in most situations; but occasionally it has been observed that aspirin and sodium salicylate may be mutually antagonistic (Ezer *et al.*, 1976).

E. Are Salicylates Stimulatory or Inhibitory?

If the net effect of salicylates is to lessen an inflammatory or other defensive response, do they achieve this directly by inhibiting a stimulatory process, or indirectly, by stimulating (or activating) an endogenous mechanism that inhibits defensive responses? If the latter, what is this endogenous inhibitory mechanism? At present, four possible mechanisms may be suggested. First, salicylates might augment adrenal activity, by releasing glucocorticoid or catecholamine antiinflammatory hormones. Second, salicylates might increase the concentration of an endogenous opioid that lessens pain and hyperalgesia. Third, salicylates might act through the recently discovered endogenous inhibitors of prostaglandin synthetase (EIPS). Fourth, salicylates might activate a counterirritant mechanism.

The suggestion that salicylates might act by augmenting glucocorticoid or epinephrine release has previously been discussed (Collier, 1969a; Domenjoz, 1971). Two facts argue strongly against such a possibility. First, the profile of pharmacological action of each hormone differs clearly from that of salicylates. Second, the adrenal hormones act systemically, whereas the salicylates act locally, as indicated, for example, by the different ratios of potency of aspirin and sodium salicylate in different pharmacological actions (see below).

The recent discovery of the endogenous opioid peptides (endorphins, enkephalins), which the opiate drugs mimic (Goldstein, 1976; Frederickson, 1977; Klee, 1977), raises the possibility that the analgesic action of aspirin derives from its stimulating or activating the release of these endogenous substances. This possibility, however, seems unlikely to be true, since morphine, which mimics them, and the opioids themselves, insofar as they have been tested, suppress responses to most types of noxious stimuli in experimental animals, whereas aspirin is effective only against a few types of nociception, such as those involving inflammatory processes (Randall and Selitto, 1957; Collier, 1964; Winter and Flataker, 1965).

The still more recent discovery that endogenous inhibitors of prostaglandin synthetase (EIPS) are present in the blood plasma and serum of adult mammals (Saeed *et al.*, 1977; Collier *et al.*, 1980) raises a third possibility—that salicylates act by increasing the level or activity of EIPS in the plasma. This again seems unlikely, however, since it would require that the ratio of potency of aspirin to sodium salicylate in different pharmacological effects would be constant. EIPS does provide, however, an endogenous mechanism that salicylates might be supposed to mimic locally.

The fourth possibility, that salicylates might act through a counterirritant mechanism, suggested by Jori and Bernardi (1966), is substantial, because salicylates can be irritant when administered systemically, and irritants can suppress, by counterirritation, some of the defensive reactions that salicylates also inhibit. Three arguments, however, diminish this possibility. First, counterirritation is only weakly evoked by oral administration of irritants, whereas salicylates are active by mouth. Second, the profile of antidefensive activities of counterirritants differs in several ways from that of salicylates. For example, the antinociceptive activity of counterirritants resembles that of morphine (Winter and Flataker, 1965; Hitchens *et al.*, 1967) which, incidentally, suggests that they may act by liberating endogenous opioid. Third, irritants, when administered at a site of inflammation, are proinflammatory, whereas salicylates, in this situation, are antiinflammatory (Goldstein *et al.*, 1966; Shanahan, 1968; Atkinson and Hicks, 1975).

To summarize this discussion, no convincing evidence has emerged that salicylates act by augmenting an endogenous mechanism restraining defensive reactions. On the contrary, there is convincing evidence, discussed below, that salicylates act locally and, in particular, that they inhibit the system of defensive reactions mediated by prostanoids and possibly also other local hormones.

F. Site of Action

The site of action of salicylates was much studied during the 1960s, and these studies were reviewed toward the end of that decade (Collier, 1969a). The conclusion was reached that salicylates exert their main effects locally, at or near the point where the defensive reaction that they inhibit is being generated. Three lines of evidence support this conclusion.

First, there are the classic cross-circulation experiments of Lim and colleagues (1964) in the dog. For example, in one series of experiments, aspirin readily suppressed nociception elicited by the injection of bradykinin into the splenic artery, when this drug was present in the blood reaching the spleen, but not when it was present in blood reaching only the head. Again, aspirin suppressed sensory action potentials in the splanchnic nerve, elicited by injecting bradykinin into the spleen.

Second, aspirin and sodium salicylate have markedly different potencies in different pharmacological actions. For example, against bradykinin-induced bronchoconstriction in the guinea pig, aspirin was considerably more potent than sodium salicylate (Collier and Shorley, 1960) whereas, in some antiinflammatory actions, their potencies were about equal.

Third, local action can be demonstrated in certain experimental situations. For example, in some isolated smooth muscle preparations, aspirin relaxed an established tone (Collier and Sweatman, 1968), presumably due to intramural generation of contractant substances, probably prostaglandins. Yet again, aspirin, taken orally, has effects on platelets in blood subsequently shed, that is, *ex vivo*.

These and other experiments argue that salicylates usually act locally rather than systemically. We should discuss further, however, two instances, fever and headache, where their therapeutic action may occur within the brain.

It appears to be established that body temperature is regulated by events occurring in the hypothalamus. The question therefore arises: do the salicylates exert their antipyretic effects within or outside the hypothalamus? It was suggested (Collier, 1969a) that salicylates might exert their antipyretic action outside the hypothalamus, either by inhibiting the release of endogenous pyrogen from leukocytes or by obstructing its passage into the brain. Three more recent experiments, however, contradict this suggestion.

First, Cashin and Heading (1968) showed that oral doses of aspirin were capable of inhibiting the fever induced by the intracerebral injection of "E" pyrogen (Organon) into mice. They considered that the injected pyrogen had a direct effect on the hypothalamus, rather than an indirect action through release of endogenous pyrogen.

Second, Feldberg and Gupta (1972) and Feldberg *et al*. (1973) showed that injection of bacterial pyrogen into a cerebral ventricle of the cat induces fever, associated with release of E prostaglandin into the cerebrospinal fluid (CSF), and that aspirin lowers this fever. This experiment sites the action of the salicylates inside the two outer membranes of the brain, but not necessarily within the inmost membrane, the pia mater, which lies between the CSF and the brain substance itself.

Third, microinjection of bacterial endotoxins into the anterior hypothalamus of the monkey produces a fever that is lowered by sodium salicylate, administered intragastrically (Myers *et al.*, 1974). Taken together, these experiments indicate that salicylates act within the brain, probably within the anterior part of the hypothalamus, to lower fever, probably elicited by the E prostaglandin produced in response to pyrogen.

Headaches are perceived centrally, but they can probably arise from more than one site, which is difficult to determine, because headache cannot be observed in experimental animals. A conventional view is that headache arises from mechanical changes in the cerebral blood vessels that could be due to vasoactive processes occurring at some distance from the blood vessels themselves. Whether or not headaches arise in this way, they can certainly arise from noxious stimulation of the envelopes of the central nervous system. For example, infection of the brain meninges or bleeding into the CSF may cause severe headache. Since we know that intravenous prostaglandins elicit headache and that prostaglandins are generated by bacterial toxins and in inflammation and tissue injury, it seems probable that prostaglandins contribute to the headaches arising from pathological changes in the brain meninges and CSF. The possibility also remains open that headache can arise from the prostaglandins that can be produced within the brain substance itself, since bacterial endotoxin induces headache, even before it produces fever (Sicuteri, 1970). It may be supposed that, wherever generation of prostaglandins produces headache, aspirin would relieve the headache by inhibiting this generation (see below).

II. Special Aspects

A. Introduction

In Section I, we reached the conclusion that the salicylates act primarily by local inhibition of defensive reactions. In Section II, we are concerned with defining (1) what biochemical processes involved in local defensive reactions the salicylates inhibit, and (2) how the salicylates exert this action.

The research done before the present decade on the mechanism of salicylate action which did not yield a clear answer has been reviewed by several authors (Whitehouse, 1965; Smith and Smith, 1966; Collier, 1969a; Domenjoz, 1971; Smith and Dawkins, 1971; Rooney *et al.*, 1973; Hichens, 1974) and hence will not be dealt with here in detail. In this article we are more concerned with current concepts and how these do, or do not, adequately explain some, if not all, of the therapeutic actions of salicylates.

B. Earlier Mechanisms Proposed

One of the earliest mechanisms proposed for salicylate action was that they uncouple oxidative phosphorylation, and thus reduce tissue levels of energy in the form of ATP. This proposal was first made by Adams and Cobb (1958) and was evaluated by Whitehouse (1965). It was based on the observations that salicylates, given to man, increased oxygen consumption (Cochran, 1952) and that the uncoupling activity of salicylates could be detected in respiring mitochondria (Brody, 1956). There are two main objections to this hypothesis: (1) 2,4-dinitrophenol is a potent uncoupler, yet is devoid of antiinflammatory activity *in vivo* (Adams and Cobb, 1958; Marks *et al.*, 1961; Whitehouse, 1965); and (2) an uncoupling action of sodium salicylate could not be demonstrated in inflamed tissues (Kalbhen *et al.*, 1967). Uncoupling of oxidative phosphorylation therefore probably does not account for the therapeutic actions of salicylates, although it might yet account for the hyperthermia of salicylate intoxication (Smith, 1963).

Another proposal was that salicylates and like-acting drugs act by inhibiting the denaturation of plasma proteins, since they inhibited heat denaturation of serum albumin (Mizushima, 1964; Mizushima and Suzuki, 1965). Hichens (1974), however, has shown that some drugs without antiinflammatory activity possess this property and, conversely, that some antiinflammatory drugs lack it. At the same time, Hichens argued that other manifestations of protein binding by these drugs were probably unrelated to their therapeutic actions.

In addition to stabilizing certain proteins, salicylates have been shown to stabilize lysosomal membranes *in vitro* (Miller and Smith, 1966; Ignarro, 1971). This action would inhibit the release of lysosomal enzymes, which are thought to participate in inflammation and in injury in rheumatoid joints (Weissmann, 1972). Despite many attempts, however, this effect has not been found to correlate with antiinflammatory action *in vivo* (Arrigoni-Martelli and Restelli, 1972; Ammendola *et al.*, 1975).

C. Interactions with Kinins and Other Mediators

The possibility that salicylates act by inhibiting the release or activity of a local hormone that elicits inflammation has long been canvassed (Winder, 1959; Collier, 1963, 1969a; Lim *et al.*, 1964; Rooney *et al.*, 1973). The available evidence appears to exclude interaction with histamine or serotonin; but aspirin does inhibit certain actions of kinins and slow-reacting substance in anaphylaxis (SRS-A) sufficiently potently to warrant serious consideration as a mechanism of action (Collier, 1963, 1969a). For example, aspirin curtailed the hypotension induced by bradykinin in several species (Turker and Kiran, 1964; Vargaftig, 1966; Collier *et al.*, 1968a). More strikingly, nonsteroidal antiinflammatory drugs suppressed bronchoconstriction induced by bradykinin or SRS-A in the guinea pig, whereas they did not antagonize the bronchoconstrictor effect of histamine, acetylcholine, serotonin, or $PGF_{2\alpha}$ (Collier and Shorley, 1960; Berry and Collier, 1964; Collier *et al.*, 1968b).

With very few exceptions, drugs outside the aspirin group did not show this activity. Moreover, the potency of the nonsteroidal antiinflammatory drugs correlated well with their therapeutic activity. When first reported, the main exception to this correlation was indomethacin, which had unexpectedly low potency. In recent tests, however, indomethacin exhibited

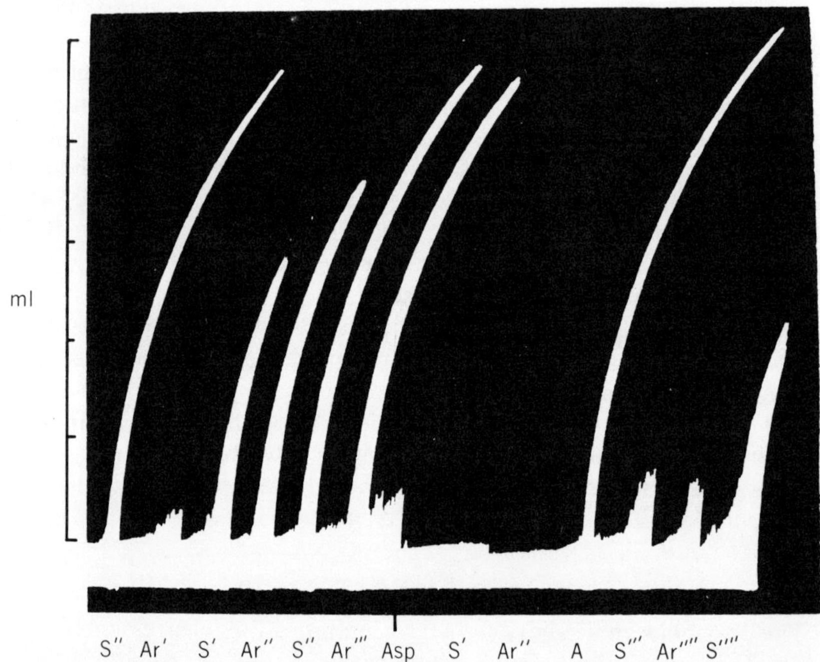

FIG. 1. Antagonism by acetylsalicylate of responses to arachidonic acid and SRS-A of the Konzett–Rössler preparation of guinea pig lungs *in vivo*. Responses are expressed as increase of air overflow volume, calibrated in milliliters; time scale, 10 seconds; guinea pig, 420 gm. S′, 9 units; S″, 18 units; S‴, 45 units; S⁗, 90 units of SRS-A. Ar′, 0.5 mg; Ar″, 1 mg; Ar‴, 2 mg; Ar⁗, 5 mg of arachidonic acid. Asp, 2 mg/kg of sodium acetylsalicylate. A, 5 μg of acetylcholine. All doses were given intravenously at 5-minute intervals. Reproduced from Berry (1966) with kind permission.

its expected high potency, the anomalous earlier result being attributed to the drug's rapid deterioration in alkaline solution (Saeed *et al.*, 1977).

In the early experiments showing that aspirin antagonizes bronchoconstriction induced by SRS-A in guinea pigs, it was also observed that aspirin was equally effective against arachidonic acid (Fig. 1), but not against several other unsaturated fatty acids (Berry, 1966; Collier, 1976). At that time, it was also shown that aspirin, although not sodium salicylate, antagonized contractions of guinea pig ileum elicited by arachidonic acid, but not by acetylcholine (Jaques, 1965). The full significance of these observations and of the failure of aspirin to antagonize $PGF_{2\alpha}$ on guinea pig lung (Berry and Collier, 1964) became evident some years later.

The antagonism of bradykinin by aspirin and like-acting drugs was, however, capricious. For example, aspirin did not antagonize bronchoconstriction induced by bradykinin in the rat nor that induced in the guinea pig by dropping bradykinin onto the pleural surface of the lungs, instead of injecting it intravenously (Bhoola *et al.*, 1962). It was, therefore, concluded that aspirin did not directly antagonize kinins, but blocked "a route leading to or from the specific receptors" (Collier *et al.*, 1966). Later it was suggested that aspirin acted by blocking the release of an intermediary substance, and it was pointed out that the prostaglandins might be involved (Collier, 1969a).

Such a substance came into view when Piper and Vane (1969) showed that isolated perfused guinea pig lungs, sensitized to ovalbumen, released on challenge with antigen, not only SRS-A, histamine, and prostaglandins E_2 and $F_{2\alpha}$, but also an unidentified substance that contracted rabbit aorta (RCS). An RCS-releasing factor (RCS-RF) was present along with RCS in the perfusate. Not only RCS-RF, but also bradykinin and SRS-A, when perfused through nonsensitized lungs, evoked a release of RCS.

Although the actions of RCS, SRS-A, and prostaglandins on the assay tissues were not inhibited by aspirin, Piper and Vane (1969) found that the release of RCS either by RCS-RF perfused through nonsensitized lungs or as a result of anaphylaxis in sensitized lungs was completely abolished by aspirin at low concentrations (1–5 μg/ml). The inhibition of release of RCS by aspirin was selective, since release of SRS-A, for example, was not inhibited. It was suspected that prostaglandin release was inhibited. Other nonsteroidal antiinflammatory agents were active, but sodium salicylate (5–100 μg/ml) was not. Furthermore, the order of potency of those drugs tested, which included indomethacin and mefenamate, was found to be similar to that observed in *in vivo* tests. This observation prompted Piper and Vane (1969) to speculate that RCS or RCS-RF might be involved in pain, fever, and inflammation. Moreover, their results helped to explain some of the effects of aspirin on bronchial muscle observed by

Collier and his colleagues. Hence, bronchoconstriction due to bradykinin and SRS-A could be interpreted as being mediated indirectly via RCS release, which was abolished by aspirin. In addition, the comparable differences in potency of aspirin and sodium salicylate on RCS release and on bronchoconstriction induced by bradykinin or SRS-A led Collier (1969b) to suggest that the release of RCS explained those *in vivo* actions in which aspirin is clearly more effective than sodium salicylate. Such actions might include analgesia and antipyresis, but would be unlikely to include antiinflammatory activity (See Section I,F).

RCS and prostaglandins were subsequently shown to be released also from chopped guinea pig lung which had been either challenged by antigen or mechanically agitated (Palmer *et al.*, 1970a) and from isolated sensitized guinea pig lungs perfused with particulate materials (Palmer *et al.*, 1970b). Vargaftig and Dao (1971) showed that RCS was also released by perfusing guinea pig lungs with arachidonic acid and the slow-reacting substance generated by cobra venom (SRS-C), and that this release was inhibited by aspirin and phenylbutazone.

Thus, by early 1971, it was becoming clear that there was some relationship between tissue damage, unsaturated fatty acids, and the release of RCS and prostaglandins. This relationship and the interaction of aspirin-like agents with this sequence of events now remained to be elucidated.

D. Inhibition of Prostanoid Biosynthesis

1. *The Prostaglandin Hypothesis Formulated*

Our understanding of the mechanism of action of aspirin-like drugs reached a deeper level when it was shown that these drugs inhibit prostaglandin synthesis in guinea pig lung homogenate (Vane, 1971), human platelets (Smith and Willis, 1971), and perfused dog spleen (Ferreira *et al.*, 1971). The essential observation had, however, been made by Piper and Vane (1969) 2 years earlier, when they showed that aspirin blocked release of RCS from guinea pig lung. These observations had been foreshadowed still earlier in the demonstrations (Fig. 1) that aspirin blocked the bronchoconstrictor action of arachidonate, but not of $PGF_{2\alpha}$ on guinea pig lungs *in vivo* (Berry and Collier, 1964; Berry, 1966; Collier, 1976) and paralleled by the observation that aminopyrine blocked the contraction of guinea pig ileum elicited by arachidonate, but not by PGE_1 *in vitro* (Jaques, 1965, 1969) (see Section II,C).

From the work described in the preceding section, Vane (1971) speculated that RCS was either a prostaglandin or had a structure intermediate between arachidonic acid and PGE_2 or $PGF_{2\alpha}$. Since the release of RCS could be antagonized by aspirin-like drugs (Piper and Vane, 1969; Vargaftig and Dao, 1971) and prostaglandin release could be equated with prostaglandin synthesis (Piper and Vane, 1971), Vane argued that these drugs might inhibit the enzymes that generate prostaglandins. He then showed that indomethacin (IC_{50}, 0.27 μg/ml), sodium aspirin (IC_{50}, 6.3 μg/ml) and, to a lesser extent, sodium salicylate inhibited the synthesis of PGE_2 and $PGF_{2\alpha}$ from arachidonic acid by cell-free homogenates of guinea pig lung (Fig. 2). Neither hydrocortisone, morphine, nor mepyramine, at 50 μg/ml, was an effective inhibitor. Furthermore, in the test preparations used, none of the aspirin-like drugs directly antagonized PGE_2 or $PGF_{2\alpha}$. Since it was already known that prostaglandins, given exogenously, could elicit fever (Milton and Wendlandt, 1970; Feldberg and Saxena, 1971a) and inflammation (Crunkhorn and Willis, 1971a) and that prostaglandins were generated during inflammation (Willis, 1969; Greaves *et al.*, 1971), Vane (1971) proposed that some of the therapeutic actions of sodium salicylate and of aspirin-like drugs are due to inhibition of the synthesis of prostaglandins. In particular, he suggested that the antipyretic and antiinflammatory actions could be explained in this way. Since, however, prostaglandins apparently did not produce pain on injection into man (Horton, 1963; Crunkhorn and Willis, 1971a), he considered

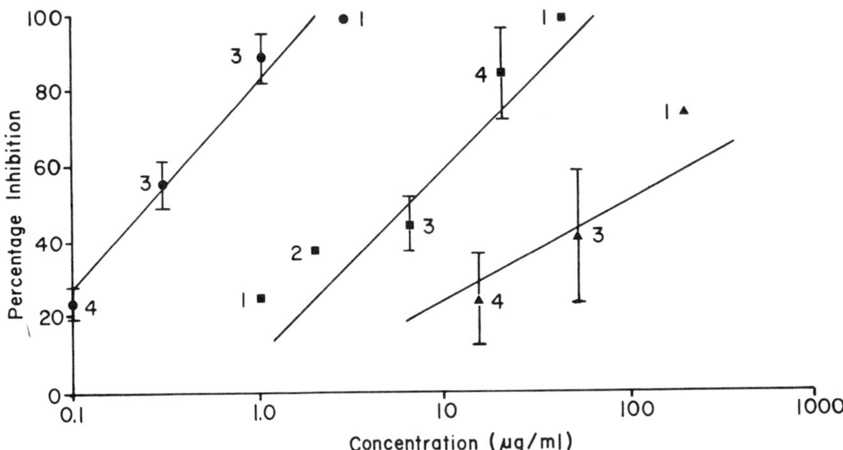

FIG. 2. Inhibitory effect *in vitro* of varying concentrations of indomethacin (●), aspirin (■), and sodium salicylate (▲) on prostaglandin synthesis (assayed as $PGF_{2\alpha}$ on rat colon) by guinea pig lung homogenates. The lines are those calculated for best fit. Numbers by the points indicate number of experiments. Reproduced from Vane (1971) with kind permission.

that the analgesic action of these drugs could be less easily explained by this hypothesis, unless another untested prostaglandin or RCS was involved.

Smith and Willis (1971) showed that platelets in the shed blood of volunteers who had taken aspirin (600 mg) or indomethacin (50 or 100 mg) could no longer produce prostaglandins when incubated with thrombin. Likewise, aspirin, indomethacin, and, to a much lesser extent, sodium salicylate, when added to platelet suspensions before addition of thrombin, inhibited prostaglandin production by the platelets. Their results likewise led them to conclude that the clinical effectiveness of aspirin and indomethacin could be explained by inhibition of prostaglandin production.

In the third of these three pioneering papers, Ferreira *et al.* (1971) showed that either aspirin or indomethacin, but neither sodium salicylate (at similar concentrations to those of aspirin) nor hydrocortisone, inhibited prostaglandin release from isolated dog spleen infused with epinephrine.

Thus, by mid-1971, aspirin-like drugs, at doses or concentrations that exert therapeutic activity, had been shown to interfere, both *in vitro* and *in vivo*, with an enzymatic process frequently occurring in stimulated tissues. Furthermore, this inhibition was characteristic of drugs of this group. Not only did these findings shed new light on the mechanism of action of aspirin-like agents, but they also showed that these drugs could be used as tools to elucidate the physiological and pathological roles of prostaglandins.

Another form of antiprostaglandin action by aspirin and like-acting drugs was first observed some time before the observation of their ability to inhibit prostaglandin synthetase. In human bronchial muscle *in vitro,* fenamates potently and phenylbutazone and aspirin less potently antagonize the contractant action of $PGF_{2\alpha}$ and PGE_2 (Collier and Sweatman, 1968; Collier and Gardiner, 1974). Indomethacin has a comparable effect on guinea pig isolated trachea (Farmer *et al.*, 1974; Gardiner and Collier, 1980a). A direct antagonism of the relaxant effect of E prostaglandins on tracheobronchial smooth muscle by fenamates and aspirin has more recently been observed (Gardiner and Collier, 1980a). To what extent this direct antagonism of prostaglandins plays a role in the action of salicylates is uncertain.

2. *Stimulation of Prostaglandin Synthetase*

Not only do drugs of the aspirin group inhibit prostaglandin synthetase, but some of them also, at noninhibitory concentrations, stimulate this enzyme system. Such stimulation, which is shown by paracetamol (Robak *et al.*, 1978; McDonald-Gibson and Collier, 1979), can be attributed to the presence in the drug molecule of a phenolic grouping (Collier *et al.*, 1976b). Salicylic acid likewise exhibited duality of actions (H.O.J. Collier, W. J. McDonald-Gibson, and S. A. Saeed, unpublished observations). It might be expected, therefore, that paracetamol and salicylic acid would have weak or paradoxical dose–response effects, arising from conflicts between stimulant and inhibitory activities.

3. *Biosynthetic Pathways of Prostaglandins*

Figure 3 shows the sequence of reactions leading to the synthesis of prostaglandins and other metabolites from arachidonic acid. The first step is the liberation of arachidonic acid from store through the action of phospholipase A_2. Depending upon various factors, including its anatomical location, arachidonic acid can then undergo various transformations by two main enzyme systems. The membrane-bound cyclooxygenase enzyme transforms arachidonic acid to the cyclic endoperoxides, PGG_2 and PGH_2 (Hamberg *et al.*, 1974b). The conversion of PGG_2 to PGH_2 is associated with the release of an oxygen-centered radical and is facilitated by a free radical scavenger, such as phenol (Egan *et al.*, 1976). These relatively unstable intermediates in prostaglandin biosynthesis, the cyclic endoperoxides, may then be converted to either: (1) stable prostaglandins (PGD_2, PGE_2, and $PGF_{2\alpha}$), or (2) to a 17-C hydroxy acid (HHT) and ma-

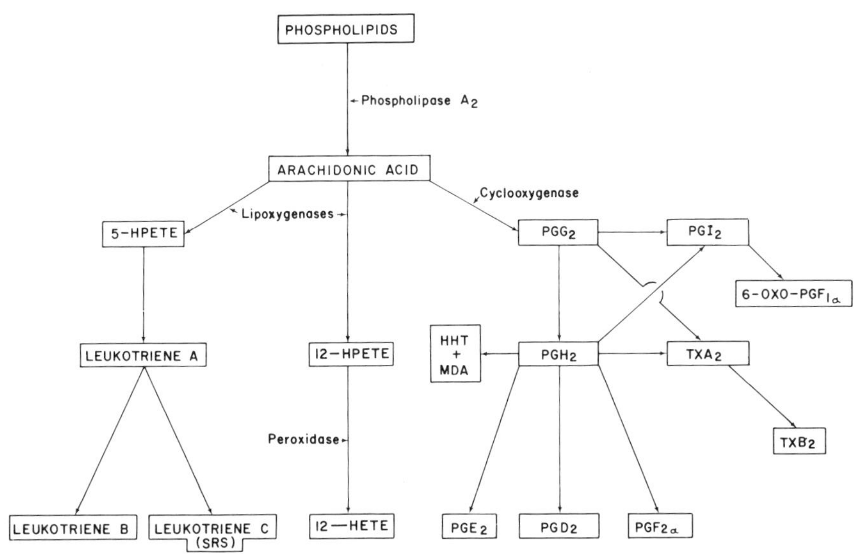

FIG. 3. A summary of the known metabolic pathways of arachidonic acid.

londialdehyde (MDA), or (3) to thromboxanes A_2 and B_2 (TXA_2, TXB_2), or (4) to prostacyclin (PGI_2) and its breakdown product, 6-oxo-$PGF_{1\alpha}$ (Hamberg and Samuelsson, 1974; Hamberg *et al.*, 1974a, 1975b; Moncada *et al.*, 1976). RCS, which Vane (1971) speculated was a possible prostaglandin intermediate, is now believed to be a mixture of PGG_2, PGH_2, and TXA_2, the latter substance being the predominant constituent (Hamberg *et al.*, 1975b; Bunting *et al.*, 1976). RCS-RF (Piper and Vane, 1969) is now thought to be a small peptide that acts by liberating arachidonate from phospholipids, probably by stimulating the phospholipase enzyme system (Nijkamp *et al.*, 1976; Blackwell *et al.*, 1978).

Arachidonic acid may also be transformed by the action of cytoplasmic lipoxygenase enzymes to the hydroxyacid 12-HETE via the unstable hydroperoxy acid 12-HPETE (Hamberg and Samuelsson, 1974; Nugteren, 1975) or to the newly discovered leukotrienes via the hydroperoxy acid 5-HPETE (Murphy *et al.*, 1979). Leukotriene C is believed to be identical to SRS.

In the prostaglandins derived from arachidonic acid (Fig. 3), the subscript "2" in their names indicates the number of double bonds in the carbon side-chains. Prostaglandins of the "1" and "3" series, derived respectively from dihomo-γ-linolenic acid and 5, 8, 11, 14, 17-eicosapentaenoic acid, are generated in a comparable way to those of the "2" series. The three unsaturated fatty acids from which these three prostaglandin series originate belong to the "essential fatty acids." If the substances formed by processes beginning with the cyclooxygenation of these three fatty acids are termed "prostanoids," this term will include not only prostaglandins, including prostacyclin, but also thromboxanes and the cyclic endoperoxides (PGG_2 and PGH_2) that are their precursors.

At what point do salicylates and like-acting drugs inhibit the synthetic pathway? It is now established that these drugs inhibit cyclooxygenase, thereby blocking the formation of the cyclic endoperoxides and hence also of the prostaglandins, thromboxanes, and prostacyclins (Takeguchi and Sih, 1972; Tomlinson *et al.*, 1972; Hamberg and Samuelsson, 1974; Hamberg *et al.*, 1974a; Kuehl *et al.*, 1977b). In short, salicylates block the formation of all prostanoids. That aspirin blocks the release of RCS (Piper and Vane, 1969), but not that of RCS-RF (Nijkamp *et al.*, 1976), is consistent with these findings. The above considerations lead to a more comprehensive restatement of the prostaglandin hypothesis—that *aspirin and like-acting drugs exert their main pharmacological effects through the inhibition of prostanoid biosynthesis.*

How do salicylates inhibit cyclooxygenase? It was first thought that they acted as competitive antagonists (Ham *et al.*, 1972; Flower *et al.*, 1973); but it has become evident that this inhibition may be irreversible

(Ku and Wasvary, 1973; Lands *et al.*, 1973; Flower and Vane, 1974a). It has been suggested that aspirin inhibits this enzyme by acetylating the active site (Roth and Majerus, 1975; Roth *et al.*, 1975; Burch *et al.*, 1978a); but this mechanism would presumably not apply to related drugs.

It has recently been shown that aspirin-like drugs also interfere with the lipoxygenase pathway of arachidonate metabolism by inhibiting the transformation of 12-HPETE to 12-HETE (Siegel *et al.*, 1979). Unlike the inhibition of cyclooxygenase, this property is shared by sodium salicylate.

4. *Biological Activity and Inhibition of Prostanoid Biosynthesis*

a. Antagonism of Bradykinin. At first sight, it seemed that the antagonism by aspirin and like-acting drugs of bronchoconstriction induced by bradykinin in the guinea pig was due to a direct blockade of kinin receptors on the smooth muscle (Collier and Shorley, 1960). When it was found, however, that aspirin also antagonized bronchoconstriction induced by SRS-A (Berry and Collier, 1964) and by ATP (Collier *et al.*, 1966), this view was abandoned. It was therefore suggested that, among other possibilities, aspirin might block the release of an unidentified bronchoactive substance through which all of these agonists act.

Vane and Ferreira (1976), reviewing the interactions between bradykinin and prostaglandins, concluded that bradykinin releases RCS, PGE_2, and $PGF_{2\alpha}$ from isolated guinea pig lungs. This implies that bradykinin would also release the cyclic endoperoxides, which have potent bronchoconstrictor actions (Hamberg *et al.*, 1975a; Wasserman, 1976). Since high doses of bradykinin are probably needed to contract bronchial muscle by direct action (Collier and James, 1966), it seems likely that the aspirin-like drugs inhibited bronchoconstriction by blocking the release of bronchoconstrictor prostanoids by bradykinin and like-acting local hormones. If so, this would account for the good correlation between this and the therapeutic effects of aspirin-like drugs (Collier *et al.*, 1968b).

b. Antinociceptive Activity. Vane (1971) thought that the analgesic activity of aspirin-like drugs could not easily be explained by inhibition of prostaglandin synthesis because prostaglandins were reported to lack algesic actions (see above). Subsequently, however, it was shown that, in man, intravenous infusions and intramuscular injections of prostaglandins caused pain (Karim, 1971; Collier *et al.*, 1972; Gillespie, 1972). Furthermore, Collier and Schneider (1972) showed that prostaglandins induced abdominal constrictions when injected intraperitoneally into mice, and that these responses were readily blocked by morphine but not by aspirin, although aspirin suppresses constrictions due to other irritants and particularly to arachidonate (Collier *et al.*, 1973). Hence these observations ful-fil the basic criterion indicating that aspirin acts by inhibiting cyclooxygenase; namely, that it blocks the effect of arachidonate, but fails to block the comparable effect of formed prostaglandins.

Although these observations indicate the feasibility of explaining the analgesic action of aspirin in terms of the inhibition of cyclooxygenase, they do not explain how the small amounts of prostaglandins liberated in tissues would participate in pain sensation, and thus how aspirin would act in practice in suppressing such sensation. An explanation has been provided by Ferreira (1972) who showed that at concentrations likely to be found in inflammation, PGE_1, infused subdermally into volunteers, produced a long-lasting hyperalgesia in which pain receptors were sensitized to bradykinin and other chemical stimuli. He postulated that aspirin-like drugs inhibited pain by blocking the endogenous release and consequent sensitizing actions of prostaglandins. This proposal was supported by studies of the effects of E prostaglandin and of aspirin on the painful responses evoked by bradykinin in the spleen and knee joint of dogs (Ferreira *et al.*, 1973; Moncada *et al.*, 1975).

Lembeck and colleagues have confirmed and extended this work, using nociception elicited by intraarterial injection of algesic substances in the rabbit ear (Juan and Lembeck, 1974, 1977; Lembeck and Juan, 1974; Lembeck *et al.*, 1976). In these experiments, nociception elicited by bradykinin was enhanced by PGE_1 and suppressed by low doses of indomethacin.

There is also evidence to suggest that products of arachidonic acid other than prostaglandins may be hyperalgesic. Thus, Helfer and Jaques (1968) reported that arachidonic acid peroxide elicits abdominal constrictions in mice. Again, Ferreira (1972) showed that, when injected intradermally into volunteers, fatty acid hydroperoxides had greater algesic potency than the parent fatty acids. Moreover, Collier *et al.* (1973) found evidence that the analgesic action of arachidonic acid, injected intraperitoneally into mice, was due to the formation of intermediates rather than of prostaglandins themselves.

The mechanism postulated by Ferreira and colleagues is consistent with or explains several earlier findings. For example, it fits the conclusion of Lim and colleagues (1964) that salicylates exert their analgesic action at peripheral sites. Also, it explains the lower analgesic potency of sodium salicylate, in terms of its correspondingly lower potency as an inhibitor of prostaglandin synthetase. Again, it explains the selectivity of aspirin against certain types of pain, such as the hyperalgesia of inflammation (Randall and Selitto, 1957; Winter and Flataker, 1965).

Despite this goodness of fit, a difficulty remains to be resolved. If hyperalgesia due to E prostaglandin lasts for several hours, how does aspirin relieve pain within half-an-hour of treatment, as it is well known to do in some circumstances? Ferreira *et al.* (1978) have suggested that, in such a case, PGI_2 is involved, since PGI_2 elicits a brief hyperalgesia (Ferreira and Nakamura, 1979). Alternatively, another short-acting prostanoid might be involved.

c. Antipyretic Activity. If inhibition of prostaglandin synthetase accounts for the antipyretic action of salicylates, what evidence is there for a pyrogenic action of prostaglandins? During the 1960s, it was established that E- and F-type prostaglandins were widely distributed in the brain (Holmes and Horton, 1968) but, at that time, no particular function could be ascribed to them. Later, however, Milton and Wendlandt (1970,1971) reported that small doses of PGE_1 or PGE_2, injected into the third ventricle of rabbits or cats, rapidly elicited fever, an observation later confirmed in other species, in particular, rats and sheep (Potts and East, 1972; Hales *et al.*, 1973). The site of action of prostaglandins was shown to be the preoptic/anterior hypothalamic region near the third ventricle (Feldberg and Saxena, 1971b; Stitt, 1973).

It was ultimately shown that, during fever induced in cats by *Shigella dysenteriae* pyrogen, prostaglandin-like activity increased in the cerebrospinal fluid (CSF) collected from either the third ventricle (Feldberg and Gupta, 1973) or the cisterna magna (Feldberg *et al.*, 1973). The major prostaglandin in CSF of fevered cats was originally thought to be PGE_1, but it was later shown, by radioimmunoassay, to be PGE_2 (Davis, cited by Feldberg, 1974).

Evidence that not only gave credence to Vane's hypothesis but also supported a positive role for prostaglandins in the mediation of pyrogen fever was the finding that paracetamol, indomethacin, and aspirin, injected intraperitoneally into cats, reduced both pyrogen-induced fever and the elevated level of prostaglandin-like activity in the CSF (Feldberg *et al.*, 1973). This observation has since been confirmed in numerous studies (Dey *et al.*, 1974; Veale and Cooper, 1974; Clark and Cumby, 1975a; Feldberg and Saxena, 1975; Laburn *et al.*, 1975). Confirmation that aspirin-like agents inhibit the release and not the pyrogenic activity of prostaglandins has been provided by the failure of these drugs to inhibit fever induced by prostaglandin itself (Milton and Wendlandt, 1971; Schoener and Wang, 1974; Clark and Cumby, 1975a; Woolf *et al.*, 1975).

Are aspirin-like agents capable of accumulating in sufficient concentration to block prostaglandin synthetase in the CNS? Lim *et al.* (1967) measured salicylate in the brain of dogs and rabbits after oral or intravenous administration of aspirin and found its concentration to be low. They concluded that the blood–brain barrier restricted the entry of salicylate into the CNS and that salicylates must act peripherally to produce antipyresis.

Subsequently, however, Rawlins *et al.* (1973) found that salicylate concentrations attainable in the anterior hypothalamic area were sufficient to inhibit prostaglandin synthetase during antipyresis.

Is the proposed mechanism compatible with the antipyretic profile of aspirin-like drugs? To date, prostanoid biosynthesis in the CNS is generally associated with pyrexia rather than with the maintenance of normothermia. Thus the reduction of pyrexia at doses of these agents which fail to modify normal body temperature is consistent with the proposed mechanism. Consistent also is the observation that sodium salicylate, which is a much weaker inhibitor of prostaglandin synthetase than aspirin (Vane, 1971), is also generally less potent as an antipyretic agent (Collier, 1969a).

Unfortunately, not all the available evidence supports the proposed mechanism of antipyresis. First, the importance of prostaglandins in fever has been questioned. For instance, E-type prostaglandins are not consistently pyrogenic in all species since, in chickens, PGE_1 and PGE_2 induced hypothermia, yet pyrogen still produced pyresis (Artunkal *et al.*, 1975). Moreover, indomethacin blocked the pyrogen fever but potentiated PGE_1 hypothermia. Also, attempts to block pyrogen fever with prostaglandin antagonists have not yielded satisfactory results. Clark and Cumby (1975b) found that the prostaglandin antagonist SC 19220 antagonized pyrogen fever in cats only at doses which produced hypothermia when given alone. Also, SC 19220, as well as the antagonist HR 54, was shown to inhibit fever induced in rabbits by PGE_2, but not by pyrogen (Cranston *et al.,* 1976) or sodium arachidonate (Laburn *et al.,* 1977). SC 19220 appears, however, to antagonize prostaglandins at only one of several types of prostaglandin receptor (Coleman *et al.*, 1980). The suggestion that prostaglandin intermediates could be mediators of fever (Piper and Vane, 1969; Laburn *et al.*, 1977) theoretically overcomes this difficulty since their synthesis would be inhibited by aspirin-like drugs, yet their activity would be unaffected by prostaglandin antagonists. However, this seems unlikely to be due to the cyclic endoperoxides since their stable analogs do not produce fever (Hawkins and Lipton, 1977). Furthermore, yeast-induced fever in rats, at least, is apparently unaffected by rendering the animals deficient in prostaglandin precursors by maintenance on a diet deficient in essential fatty acids (Frens *et al.*, 1978). However, it remains to be demonstrated that this procedure lowers CNS levels of prostaglandins or their intermediates sufficiently to impair fever production.

Further evidence against the proposed mechanism has been obtained by the demonstration that sodium salicylate, while failing to inhibit the fever, nevertheless blocked the rise in CSF prostaglandin-like activity produced in rabbits by infused endogenous pyrogen (Cranston *et al.*,

1975). Likewise, Myers (1976) reported that a low dose of aspirin perfused into the cat hypothalamus, although sufficient to inhibit prostaglandin synthetase in this organ, failed to inhibit bacterial fever.

In conclusion, it is clear from the above that the proposed mechanism of antipyretic action of aspirin-like agents involving prostanoid synthesis cannot yet be fully accepted until the difficulties outlined above are resolved. The postulation of a second, subsidiary mechanism of fever, not involving prostanoid production, may be needed to explain all the phenomena observed.

d. Antiinflammatory Activity. If inhibition of prostaglandin synthetase provides a valid explanation of the antiinflammatory activity of salicylates, the appropriate criteria given in Section I,B should be satisfied. First, prostaglandins (including their biosynthetic intermediates) should induce inflammation or enhance that induced by other local hormones; also, prostaglandins should increase in inflamed tissues; and, furthermore, prostaglandin antagonists should reduce inflammation. Second, aspirin and sodium salicylate should lessen inflammation *in vivo* with potencies and time-courses corresponding with their ability to inhibit prostaglandin synthetase *in vitro,* taking into account the rapid conversion of aspirin to salicylate *in vivo.* Third, salicylates should lower tissue levels of prostaglandins and exogenous prostaglandin should reverse the antiinflammatory effect of salicylates. The extent to which all these criteria are met is not fully known; but the evidence for and against the prostaglandin hypothesis is discussed in the next three subsections.

i. Prostanoids and inflammation. Earlier work examining the role of prostanoids in inflammation has been concerned with prostaglandins themselves, in particular, PGE_1, PGE_2, and $PGF_{2\alpha}$. It is only relatively recently that the role of other prostanoids (cyclic endoperoxides, thromboxanes, and PGI_2) has been evaluated. The latter will be discussed separately at the end of this subsection.

Prostaglandins have been detected in a variety of inflammatory lesions such as those elicited by carrageenin in rat hind paws (Willis, 1969) and in the pleural (Capasso *et al.*, 1975; Vinegar *et al.*, 1976) and peritoneal (Velo *et al.*, 1973) cavities of rats. Also, the synovial fluid from either the challenged joints of rabbits with monoarticular arthritis (Blackham *et al.*, 1974) or human rheumatoid joints (Robinson and Levine, 1974; Higgs *et al.*, 1974) contains prostaglandins.

As well as being present at inflammatory sites, when injected, prostaglandins induce erythema (Solomon *et al.,* 1968; Juhlin and Michaelsson, 1969) and edema (Horton, 1963; Kaley and Weiner, 1968; Crunkhorn and Willis, 1969). E-type prostaglandins are more potent in this respect than F-type prostaglandins (Crunkhorn and Willis, 1971a). Certain prostaglandins have also been reported to be chemotactic. *In vitro,* PGE_1 is chemotactic for polymorphonuclear leukocytes (PMNLs) of some species (Kaley and Weiner, 1971; McCall and Youlten, 1973; Higgs *et al.*, 1975) but is apparently devoid of any such activity *in vivo* (Arora *et al.*, 1970; Sondergaard and Wolf-Jurgensen, 1972).

Of greater importance, however, is the ability of prostaglandins to enhance inflammatory edema induced by other mediators. For instance, PGE_1 potentiates the increased vascular permeability responses induced by bradykinin in rats (Thomas and West, 1973) and guinea pigs (Williams and Morley, 1973). Furthermore, PGE_1 potentiates carrageenin paw edema in rats (Moncada *et al.*, 1973; Lewis *et al.*, 1974; Komoriya *et al.*, 1978; Ford-Hutchinson *et al.*, 1978) but not the increased synovial blood flow induced by low doses of bradykinin injected into dog joints (Dick *et al.*, 1976). It has been suggested that the enhancing effects of prostaglandins on the permeability-increasing action of other mediators observed in rodents result from increased blood flow (Williams and Morley, 1973; Williams, 1976; Johnston *et al.*, 1976). Moreover, this sensitizing action has been put forward to explain why antiinflammatory drugs fail to block inflammation totally (Moncada *et al.*, 1973).

Supportive evidence that prostaglandins play an active role in inflammation has been obtained by Ferreira *et al.* (1974) who showed that the inflammatory response to carrageenin in rats immunized against PGE_1 was significantly diminished. Furthermore, carrageenin paw edema is also inhibited in rats rendered deficient in prostaglandin precursors by maintenance on a diet deficient in essential fatty acids (Bonta *et al.*, 1977a).

Prostaglandins are reportedly antiinflammatory as well as proinflammatory; for example, locally administered prostaglandins inhibit, and dietary deprivation of fatty acid precursors of prostaglandins stimulates, proliferation of granulomata in rats (DiPasquale *et al.*, 1973; Bonta *et al.*, 1977b; Bonta and Parnham, 1979). Again, $PGF_{2\alpha}$ inhibits the inflammatory actions of E-type prostaglandins (Willoughby, 1968; Crunkhorn and Willis, 1971b). Indeed, the observed increases in $PGF_{2\alpha}$ concentrations in inflammatory exudates which coincided with a waning of inflammation (Velo *et al.,* 1973) have prompted the suggestion that the local control of inflammation might result from the preferential biosynthesis of one particular prostaglandin (Velo *et al.,* 1973; Zurier, 1974).

E-type prostaglandins are reportedly antiinflammatory in their own right, thereby implying that they may have a modulatory rather than an active role in inflammation. When administered systemically, PGE_1 and PGE_2 inhibited carrageenin paw edema and adjuvant-induced arthritis in rats (Glenn and Rohloff, 1972). Moreover, the instillation of PGE_1 and PGE_2 into carrageenin air-blebs reduced the rate of influx of inflammatory cells (Zurier *et al.*, 1973). The inhibitory effect of PGE_1 on sponge-induced granulomata in rats is apparently dependent on the time of administration (Bonta and Parnham, 1979). *In vitro* prostaglandins inhibit mediator release from various cells and tissues (Weissmann *et al.*, 1971; Lichtenstein and DeBernardo, 1971; Orange *et al.*, 1971; Bray *et al.*, 1974), but such an action appears to be concentration dependent; whereas low concentrations enhance antigen-induced histamine release from human lung tissue, high concentrations suppress it (Tauber *et al.*, 1973).

Since the inflammatory role of prostaglandins is by no means proven and since aspirin-like drugs inhibit the formation of all prostanoids, Kuehl *et al.* (1977b) have argued that prostaglandin intermediates also need to be considered as potential inflammatory mediators. Intermediates so far considered to have a mediatory role include the endoperoxide PGG_2 (Kuehl *et al.*, 1977b), TXB_2 (Boot *et al.*, 1976; Kitchen *et al.*, 1978; Higgs and Salmon, 1979; Murota *et al.*, 1979), PGI_2 (Ford-Hutchinson *et al.*, 1978; Higgs *et al.*, 1978; Komoriya *et al.*, 1978; Murota *et al.*, 1978, 1979; Higgs and Salmon, 1979; Williams, 1979), and HHT (Goetzl and Gorman, 1978). Thromboxanes and PGI_2, while also having a possible role in acute inflammation (Higgs and Salmon, 1979), may have a more important role in chronic inflammation (Murota *et al.*, 1979). These latter authors have shown that rat carrageenin granuloma homogenates convert arachidonic acid to 6-keto $PGF_{1\alpha}$ (the breakdown product of PGI_2) and TXB_2 but not to PGE_2, $PGF_{2\alpha}$, or PGD_2. Moreover, in this study, TXB_2 initiated granuloma formation *in vitro* whereas PGI_2 enhanced local vascular permeability in the granuloma pouch. PGI_2, like PGE_1 and PGE_2, is also capable of enhancing increased vascular permeability induced by other potential inflammatory mediators (Ford-Hutchinson *et al.*, 1978; Higgs *et al.*, 1978; Komoriya *et al.*, 1978; Williams, 1979).

Another product of arachidonic acid oxidation that may have an inflammatory role is 12-HETE (see Section II,D,2). This substance is potently chemotactic for neutrophilic PMNLs and, until recently, it was believed that its formation was not well blocked by either indomethacin or, presumably, other like-acting drugs (Turner *et al.*, 1975). However, as mentioned above, Siegel *et al.* (1979) have recently shown that aspirin-like drugs inhibit the formation of 12-HETE from 12-HPETE but have no direct effect on lipoxygenase activity.

ii. Antiinflammatory action of salicylates. If inhibition of prostanoid biosynthesis adequately explains the antiinflammatory activity of salicylates, how well do these actions correlate? One of the earliest attempts to correlate these actions was that of Flower *et al.* (1972). They showed that the inhibitory potency of a variety of nonsteroidal antiinflammatory agents on a cell-free dog spleen synthetase preparation correlated well with their *in vivo* antiinflammatory potency measured in the carrageenin rat paw edema test. Two aspirin analogs devoid of *in vivo* antiinflammatory activity also lacked antisynthetase activity. Furthermore, antisynthetase IC_{50}s for clinically used drugs were in general less than the peak plasma concentrations achieved after therapeutic dosage, even after taking protein binding into account.

Support for the hypothesis was further boosted when it was reported that an enantiomer of naproxen, which had much less antiinflammatory and antipyretic activity than naproxen itself, had correspondingly less *in vitro* antisynthetase activity (Tomlinson *et al.*, 1972). Similar results were obtained for two pairs of enantiomers of indomethacin analogs (Ham *et al.*, 1972).

In vivo evidence in support of the hypothesis is the reported lowering of prostaglandin levels in inflammatory exudates by antiinflammatory doses of aspirin-like drugs. Thus, these drugs lower prostaglandin levels in exudates from either carrageenin air-blebs (Willis *et al.*, 1972; McCall and Youlten, 1974; Whelan, 1974; Atkinson and Leach, 1978) or subcutaneous sponge implants (Walker *et al.*, 1976; Higgs *et al.*, 1976) in rats, and in synovial fluid from either the challenged joints of rabbits with monoarticular arthritis (Blackham *et al.*, 1974) or human rheumatoid joints (Higgs *et al.*, 1974; Robinson and Levine, 1974). Moreover, Crook *et al.* (1976) found that rheumatoid synovium from patients treated with aspirin was unable to synthesize prostaglandins.

iii. Difficulties and objections. Not all the available experimental evidence supports the hypothesis; indeed, several difficulties have yet to be overcome. One of the earliest papers to question the hypothesis reported that an analog of fenclozic acid, ICI 54,501, was equipotent with fenclozic acid as an inhibitor of guinea pig lung synthetase *in vitro* but lacked *in vivo* antiinflammatory activity (Sykes and Maddox, 1972). A metabolic explanation of this anomaly was unlikely since expected plasma levels of ICI 54,501 were reportedly obtained following oral administration.

An apparent anomaly is sodium salicylate. This drug is a very weak inhibitor of prostaglandin synthetase *in vitro* (Vane, 1971) yet it is equipotent with aspirin as an antiinflammatory agent *in vivo* (Collier, 1969a; Smith *et al.*, 1975). Attempts to accommodate this observation to the prostaglandin hypothesis have largely revolved around the idea that sodium salicylate may exert its *in vivo* activity via transformation to a metabolite with antisynthetase activity. This suggestion was originally prompted by the finding that, *in vivo,* sodium salicylate was as effective as aspirin in lowering prostaglandin levels in carrageenin air-bleb exudate (Willis *et al.*, 1972). Furthermore, Hamberg (1972) reported that sodium salicylate was at least as effective as aspirin in reducing the basal excretion of 7α-hydroxy-5,11-diketotetranorprotane-1,16-dioic acid (PM), the major urinary metabolite of PGE_1 and PGE_2 in man. Salicylate metabolites, such as gentisic acid and its isomers, were subsequently found to be as active as aspirin (in relative molar terms) as synthetase inhibitors (Flower and Vane, 1974b). Moreover, the observation that aspirin, but not salicylic acid, inhibits inflammation when administered locally (Vinegar, cited by Vane, 1974) supports the view that salicylic acid requires metabolic activation.

Certain facts, however, are inconsistent with this metabolite hypothesis. For instance, if sodium salicylate is equipotent with aspirin as an antiinflammatory agent because of metabolic transformation to a synthetase inhibitor, it should also be equipotent with aspirin in other actions resulting from synthetase inhibition (e.g., antinociceptive activity), but this is clearly not the case, as has already been discussed. This objection can, of course, be countered by postulating that the metabolite is extremely potent and possesses an unusually high specificity of action. However, the salicylate metabolites examined so far are no more potent than aspirin (Flower and Vane, 1974b) and, at any rate, they are considered to contribute little to the overall activity of salicylates (Lim, 1966). This view is consistent with the finding that, whereas aspirin inhibits the potentiation of carrageenin rat paw edema by arachidonic acid, sodium salicylate does not (Smith *et al.*, 1975). Thus, on balance, a metabolic activation of salicylic acid seems unlikely.

An alternative explanation of the above discrepancy may be sought in the fact that aspirin is quickly deacetylated *in vivo*. Therefore, in actions that need a persistent presence of drug or are located at poor accessible sites, most of the acetylsalicylate will have been converted to salicylate before it acts. This might apply, for example, in rheumatic joints, in which aspirin and sodium salicylate would hence be of approximately equal potency. On the contrary, in actions that are rapid, in sites readily accessible to aspirin, such as the inhibition of platelet prostanoid synthesis of bradykinin-induced bronchoconstriction in the guinea pig, aspirin might be expected to act as the acetylsalicylate ion, and hence to be more potent than sodium salicylate. In short, to explain some of the discrepancies observed, we need not postulate that sodium salicylate is activated if we take into account that aspirin is readily deacetylated *in vivo*.

The recent finding that sodium salicylate and aspirin equipotently inhibit the generation of chemotactic 12-HETE from 12-HPETE in the lipoxygenase pathway of arachidonic acid metabolism (Siegel *et al.*, 1979) may now help to overcome the anomalous position of sodium salicylate while, at the same time, tending to diminish the importance of the cyclooxygenase pathway to the antiinflammatory activity of salicylates.

Paracetamol is also anomalous. This compound has slight or no antiinflammatory activity, yet it is both analgesic and antipyretic and also has antisynthetase activity in a variety of tissues (Flower and Vane, 1972, 1974b; Flower *et al.*, 1973; Collier, 1974b; Robak *et al.*, 1978; McDonald-Gibson and Collier, 1979). The same can be said of amidopyrine and phenazone (Collier, 1974a; H. O. J. Collier, W. J. McDonald-Gibson, and S. A. Saeed, unpublished observations). Since synthetases from different tissues appear to have differing drug susceptibilities (Vane, 1972; Bhattacherjee and Eakins, 1973; Flower and Vane, 1974b), it might be argued, however, that paracetamol lacks antiinflammatory activity because it fails to inhibit those synthetases activated during inflammation. This argument appears to be untenable since paracetamol, directly or indirectly, significantly reduces prostaglandin levels in rat inflammatory exudate (Walker *et al.*, 1976).

The finding that aspirin-like drugs can markedly reduce prostaglandin levels in inflammatory exudates *in vivo* at doses which have little or no antiinflammatory activity is also inconsistent with the prostaglandin hypothesis. In particular, Walker *et al.* (1976), using a sponge implantation technique in rats, showed that a marginally active acute antiinflammatory dose of indomethacin (1 mg/kg po) produced almost total inhibition of prostaglandin release. Furthermore, since indomethacin blocks the cyclooxygenase stage of prostanoid biosynthesis (Horodniak *et al.*, 1974; Kuehl *et al.*, 1977b), the production of inflammatory prostaglandin intermediates (e.g., PGG_2) was, presumably, also suppressed in these experiments. This difficulty diminishes, however, if it is supposed that prostanoids, even at low concentrations, can enhance the inflammatory effect of another mediator.

A similar situation appears to exist in man since aspirin, after a single dose of 600 mg, blocks prostaglandin synthetase *in vivo* in both platelets (Smith and Willis, 1971) and rheumatoid synovium (Crook *et al.*, 1976), yet much higher doses (at least 3.6 gm per day) are required to produce clinically detectable antiinflammatory activity. The antiinflammatory activity of aspirin-like drugs may therefore be mediated via an additional or alternative mechanism which only becomes operative at doses in excess of those required to suppress prostaglandin synthetase.

That aspirin inhibited equally carrageenin paw edema elicited in both normal rats and those rendered deficient in prostaglandin precursors by maintenance on a diet deficient in essential fatty acids (Bonta *et al.*, 1977a) also suggests that an alternative mechanism of action may operate. However, the possibility was not ruled out that deficient rats could have been more sensitive to prostaglandins or their bioactive precursors, thus masking any effect prostaglandin precursor depletion may have had on drug activity.

In a rat study designed to examine the relationship between inhibition of prostaglandin synthetase *in vivo* and antinociceptive or antiinflammatory activity among several nonnarcotic analgesics, it was found that only the antinociceptive activity correlated with effects on prostaglandin synthetase (Deraedt *et al.*, 1976).

Finally, it is worth considering data presented some years ago which indicate that the antiinflammatory activity of aspirin-like drugs probably does not arise from a single mechanism. In particular, Winter (1965) reported that aspirin inhibited both carrageenin- and formalin-induced rat paw edema whereas flufenamic acid and indomethacin affected only the former. Furthermore, in contrast to aspirin, indomethacin was only weakly active as an inhibitor of yeast edema. These findings imply that aspirin has additional components to its mechanism of action not possessed by either flufenamic acid or indomethacin, yet all inhibit prostaglandin synthetase.

Allied to these observations is the apparent divergence of effect of drugs such as indomethacin and phenylbutazone on the hyperesthesia and edema produced by yeast in the rat paw. Both of these drugs inhibit yeast-induced hyperesthesia (Atkinson and Cowan, 1974) but they only weakly inhibit yeast edema (Winter, 1965). Likewise, aspirin more potently inhibits yeast-induced hyperesthesia than the edema (Gilfoil *et al.*, 1963). Furthermore, in man, aspirin is more potent as an analgesic than as an antiinflammatory agent. These results do not support the view that the analgesic and antiinflammatory activities are both entirely due to inhibition of prostanoid biosynthesis; rather they indicate that at least one other mechanism may operate in one case.

In conclusion, while inhibition of prostanoid synthesis has become an attractive, unifying explanation of the antiinflammatory activity of aspirin-like drugs, it is clear from the foregoing that it does not explain all aspects of the antiinflammatory action of salicylates. It is therefore necessary to construct one or more subsidiary or alternative hypotheses to overcome the difficulties that have emerged (see Section II,E).

e. Aspirin and Platelet Aggregation. Aspirin inhibits the blood platelet aggregation response induced by either epinephrine or ADP, as demonstrated both *in vitro* and *ex vivo* (Weiss *et al.*, 1968; Zucker and Peterson, 1968; O'Brien, 1968), that is, under conditions in which the formation and/or action of thrombin is blocked. Following the discovery that indomethacin and aspirin inhibited prostaglandin synthetase in human platelets (Smith and Willis, 1971), the possibility was raised that the inhibition of platelet aggregation by aspirin-like drugs might result from inhibition of prostaglandin synthetase.

If prostanoid synthesis promotes platelet aggregation, then prostaglandins are not themselves involved. PGE_2 induces neither aggregation nor the platelet release reaction on its own, whereas arachidonic acid does so (Vargaftig and Zirinis, 1973; Silver *et al.*, 1973). Furthermore, PGE_1 is a potent inhibitor of platelet aggregation (Kloeze, 1967, 1969). Nevertheless, PGE_2 appears to potentiate both ADP- and collagen-induced aggregation (Shio and Ramwell, 1972) by sensitizing platelets to other aggregating agents (Willis *et al.*, 1974).

Consequently, other prostanoids have been investigated as potential aggregating agents and it is now believed that thromboxane A_2 plays a major role in the process. It is a potent, but labile, irreversible platelet aggregator which also promotes the release of serotonin from platelets and which is produced in large amounts during platelet aggregation induced by various agents (Hamberg and Samuelsson, 1974). Its formation during clotting is thought to result from the liberation of arachidonic acid from the platelet phosphatide fraction by the action of phospholipase A_2, thereby triggering cyclooxygenase activity (Blackwell *et al.*, 1977).

How well does inhibition of platelet aggregation and ADP release by aspirin-like drugs correlate with their inhibitory effects on prostanoid biosynthesis? In one study to assess this correlation, platelets were obtained from volunteers before and at intervals after they had ingested single doses of either aspirin, indomethacin, or sodium salicylate, and were then examined for both aggregation and prostanoid synthesis (Kocsis *et al.*, 1973). Sodium salicylate had no effect on aggregation, nor any consistent effect on prostaglandin synthetase in platelets *ex vivo*. Aspirin and indomethacin inhibited both processes, there being a temporal relationship in both cases. Furthermore, aspirin's action lasted several days. This close correlation was subsequently confirmed when it was found that *in vivo* inhibition by indomethacin and aspirin of aggregation or rat platelets deficient in arachidonic acid was reduced compared with normal platelets (Vincent *et al.*, 1975). However, aspirin's activity was reduced to a smaller degree, which the authors suggested was indicative of additional mechanisms not involving prostanoids. The acetylation of platelet proteins by aspirin may be one such mechanism (Mills *et al.*, 1974; Roth and Majerus, 1975), although one of these proteins is believed to be a subunit of fatty acid cyclooxygenase (Roth *et al.*, 1977), while the nonspecific acetylation of other platelet proteins is currently of unknown biological significance (Burch and Majerus, 1979). Nevertheless, this irreversible acetylation of platelet proteins and the inability of platelets to synthesize proteins are observations which probably account for the extended effects of aspirin on platelets, the length of action corresponding closely to the lifespan of the platelet. The acetylation of platelet proteins by aspirin appears, however, to be of little importance *in vivo*, particularly since aspirin does not inhibit thrombin-induced platelet aggregation (Majerus, 1976).

Thus, there is good evidence to support the proposal that aspirin-like drugs inhibit *in vitro* blood platelet aggregation via inhibition of prostanoid biosynthesis. The interaction of aspirin with platelets has provided the basis for determining its usefulness as a potential antithrombotic agent (Verstraete, 1976; Weiss, 1976). However, to date, the results from clinical trials have been disappointing or, at best, inconclusive (Verstraete, 1976; Packham and Mustard, 1977). Moreover, several, but not all, animal studies have failed to demonstrate any effect of aspirin on bleeding times or on experimental thrombosis (Didisheim, 1968; Dejana *et al.*, 1979). There are several explanations to account for the apparent lack of aspirin's antiplatelet effects *in vivo,* most notably, the relatively recent discovery and identification of the prostanoid PGI_2 which has an opposing role to that of thromboxane A_2. Moncada *et al.* (1976) reported that the microsomes prepared from rabbit or pig aortas converted the cyclic endoperoxides PGG_2 and PGH_2 to an unstable substance which potently inhibited platelet aggregation. They called this substance PGX but it was later renamed prostacyclin (now designated PGI_2) following the elucidation of its structure (Johnson *et al.*, 1976). PGI_2 was later shown to be produced by human arterial and venous tissues (Moncada *et al.*, 1977). The discovery of PGI_2 prompted the suggestion that its generation by normal blood vessel walls enabled them to resist platelet adhesion and that a balance between proaggregatory thromboxane A_2 formed by platelets and antiaggregatory PGI_2 formed by vessels could be important for thrombus formation (Moncada *et al.*, 1976). Thus inhibition of endoperoxide formation by aspirin will in turn lead to inhibition of both thromboxane A_2 and PGI_2 synthesis, a realization that has prompted questioning of the rationale for the use of aspirin as an antithrombotic agent. However, it has been shown that cyclooxygenase in cultured smooth muscle cells from human aorta is less easily inactivated by aspirin than the platelet enzyme (Baenziger *et al.*, 1977), thereby raising the theoretical possibility that a dose of aspirin may be found which inhibits only the platelet enzyme (Burch *et al.*, 1978b; Masotti *et al.*, 1979). Nevertheless, while rat arterial cyclooxygenase is likewise less sensitive than the platelet enzyme, the rat venous enzyme is equally sensitive and no dose of aspirin preferentially inhibits the platelet enzyme without some measure of effect also on vascular cyclooxygenase (Villa *et al.*, 1979).

It is obvious that the potential usefulness of aspirin as an antithrombotic agent presupposes that prostanoids play a positive role in blood clotting *in vivo*. However, the following observations contradict such a role: patients with cyclooxygenase deficiency have only a mild bleeding syndrome (Malmsten *et al.*, 1975); the ingestion of aspirin by normal individuals induces only a mild prolongation of the bleeding time (Mielke *et al.*, 1969); and aspirin fails to inhibit platelet aggregation induced by either thrombin (Majerus, 1976) or high concentrations of collagen (Weiss *et al.*, 1968).

Although, therefore, aspirin does not materially modify normal platelet aggregation, it might nonetheless suppress a pathological tendency toward platelet aggregation in a particular situation where excessive quantities of TXA_2 might be liberated by a diseased vasculature. In so doing, aspirin would parallel in action its effect on fever, in which it lowers pathologically raised but not normal body temperature. Aspirin may therefore be useful in restraining a pathological tendency toward platelet aggregation, provided it is given at an appropriately low dose that does not greatly impair PGI_2 formation. For this purpose, a dose of about 160 mg per day has been suggested (Harter *et al.*, 1979; Masotti *et al.*, 1979).

f. Gastrointestinal Effects. i. Potentially useful effects of salicylates. Drugs of the aspirin group may have two different kinds of effect on gastrointestinal (GI) function. On the one hand, as is well known, these drugs can cause mucosal erosions by a local mechanism. On the other hand, as is less well known, salicylates can have potentially useful effects on GI function. Thus, there is evidence that aspirin inhibits diarrhea due to *E. coli* endotoxin in dogs (Collier, 1974b), and diarrhea and abdominal pain due to radiotherapy in women (Mennie *et al.*, 1975). Again, some cases of persistent diarrhea, for example, in irritable bowel syndrome, have been successfully treated with aspirin or indomethacin (Smythies and Russell, 1974; Luderer *et al.*, 1976; Rask-Madsen and Bukhave, 1978; Rask-Madsen, 1980). Furthermore, in five or six cases, aspirin, indomethacin, or ibuprofen prevented nausea, vomiting, abdominal pain, and diarrhea caused by food intolerance (Buisseret *et al.*, 1978). This has been confirmed in further cases (Lieb, 1978; L. J. F. Youlten, personal communication). Indomethacin also increases the pressure of the lower esophageal sphincter in normal volunteers and might therefore ameliorate heartburn (Dilawari *et al.*, 1975). Since we are concerned with the mechanism of the therapeutic action of salicylates, we shall consider the evidence that their potentially useful effects are due to inhibition of prostanoid production.

ii. Production of prostanoids by GI tissue. That GI tissue can produce prostanoids is well established. The isolated whole stomach of the rat, stimulated in various ways, produces prostaglandins E_1, $F_{1\alpha}$, E_2, and $F_{2\alpha}$ (Bennett *et al.*, 1967; Coceani *et al.*, 1967; Ramwell and Shaw, 1968). Not only external stimuli, but even peristalsis, can liberate prostaglandins (Bennett *et al.*, 1967). Rat stomach homogenates, incubated with arachidonic acid as substrate and norepinephrine as cofactor, produce PGE_2, $PGF_{2\alpha}$, and 6(9)-oxy PGF (Pace-Asciak and Wolfe, 1971; Pace-Asciak, 1973). From arachidonic acid, the microsomes of rat stomach produce

PGI_2 (Gryglewski *et al.*, 1976) and human stomach microsomes produce PGE_2 and $PGF_{2\alpha}$ (Peskar, 1977).

Leduc and Needleman (1979) have made a comprehensive analysis of the capacity of microsomes of the dog stomach and intestine to produce prostanoids from arachidonate. PGI_2 is the main product of the muscular layers; other products are PGD_2, PGE_2, $PGF_{2\alpha}$, and TXA_2. The mucosal microsomes mainly produce PGI_2 and TXA_2, with lesser amounts of PGD_2, PGE_2, and $PGF_{2\alpha}$.

Application of an artery clip to many parts of the alimentary canal of the rat (Collier, 1974b) and to isolated pieces of human stomach (Bennett *et al.*, 1977) cause prostaglandin release. Treatment of whole rabbits with *E. coli* endotoxin (Herman and Vane, 1975) or of whole mice with X-rays (Eisen *et al.*, 1977; Borowska *et al.*, 1979) enhances the ability of the jejunum, subsequently isolated, to produce prostaglandins. A fall in 15-hydroxy prostaglandin dehydrogenase in the jejunum after whole body irradiation may be associated with its increased capacity to produce prostaglandins (Walker and Eisen, 1979). In a few cases of food intolerance, high prostaglandin levels in blood and feces were observed after challenge (Buisseret *et al.*, 1978).

iii. Inhibition of the prostaglandin synthetase of GI tissue. The inhibition by salicylates of prostaglandin production by GI tissue has been less widely studied: but aspirin at 1 m*M* (180 μg/ml) has been found to inhibit by 50% the production of prostaglandins by homogenate of the whole stomach of the rat (McDonald-Gibson and Collier, 1979). The potency with which salicylates inhibit prostaglandin synthetase in rat stomach fundus has also been indirectly determined (Collier, 1974b; McDonald-Gibson and Collier, 1979), in terms of the drug concentration needed to inhibit by 50% (IC_{50}) the tone of the rat fundic strip, which is thought to be generated by continued intramural production of prostaglandin (Eckenfels and Vane, 1972). In two series of experiments on the rat fundic strip (Collier *et al.*, 1976a; McDonald-Gibson and Collier, 1979), the following IC_{50} values were obtained: aspirin, 0.5 ± 0.01 and 2.15 ± 0.16 m*M*; sodium salicylate, 1.53 ± 0.03 m*M*; paracetamol, 6.36 ± 1.30 m*M*. Such concentrations may well be reached in GI tissue during oral treatment.

iv. Effects of prostaglandins on GI function. Prostaglandins E_1, E_2, and $F_{2\alpha}$ have a wide range of disagreeable effects on the alimentary canal. In man, administration of exogenous prostaglandins causes nausea, vomiting, bile reflux, abdominal colic, accumulation of fluid in the intestine, increased intestinal propulsion, and diarrhea (Horton *et al.*, 1968; Misiewicz *et al*; 1969; Filshie, 1971; Barr and Naismith, 1972; Craft, 1972). Intravenous infusion of 0.8 μg/kg/minute of $PGF_{2\alpha}$ (Cummings *et al.*, 1973) or intrajejunal infusion of 0.9 μg/kg/minute of PGE_1 in volunteers

(Matuchansky and Bernier, 1973; Matuchansky *et al.*, 1976) increased the secretion of fluids and electrolytes into the lumen of the small intestine and in some instances produced diarrhea, nausea, and vomiting.

v. Conclusion. The foregoing evidence shows that: (1) aspirin and like-acting drugs inhibit certain diarrheas and associated symptoms; (2) intestinal tissue produces increased prostaglandins in response to some of the stimuli that cause diarrhea (*E. coli* endotoxin, X-rays, and challenge with food to which the subject is intolerant); (3) aspirin inhibits prostaglandin synthetase in intestinal tissue at concentrations likely to be attainable *in vivo* in the GI tract; and (4) prostaglandins readily elicit diarrhea. All this evidence is consistent with the hypothesis that the potentially useful antidiarrheal action of aspirin is due to inhibition of prostaglandin synthetase (Collier, 1974b, 1977; Rask-Madsen, 1980).

E. Alternative Current Hypotheses

It is evident from the preceding section that inhibition of prostanoid biosynthesis does not fully explain all the therapeutic actions of salicylates, particularly their antiinflammatory properties. Consequently, several workers have pursued additional or alternative mechanisms which may explain their activity. The current major lines of research are discussed below.

1. *Effects on Lymphocyte Function*

Lymphocytes play an important role in experimental immunogenic inflammation (Whitehouse, 1971) and, possibly, also in rheumatic disorders (Vaughan and Chihara, 1975). They may also have a role in nonimmunogenic inflammation (Ribeiro dos Santos *et al.*, 1976; Garcia Leme *et al.*, 1977). *In vitro* studies have shown that aspirin-like drugs can labilize lymphocyte membranes (Famaey and Whitehouse, 1973) and modify the uptake of various cations by lymphoid cells (Famaey and Whitehouse, 1976). Moreover, aspirin, at therapeutic concentrations, reversibly binds to human peripheral blood lymphocytes (Anthony and Panush, 1978). Furthermore, these drugs inhibit lymphocyte responses to mitogens *in vitro* (Smith and Forbes, 1967; Forbes and Smith, 1967; Opelz *et al.*, 1973; Twomey *et al.*, 1974), while their effects on lymphocyte transformation following *in vivo* administration remain controversial (Crout *et al.*, 1975; Duncan *et al.*, 1977). Nevertheless, the relevant question arises: is the antiinflammatory activity of aspirin-like drugs mediated via inhibition of lymphocyte function? That aspirin-like agents have little effect on immunopathological conditions such as experimental allergic encephalomyelitis in rats (Rosenthale and Nagra, 1967) and tuberculin sensitivity in guinea pigs (Floersheim, 1965) and rats (Bramm *et al.*, 1979) suggests that the answer to this question is no. On the other hand, aspirin reportedly inhibits Arthus reactions in rabbits (Goldlust and Schreiber, 1975) and guinea pigs (Blackham *et al.*, 1975). Furthermore, lymphocytes from rats treated with aspirin-like drugs failed to produce their restorative effect on the depressed inflammatory responses observed in leukopenic rats (Garcia Leme *et al.*, 1977). Hence, inhibition of lymphocyte function appears to be one feature of the antiinflammatory activity of salicylates and like-acting drugs that might be explored.

In view of the effects of aspirin on both lymphocytes and prostaglandin biosynthesis in rheumatoid joints, Morley (1974, 1975) has proposed that the antirheumatic activity of aspirin results from its interaction with a postulated pathogenic event involving lymphocytes and prostaglandins. From observations that PGE_1 inhibits lymphokine secretion by lymphocytes and that macrophages secrete prostaglandins (Bray *et al.*, 1974),

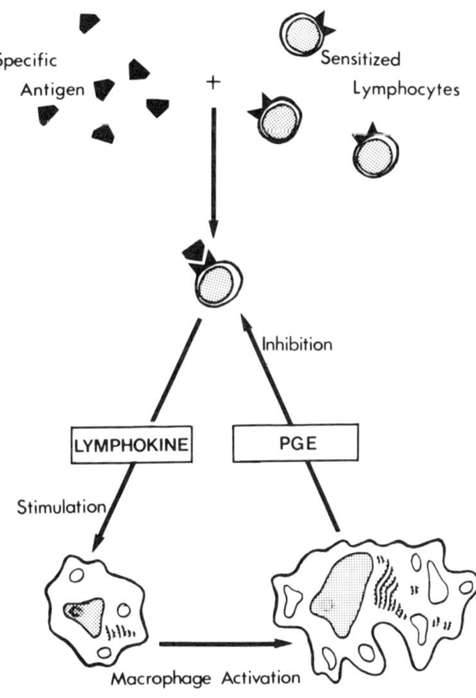

FIG. 4. Negative feedback mechanism operating in normal individuals whereby PGE production by activated macrophages restrains lymphokine secretion. Reproduced from Morley (1974) with kind permission.

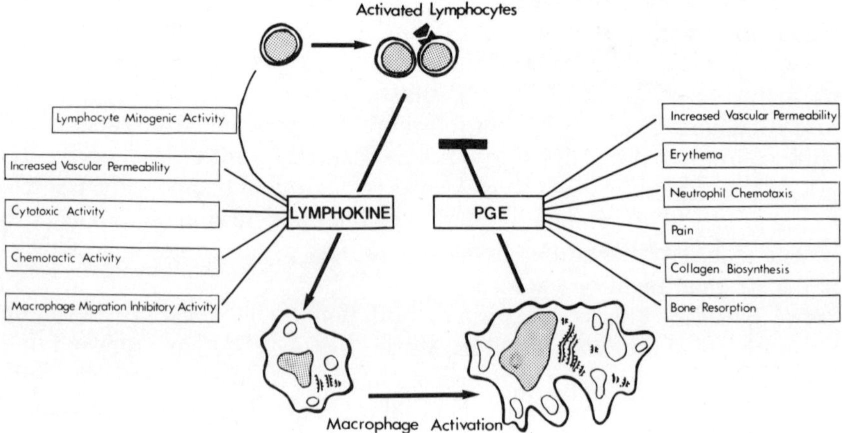

FIG. 5. Proposed mechanism involving defective lymphocyte reactivity, which leads to hypersecretion of both lymphokines and PGE, suggested to occur in rheumatoid arthritis. Reproduced from Morley (1974) with kind permission.

Morley (1974) proposed that, in normal individuals, the secretion of lymphokine, evoked by the reaction of antigen with sensitized lymphocytes, induces macrophages to secrete E-type prostaglandins which then act on the lymphocyte to restrain further lymphokine production (Fig. 4). In rheumatoid arthritis, however, this negative feedback mechanism breaks down because of defective lymphocyte reactivity to prostaglandins so that lymphokine secretion then becomes persistent, as does also the production of prostaglandins, thereby leading to joint inflammation (Fig. 5). Evidence supporting the existence of such a feedback system comes from a study in which activated lymphocytes provoked prostaglandin synthesis by macrophages and E-type prostaglandins inhibited lymphokine secretion (Gordon *et al.*, 1976). Moreover, the cyclic AMP responses to PGE_1 in mononuclear cells from rheumatoid sera and synovia were depressed (Zurier *et al.*, 1977), an observation that provides evidence of defective reactivity to prostaglandins by lymphoid cells in rheumatoid arthritis. Thus, Morley (1976) has suggested that, in addition to inhibiting prostaglandin synthesis by lymphokine-stimulated macrophages, aspirin may also reduce rheumatoid joint inflammation by inhibiting lymphocyte activation.

2. *Inhibition of Leukocyte and Platelet Migration*

A key event in any inflammatory reaction, whether acute or chronic, is the marked influx of leukocytes from the blood into the inflammatory lesion. Could aspirin-like drugs reduce inflammation by inhibiting the migration of these inflammatory cells? Northover (1964) failed to show an inhibitory effect of aspirin-like drugs on PMNL migration induced in the peritoneal cavity of mice injected with acetic acid. This finding was subsequently confirmed in a study on carrageenin rat paw edema (Di Rosa *et al.*, 1971), although in this study, inhibition of monocyte migration was observed. These results were essentially confirmed using dextran pleurisy in rats (Di Rosa *et al.*, 1972). Nevertheless, some workers have shown that aspirin-like drugs will inhibit both PMNL and monocyte migration in other rat pleurisy models. Vinegar *et al.* (1973), studying carrageenin pleurisy, found that aspirin given orally inhibited neutrophilic migration, but were unable to show such an effect by locally administered aspirin in a later study (Vinegar *et al.*, 1976). In this particular study, orally administered indomethacin failed to inhibit neutrophilic migration at doses that nevertheless blocked edema formation. In contrast, Blackham and Owen (1975) found that inhibition of exudate formation by aspirin-like drugs in rat carrageenin pleurisy correlated with inhibition of PMNL but not monocyte migration. More recently, the antiinflammatory activity of aspirin-like drugs was shown to correlate to a greater degree with inhibition of leukocyte migration than with reduction of prostaglandin levels in a sponge implant model in rats (Walker *et al.*, 1976).

Thus no clear picture emerges as to whether inhibition of leukocyte migration participates in the antiinflammatory activity of aspirin-like drugs. Warne and West (1978) found that the inhibitory action of salicylates on mononuclear cell migration, in both rat carrageenin pleurisy and a sponge implantation model, varied according to the time of year, an observation which they suggested may explain some of the conflicting literature reports. Perhaps these inconsistencies can also be rationalized, at least partly, by supposing that these drugs act by influencing processes that ultimately provoke migration. Such processes may vary according to the inflammatory stimulus and/or its injection site. For instance, aspirin-like drugs inhibit neutrophil adherence (Stecher and Chinea, 1978), a process which occurs prior to migration into the inflammatory site. Furthermore, there is evidence that platelets may play an important role in inflammation and that aspirin-like drugs may inhibit inflammation through their interaction with platelets. Blood platelets were observed migrating into exudates induced by subcutaneous sponge implants in rats (Smith *et al.*, 1976). The administration of antiplatelet serum reduced both platelet and leukocyte migration as well as exudate prostaglandin levels. Indomethacin and sodium salicylate likewise inhibited all three parameters and also the thrombocytopenia observed 15 minutes following sponge implantation. However, an antiinflammatory fraction found in human plasma (Smith and Ford-Hutchinson, 1975) inhibited leukocyte migration only.

These results suggested that platelets are the source of prostaglandins in the sponge exudate and that they may initiate leukotaxis possibly by generating chemotactic factors such as C5a (Weksler, 1974). In this connection, Walker (1979) has shown that aggregated rat platelets are capable of generating chemotactic activity via complement activation. Moreover, the chemotactic metabolite of arachidonic acid, 12-HETE, is generated by platelets (Turner *et al.*, 1975), and its formation from 12-HPETE is inhibited by aspirin-like drugs (Siegel *et al.*, 1979).

As further general support for a possible role of platelets in inflammation, Vincent *et al.* (1978) found that platelets accumulate at the site of carrageenin paw edema in rats, a process which apparently occurs prior to leukocyte migration. However, it should also be mentioned that the active migration of platelets, at least into implanted sponge exudates, has been questioned (Bolam and Smith, 1977).

3. *Inhibition of Superoxide Anion Production*

Phagocytosis by migrated leukocytes is important in the development of inflammatory responses. In addition to releasing hydrolytic enzymes and other potential inflammatory mediators, phagocytosing leukocytes generate the so-called superoxide anion ($O_2^-\cdot$) (Babior *et al.*, 1973), a powerful oxidation–reduction agent produced by certain oxidative enzymes, notably xanthine oxidase (Misra and Fridovich, 1972). One possible physiological role of $O_2^-\cdot$ is that of a bactericidal agent (Babior *et al.*, 1973). Of greater importance, as far as inflammation is concerned, is the finding that $O_2^-\cdot$, when reacted with hydrogen peroxide to yield the hydroxyl radical OH·, depolymerizes purified hyaluronic acid and bovine synovial fluid (McCord, 1974). Superoxide dismutase (SOD), the naturally occurring protective enzyme that scavenges $O_2^-\cdot$, was found to protect synovial fluid against depolymerization. It was suggested that $O_2^-\cdot$ production could account for the deterioration of synovial fluid in arthritic joints, and that SOD might be antiinflammatory under certain conditions. SOD has since been shown to inhibit the "prostaglandin phase" of carrageenin rat paw edema and hence $O_2^-\cdot$ may also mediate this inflammatory reaction (Oyanagui, 1976a).

Aspirin-like drugs inhibit the production of $O_2^-\cdot$ by guinea pig macrophages in peritoneal exudate induced by paraffin oil (Oyanagui, 1976b), by nonstimulated peritoneal exudate cells from guinea pigs (Oyanagui, 1978), by a xanthine–oxidase system (de Alvare *et al.*, 1976; Puig-Parellada and Planas, 1978), by human phagocytes in contact with aggregated IgG fixed to micropore filters (Lehmeyer and Johnston, 1978), and by human peripheral neutrophils activated by a synthetic chemotactic factor (Simchowitz *et al.*, 1979). In contrast, aspirin itself has little or no effect in most of these systems, whereas copper (II) salicylate is reported to interact with $O_2^-\cdot$ generated by a xanthine–oxidase system (de Alvare *et al.*, 1976). However, since cupric ions themselves are known to catalyze superoxide dismutation (Brigelius *et al.*, 1974, 1975), the activity observed in this study may not necessarily have been due to the salicylate ion per se. Nevertheless, Amphlett *et al.* (1968) state that salicylates react very readily with hydroxyl radicals and, since the *ortho*-hydroxy group of the salicylate molecule is involved in this reaction, it would seem likely that the deacetylation of aspirin (which occurs readily *in vivo*) is necessary before the scavenging of hydroxyl radicals generated from $O_2^-\cdot$ can occur. Also important in determining aspirin's activity may be the tissue examined and/or the mode of $O_2^-\cdot$ generation since aspirin was apparently effective against $O_2^-\cdot$ production in paraffin oil-induced macrophages (Oyanagui, 1976b) but not that produced in unstimulated peritoneal exudate cells (Oyanagui, 1978).

The biosynthesis of prostanoids from arachidonic acid is associated with the production of an oxygen-centered radical, possibly a hydroxyl-like radical derived from $O_2^-\cdot$ (Panganamala *et al.*, 1974a,b). Since phagocytosing PMNLs (Higgs and Youlten, 1972; McCall and Youlten, 1973; Zurier and Sayadoff, 1975) and inflammatory exudate-derived macrophages (Bray *et al.*, 1974; Bray and Gordon, 1976) synthesize prostanoids, the question therefore arises: is the radical produced during phagocytosis the same as that generated during prostanoid synthesis? The answer is probably no, owing to reported differences in the half-life of each radical (Kuehl *et al.*, 1977a). If these radicals are of different origin, then an interaction with nonprostanoid-derived $O_2^-\cdot$ must be considered as a possible additional mechanism of antiinflammatory action of aspirin-like drugs.

4. *Displacement of Endogenous Nonsteroidal Antiinflammatory Substances from Plasma Proteins*

During the last decade or so, there has been much interest in endogenous antiinflammatory substances of nonadrenal origin, particularly as regards their possible role in counterirritant phenomena (Atkinson and Hicks, 1975; Lewis, 1977). More recently, attention has been directed toward their possible involvement in mediating the antiinflammatory action of aspirin-like drugs. Although structurally speaking, the aspirin-like drugs are a heterogeneous group, they all bind extensively to plasma proteins, and there has been much controversy as to whether the bound or free fractions are responsible for their therapeutic activity.

In 1969, McArthur and Dawkins (1969) showed that, *in vitro,* sodium salicylate displaced L-tryptophan from its binding sites on human serum proteins. This was later demonstrated for other antirheumatic drugs (McArthur *et al.*, 1971a) but drugs without antirheumatic activity which bind equally well to plasma proteins did not exhibit this effect (Smith *et al.*, 1971). Furthermore, the displacement of L-tryptophan occurred in rheumatoid patients treated with antirheumatic agents, treatment withdrawal in one patient causing a reversal of this effect (McArthur *et al.*, 1971b). It was proposed that, in rheumatoid patients, an antiinflammatory substance, mimicked by L-tryptophan, becomes bound to an abnormal extent to plasma proteins and that aspirin-like drugs, by binding to these proteins, displace this substance in such a way that the bound: free ratio pertaining in normal individuals is reestablished (Smith and Dawkins, 1971). It was later shown that the total plasma L-tryptophan concentrations in rheumatoid patients were significantly higher than those in normal individuals and that the concentration and percentage of unbound L-tryptophan were both significantly lower in rheumatoid patients (Aylward and Maddock, 1973).

Support for this hypothesis was obtained when human serum was found to contain a protein-bound peptide-like substance with marked antiinflammatory activity (McArthur *et al.*, 1972). Further work, which has been reviewed by Smith and Ford-Hutchinson (1975), showed that this substance was associated with a plasma fraction containing L-tryptophan. Removal of this amino acid did not reduce the antiinflammatory activity of the fraction which appeared to be associated with substances of molecular weight of <1000 that were not linear peptides. The fraction had a wide antiinflammatory spectrum but, unlike the aspirin-like agents, it did not possess antipyretic or antinociceptive properties. Moreover, unlike these drugs, it inhibited Arthus reactions but not cotton pellet- or sponge-induced granuloma formation in rats. It is therefore questionable whether this substance is responsible for the therapeutic activity of aspirin-like drugs. In addition, the foregoing work has recently been overshadowed by the finding that many of the endogenous antiinflammatory substances discovered in biological fluids may be artifacts of the extraction procedures used for their isolation, arising from contamination with bacterial endotoxin which can mimic the pharmacological actions of these substances (Maguire and Wallis, 1977).

5. *The Pharmacokinetic Hypothesis*

Brune (1974) has put forward the intriguing proposal that the antiinflammatory action of aspirin-like drugs may result from their ability to accumulate at sites of inflammation, where they may exert a variety of actions, rather than from a single specific action at some hypothetical receptor. The capacity of these drugs to bind onto plasma proteins, which are subsequently extravasated at inflammatory sites, would be expected to promote their accumulation at such sites. Moreover, because of their acidity (all have pK_a values of approximately 4), these drugs, through enhanced lipophilicity, should more easily penetrate the membranes of cells in the acidic environment of the inflammatory lesion to produce pharmacological/toxicological actions leading to inhibition of inflammation. Brune also suggested that the toxicological profiles of aspirin-like drugs could be explained on a similar basis; they would tend to accumulate in gastric mucosal and renal tubular epithelial cells, both of which border acidic compartments, to produce gastric damage and nephrotoxicity, respectively.

Support for this hypothesis has been obtained from autoradiographic studies in rats in which ^{14}C-labeled phenylbutazone was shown to accumulate at subcutaneous carrageenin injection sites, as well as in the liver, small intestine, and kidney (Graf *et al.*, 1975). In contrast, the basic drug, antipyrine (phenazone), showed no such accumulation. *In vitro* studies have also shown that an acidic environment promotes enhanced accumulation of phenylbutazone within PMNLs (Brune and Graf, 1978). However, that the specific accumulation of acidic antiinflammatory drugs at inflammatory sites is due to plasma protein binding is somewhat in doubt, since it has recently been shown that extensive binding may actually retard the penetration of such drugs into inflammatory exudates (Doherty *et al.*, 1977).

III. General Summary and Conclusions

A. The Argument Summarized

We began this analysis of the molecular mechanism of action of salicylates with the aim of interpreting the therapeutic effects of these drugs in terms of their interactions with biochemical processes in cells or tissues. We expected that such interactions might result from the binding of the drug molecule with one or more types of macromolecule that conducts such processes. Such binding might be expected to occur, for example, at the active site of an enzyme, at the receptor for a neurohumoral transmitter, or at some comparable point. We considered that our primary task, however, was to identify, if possible, the biochemical process or processes whose modification by salicylates led to the therapeutic effects of these drugs and to examine how these effects occurred. This task was pursued along two main lines, emerging from the questions: (1) what is the character of the therapeutic actions of salicylates; and (2) what potent effect(s) of salicylates at a molecular level might give rise to actions of this character?

To answer the first question, we argued that, despite the number and variety of the actions of salicylates, most of these could be regarded as the inhibition of a bodily defensive reaction that had become excessive, unbalanced, or misguided. In short, we continue to hold the view, first proposed 15 years ago (Collier, 1963), that salicylates are "antidefensive" drugs (see Section I,C). This description applies not only to the conventional uses of salicylates as antipyretic, analgesic, and antirheumatic drugs, but also to new potential uses; for example, the suppression of diarrhea and associated symptoms of gastrointestinal distress arising from intolerance to particular foods (Buisseret *et al.*, 1978) or from radiotherapy (Mennie *et al.*, 1975), or, again, of threatened thrombosis (Harter *et al.*, 1979). The description applies, moreover, to some toxic effects of nonsteroidal antiinflammatory drugs. Thus, the ulceration of the small intestine of the rat due to large doses of indomethacin appears to arise from inhibition of a defensive mechanism controlling bacterial invasiveness, since indomethacin does not induce these ulcers in germ-free rats (Robert and Asano, 1977).

It is consistent with the concept that salicylates are antidefensive drugs and that they act therapeutically against pathological processes in the body that have become excessive or misguided rather than against normal physiological processes. It follows that, in the analysis of salicylate action, we are concerned with mechanisms by which pathological processes are mediated or controlled (see Section I,C).

The considerations advanced in Section I,E indicate that salicylates act by inhibiting one, or possibly more than one, local hormonal mechanism mediating defense. Since salicylates affect so many biological systems, this mechanism should be widely distributed through the body.

To the second of our two questions (what potent effect(s) of salicylates at a molecular level might give rise to their therapeutic actions?) many answers have, over the years, been suggested. Some of these suggestions are discussed in Sections I,E and II,E. Most of them need not be considered again, because they show relatively poor fit with the experimental data or because too little is yet known about them for definite conclusions to be reached. There remain, however, two effects of salicylates, both on the metabolism of long-chain unsaturated fatty acids, such as arachidonic acid, that may explain the therapeutic actions of salicylates. These two effects, which we will consider in turn, are: (1) the inhibition of fatty acid cyclooxygenase; and (2) the inhibition of conversion of 12-HPETE to 12-HETE on the lipoxygenase pathway of fatty acid metabolism.

The inhibition of the cylcooxygenase of the prostaglandin synthetase system presumably arises through interaction of the drug molecule with the active site of the enzyme that normally processes a fatty acid substrate. The cyclooxygenase forms the cyclic endoperoxides, which in turn give rise to thromboxanes, prostacyclins, or prostaglandins, according to relative activities of other enzymes of the synthetase system (Fig. 3). Salicylic acid is also an inhibitor of cyclooxygenase, but acts with notably less potency than does aspirin.

Salicylates thus block, with greater or lesser potency, the formation of all local hormones of the prostanoid group. They do so at concentrations obtainable in plasma during therapy and their effects can largely be reversed by exogenous prostaglandins. Prostanoids are produced by every tissue of the body. Many of their actions are such as would fulfill a defensive purpose (Collier, 1971, 1974b). For example, prostanoids induce or cooperate with other local hormones in inducing pain, vasodilation, edema, vomiting, diarrhea, and cough. Moreover, prostanoids are liberated in parts of the body when exposed to assaults against which defense might be expected—by mechanical injury, bacterial toxins, allergens, or other noxious chemicals, and UV- or X-radiation. Thus, the general hypothesis appears to be well supported that salicylates mainly act at a molecular level by inhibiting the cyclooxygenase of prostaglandin synthetase. This hypothesis is essentially that proposed in 1971 by the group at the Royal College of Surgeons in London, headed by J. R. Vane (Vane, 1971; Smith and Willis, 1971; Ferreira *et al.*, 1971). This hypothesis may now be more comprehensively expressed as the "inhibition of prostanoid biosynthesis."

The second possible mechanism so far put forward, which would supplement the inhibition of prostanoid biosynthesis, is based on the observation of Siegel *et al.* (1979) that salicylates inhibit conversion of 12-HPETE to 12-HETE on the lipoxygenase pathway of arachidonate metabolism (Fig. 3). As a result of this observation, these authors proposed that "at least some of the pharmacological actions that these drugs have in common may be related to their ability to influence arachidonate metabolism via the lipoxygenase pathway." The obstacles that the prostanoid hypothesis has encountered and the escape routes offered by the HETE hypothesis will be briefly considered in the next section.

B. Objections Answered and Unanswered

One of the questions raised by the above argument concerns the defensive action of prostanoids and the antidefensive character of salicylates. If different prostanoids liberated in the same area of the body by the same stimulus have opposed actions, how can both be defensive? This question can probably be answered by a careful scrutiny of the defense strategy involved.

For instance, cutting an artery causes both TXA_2, which aggregates platelets, and PGI_2, which inhibits aggregation, to be produced. Study of the exact sites of production, however, reveals that TXA_2 is produced by the platelets and thus may contribute to the formation of a plug of platelets that stems the escape of blood, though its role is probably minor compared to that of thrombin. PGI_2, however, is mainly produced by the intima of the artery and thus helps to prevent platelets sticking to the lining of the artery, with consequent blockage of the lumen (J. R. Vane, personal communication). Thus, production of two prostaglandins of opposed actions in response to local injury can be a coordinated defensive operation.

Other instances of antagonism between prostanoids are also known. For example, PGE_1 antagonizes the bronchoconstrictor action of $PGF_{2\alpha}$, although both are irritants in the airways (Sweatman and Collier, 1968; Gardiner and Collier, 1980b). Again, $PGF_{2\alpha}$ antagonizes the hyperalgesic action of PGE_1 (Juan and Lembeck, 1977). It therefore seems reasonable to postulate that prostanoids can have the secondary function of controlling the excessive or misguided activity of other prostanoids (Collier, 1980).

A second objection to the above hypothesis is that, whereas sodium salicylate is considerably less potent than aspirin as an inhibitor of prostaglandin synthetase, it is about equipotent with aspirin as an antirheumatic, although it is somewhat less potent than aspirin as an antipyretic and relatively still less potent as an analgesic. Thus, two dose levels of aspirin are used in therapy, a high level for rheumatism and a low level for pain or fever, whereas sodium salicylate is usually given only at the higher level, as an antirheumatic.

The route of escape from this difficulty proposed by Flower and Vane (1974b)—that sodium salicylate is activated *in vivo*—has gained little experimental support. An alternative route, for which there is some evidence, is that the pharmacological activity of aspirin is quickly reduced *in vivo* by its conversion to salicylate. Hence, aspirin would be equiactive with salicylate in conditions in which its action is slow, but more active where its action is fast. Thus, we would expect aspirin to be about equal with salicylate against the chronic inflammation of rheumatoid arthritis, but more active against platelet aggregation and bradykinin-induced bronchoconstriction in the guinea pig. This expectation appears to fit the experimental findings; but the relatively weak action of salicylate against cyclooxygenase remains a difficulty. This analysis fits the superior activity of aspirin against headache and menstrual pain; the action of salicylates in chronic pain may be allied to their antiinflammatory action.

A third objection to Vane's hypothesis is that certain inhibitors of prostaglandin synthetase, such as paracetamol, amidopyrine, and phenazone, lack antiinflammatory action, although they are antipyretic and analgesic. The finding that paracetamol is more active against prostaglandin synthetase from rabbit brain than from dog spleen (Flower and Vane, 1972) would explain a central antipyretic or analgesic action of paracetamol, but not a local analgesic action that might occur in the same site as the inflammation that it did not inhibit. Moreover, paracetamol, although a weaker inhibitor of prostaglandin synthetase than is aspirin, does reduce prostaglandin levels in inflammatory exudate in the rat (Walker *et al.*, 1976). It thus appears that another factor is also involved. It does not seem likely that this factor is merely the production of a different spectrum of prostaglandins, since inhibition of cyclooxygenase blocks formation of all prostanoids.

The paradox of paracetamol seems most simply explained by the postulate that, in their antiinflammatory action, salicylates modify a second biochemical process. The best candidate for this second process at present seems to be the conversion of 12-HPETE to 12-HETE (Siegel *et al.*, 1979). If so, it would be required that paracetamol, unlike salicylates, fails to inhibit the conversion. Unfortunately, Siegel *et al.* (1979) have not reported this decisive point.[2]

A further postulate is needed to complete the picture. It is that other processes not mediated by metabolites of long-chain fatty acids, nor inhibited by salicylates, also contribute to inflammatory and allied defensive reactions. The existence of such processes would explain the less than complete effectiveness of salicylates in controlling pain and inflammation.

C. Final Conclusion

From this analysis of the mechanism of action of salicylates, we conclude that inhibition of the cyclooxygenase of prostaglandin synthetase explains those actions of salicylates in which aspirin is more potent than sodium salicylate, including certain forms of analgesia, inhibition of platelet aggregation, antagonism of bradykinin-induced bronchoconstriction in the guinea pig, and possibly antipyresis. This mechanism alone does not, however, appear fully to explain the antiinflammatory action of salicylates, in which aspirin and sodium salicylate are about equipotent and

[2] Since the completion of this review, M. I. Siegel, R. T. McConnell, N. A. Porter, and P. Cuatrecasas (1980. *Proc. Natl. Acad. Sci. U.S.A.* **77**, 308–312) have reported that paracetamol (acetaminophen) fails to inhibit, in platelets, the conversion of 12-HPETE to 12-HETE. This finding supports the proposal that the inhibition of production of 12-HETE contributes to the antiinflammatory action of salicylates.

which certain other antipyretic and analgesic inhibitors of prostaglandin synthetase do not possess. It seems best to suppose, therefore, that, in inhibiting inflammation, salicylates act by two mechanisms, one of which is the inhibition of cyclooxygenase. It is the task of future research on salicylate mechanisms to test this hypothesis and, if possible, to identify the second mechanism involved. The best candidate mechanism now in sight is the inhibition of the conversion of 12-HPETE to 12-HETE; but the critical experiment with paracetamol does not appear to have been done.[2]

References

Adams, S. S., and Cobb, R. (1958). *Nature (London)* **181,** 773–774.

Ammendola, G., Di Rosa, M., and Sorrentino, L. (1975). *Agents Actions* **5,** 250–255.

Amphlett, C. B., Adams, G. E., and Michael, B. D. (1968). *In* "Advances in Chemistry Series No. 81" (R. F. Gould, ed.), pp. 231–250. American Chemical Society, Washington, D.C.

Anthony, C. R., and Panush, R. S. (1978). *Clin. Exp. Immunol.* **31,** 482–489.

Arora, S., Lahiri, P. K., and Sanyal, R. K. (1970). *Int. Arch. Allergy Appl. Immunol.* **39,** 186–191.

Arrigoni-Martelli, E., and Restelli, A. (1972). *Eur. J. Pharmacol.* **19,** 191–198.

Artunkal, A., Marley, E., and Stephenson, J. D. (1975). *Br. J. Pharmacol.* **54,** 250P–251P.

Atkinson, D. C., and Cowan, A. (1974). *J. Pharm. Pharmacol.* **26,** 727–729.

Atkinson, D. C., and Hicks, R. (1975). *Agents Actions* **5,** 239–249.

Atkinson, D. C., and Leach, E. C. (1978). *Agents Actions* **8,** 263–267.

Aylward, M., and Maddock, J. (1973). *J. Pharm. Pharmacol.* **25,** 570–572.

Babior, B. M., Kipnes, R. S., and Curnutte, J. T. (1973). *J. Clin. Invest.* **52,** 741–744.

Baenziger, N. L., Dillinder, M. J., and Majerus, P. W. (1977). *Biochem. Biophys. Res. Commun.* **78,** 294–301.

Barr, W., and Naismith, W. C. M. K. (1972). *Br. Med. J.* **2,** 188–191.

Benitz, K. -F., and Hall, L. M. (1963). *Arch. Int. Pharmacodyn. Ther.* **144,** 185–195.

Bennett, A., Friedman C. A., and Vane, J. R. (1967). *Nature (London)* **216,** 873–876.

Bennett, A., Stamford, I. F., and Stockley, H. L. (1977). *Br. J. Pharmacol.* **61,** 579–586.

Berry, P. A. (1966). Ph. D. Thesis, Council for National Academic Awards, London.

Berry, P. A., and Collier, H. O. J. (1964). *Br. J. Pharmacol. Chemother.* **23,** 201–216.

Bhattacherjee, P., and Eakins, K. E. (1973). *Pharmacologist* **15,** 209–215.

Bhoola, K. D., Collier, H. O. J., Schachter, M., and Shorley, P. G. (1962). *Br. J. Pharmacol. Chemother.* **19,** 190–197.

Bizzi, A., Garattini, S., and Veneroni, E. (1965). *Br. J. Pharmacol. Chemother.* **25,** 187–196.

Blackham, A., and Owen, R. T. (1975). *J. Pharm. Pharmacol.* **27,** 201–203.

Blackham, A., Farmer, J. B., Radziwonik, H., and Westwick, J. (1974). *Br. J. Pharmacol.* **51,** 35–44.

Blackham, A., Radziwonik, H., and Shaw, I. H. (1975). *Agents Actions* **5,** 519–527.

Blackwell, G. J., Duncombe, W. G., Flower, R. J., Parsons, M. F., and Vane, J. R. (1977). *Br. J. Pharmacol.* **59,** 353–366.

Blackwell, G. J., Flower, R. J., Nijkamp, F. P., and Vane, J. R. (1978). *Br. J. Pharmacol.* **62,** 79–89.

Bolam, J. P., and Smith, M. J. H. (1977). *J. Pharm. Pharmacol.* **29,** 674–676.

Bonta, I. L. (1969). *Acta Physiol. Pharmacol. Neerl.* **15,** 188–222.

Bonta, I. L., and Parnham, M. J. (1979). *Br. J. Pharmacol.* **65,** 465–472.

Bonta, I. L., Bult, H., Vincent, J. E., and Zijlstra, F. J. (1977a). *J. Pharm. Pharmacol.* **29,** 1–7.

Bonta, I. L., Parnham, M. J., and Adolfs, M. J. P. (1977b). *Prostaglandins* **14,** 295–307.

Boot, J. R., Dawson, W., and Kitchen, E. A. (1976). *J. Physiol. (London)* **257,** 47P–48P.

Borowska, A., Sierakowski, S., Mackowiak, J., and Wisniewski, K. (1979). *Experientia* **35,** 1368–1370.

Bramm, E., Binderup, L., and Arrigoni-Martelli, E. (1979). *Acta Pharmacol. Toxicol.* **44,** 75–80.

Bray, M. A., and Gordon, D. (1976). *Br. J. Pharmacol.* **57,** 466P–467P.

Bray, M. A., Gordon, D., and Morley, J. (1974). *Br. J. Pharmacol.* **52,** 453P.

Brigelius, R., Spöttl, R., Bors, W., Lengfelder, E., Saran, M., and Weser, U. (1974). *FEBS Lett.* **47,** 72–75.

Brigelius, R., Hartmann, H. J., Bors, W., Saran, M., Lengfelder, E., and Weser, U. (1975). *Hoppe-Seylers Z. Physiol. Chem.* **356,** 739–745.

Brody, T. M. (1956). *J. Pharmacol. Exp. Ther.* **117,** 39–51.

Brune, K. (1974). *Agents Actions* **4,** 230–232.

Brune, K., and Graf, P. (1978). *Biochem. Pharmacol.* **27,** 525–530.

Buisseret, P. D., Youlten, L. J. F., Heinzelmann, D. I., and Lessof, M. H. (1978). *Lancet* **1,** 906–908.

Bunting, S., Moncada, S., and Vane, J. R. (1976). *Br. J. Pharmacol.* **57,** 462P–463P.

Burch, J. W., and Majerus, P. W. (1979). *Semin. Hematol.* **16,** 196–207.

Burch, J. W., and Baenziger, N. L., Stanford, N., and Majerus, P. W. (1978a). *Proc. Natl. Acad. Sci. U.S.A.* **75,** 5181–5184.

Burch, J. W., Stanford, N., and Majerus, P. W. (1978b). *J. Clin. Invest.* **61,** 314–319.

Capasso, F., Dunn, C. J., Yamamoto, S., Willoughby, D. A., and Giroud, J.-P. (1975). *J. Pathol.* **116,** 117–124.

Cashin, C. H., and Heading, C. E. (1968). *Br. J. Pharmacol.* **34,** 148–158.

Chenoweth, M. B. (1956). *Pharmacol. Rev.* **8,** 57–87.

Clark, W. G., and Cumby, H. R. (1975a). *J. Physiol. (London)* **248,** 625–638.

Clark, W. G., and Cumby, H. R. (1975b). *Prostaglandins* **9,** 361–368.

Coceani, F., Pace-Asciak, C., Volta, F., and Wolfe, L. S. (1967). *Am. J. Physiol.* **213,** 1056–1064.

Cochran, J. B. (1952). *Br. Med. J.* **2,** 964–967.

Coleman, R. A., Kennedy, I., and Levy, G. P. (1980). *Br. J. Pharmacol.* **69,** 266P–267P.

Collier, H. O. J. (1963). *Sci. Am.* **209,** 97–108.

Collier, H. O. J. (1964). *In* "Evaluation of Drug Activities: Pharmacometrics" (D. R. Laurence and A. L. Bacharach, eds.), pp. 183–203. Academic Press, New York.

Collier, H. O. J. (1968). *Sci. Basis Med. Annu. Rev.* pp. 308–335.

Collier, H. O. J. (1969a). *Adv. Pharmacol. Chemother.* **7,** 333–405.

Collier, H. O. J. (1969b). *Nature (London)* **223,** 35–37.

Collier, H. O. J. (1971). *Nature (London)* **232,** 17–19.

Collier, H. O. J. (1974a). *In* "Prostaglandin Synthetase Inhibitors" (H. J. Robinson and J. R. Vane, eds.), p. 76. Raven, New York.

Collier, H. O. J. (1974b). *In* "Prostaglandin Synthetase Inhibitors" (H. J. Robinson and J. R. Vane, eds.), pp. 121–133. Raven, New York.

Collier, H. O. J. (1976). *In* "Chemistry and Biology of the Kallikrein-Kinin System in Health and Disease, Fogarty International Center Proceedings No. 27" (J. J. Pisano and K. F. Austen, eds.), pp. 495–503. U.S. Gov. Printing Office, Washington, D.C.

Collier, H. O. J. (1977). *In* "Comments on Proposals to Establish a Monograph for OTC Internal Analgesic, Antipyretic and Antirheumatic Products." Appendix C, Submission to U.S. FDA by Miles Laboratories, No. 77N-0094.

Collier, H. O. J. (1980). *In* "Prostaglandin Synthetase Inhibitors in Clinical Medicine" (P. W. Ramwell, ed.), pp. 87–105. Liss, New York.
Collier, H. O. J., and Gardiner, P. J. (1974). *In* "Evaluation of Bronchodilator Drugs" (D. M. Burley, S. W. Clarke, M. F. Cuthbert, J. W. Paterson, and J. H. Shelley, eds.), pp. 17–25. Trust for Education and Research in Therapeutics, London.
Collier, H. O. J., and James, G. W. L. (1966). *J. Physiol. (London)* **185,** 71P–72P.
Collier, H. O. J., and Schneider, C. (1972). *Nature (London) New Biol.* **236,** 141–143.
Collier, H. O. J., and Shorley, P. G. (1960). *Br. J. Pharmacol. Chemother.* **15,** 601–610.
Collier, H. O. J., and Sweatman, W. J. F. (1968). *Nature (London)* **219,** 864–865.
Collier, H. O. J., James, G. W. L., and Schneider, C. (1966). *Nature (London)* **212,** 411–412.
Collier, H. O. J., Dinneen, L. C., Perkins, A. C., and Piper, P. J. (1968a). *Naunyn-Schmiedebergs Arch. Exp. Pathol. Pharmakol.* **259,** S159.
Collier, H. O. J., James, G. W. L., and Piper, P. J. (1968b). *Br. J. Pharmacol.* **34,** 76–87.
Collier, J. G., Karim, S. M. M., Robinson, B., and Somers, K. (1972). *Br. J. Pharmacol.* **44,** 374P–375P.
Collier, H. O. J., Saeed, S. A., Schneider, C., and Warren, B. T. (1973). *Adv. Biosci.* **9,** 413–418.
Collier, H. O. J., Francis, A. A., McDonald-Gibson, W. J., and Saeed, S. A. (1976a). *Prostaglandins* **11,** 219–225.
Collier, H. O. J., McDonald-Gibson, W. J., and Saeed, S. A. (1976b). *Br. J. Pharmacol.* **58,** 193–199.
Collier, H. O. J., Denning-Kendall, P. A., McDonald-Gibson, W. J., and Saeed, S. A. (1980). *In* "Hemostasis, Prostaglandins and Renal Disease" (G. Remuzzi, G. Mecca and G. de Gaetano, eds.), pp. 257–267. Raven, New York.
Craft, I. (1972). *Br. Med. J.* **2,** 191–194.
Cranston, W. I., Hellon, R. F., and Mitchell, D. (1975). *J. Physiol. (London)* **248,** 27P–29P.
Cranston, W. I., Duff, G. W., Hellon, R. F., Mitchell, D., and Townsend, Y. (1976). *J. Physiol. (London)* **259,** 239–249.
Crook, D., Collins, A. J., Bacon, P. A., and Chan, R. (1976). *Ann. Rheum. Dis.* **35,** 327–332.
Crout, J. E., Hepburn, B., and Ritts, R. E. (1975). *New Engl. J. Med.* **292,** 221–223.
Crunkhorn, P., and Willis, A. L. (1969). *Br. J. Pharmacol.* **36,** 216P–217P.
Crunkhorn, P., and Willis, A. L. (1971a). *Br. J. Pharmacol.* **41,** 49–56.
Crunkhorn, P., and Willis, A. L. (1971b). *Br. J. Pharmacol.* **41,** 507–512.
Cummings, J. H., Newman, A., Misiewicz, J. J., Milton-Thompson, G. J., and Billings, J. A. (1973). *Nature (London)* **243,** 169–171.
de Alvare, L. R., Goda, K., and Kimura, T. (1976). *Biochem. Biophys. Res. Commun.* **69,** 687–694.
Dejana, E., Quintana, A., Callioni, A., and de Gaetano, G. (1979). *Thromb. Res.* **15,** 199–207.
Deraedt, R., Jouquey, S., Benzoni, J., and Peterfalvi, M. (1976). *Arch. Int. Pharmacodyn. Ther.* **224,** 30–42.
Dey, P. K., Feldberg, W., Gupta, K. P., Milton, A. S., and Wendlandt, S. (1974). *J. Physiol. (London)* **241,** 692–646.
Dick, W. C., Grennan, D. M., and Zeitlin, I. J. (1976). *Br. J. Pharmacol.* **56,** 313–316.
Didisheim, P. (1968). *Throm. Diath. Haemorrh.* **20,** 257–266.
Dilawari, J. B., Newman, A., Poleo, J., and Misiewicz, J. J. (1975). *Gut* **16,** 137–143.
DiPasquale, G., Rassaert, C., Richter, R., Wielaj, P., and Tripp, L. (1973). *Prostaglandins* **3,** 741–757.
Di Rosa, M., Papdimitriou, J. M., and Willoughby, D. A. (1971). *J. Pathol.* **105,** 239–256.
Di Rosa, M., Sorrentino, L., and Parente, L. (1972). *J. Pharm. Pharmacol.* **24,** 575–576.

Doherty, N. S., Anttila, M., and Dean, P. B. (1977). *Ann. Rheum. Dis.* **36,** 244–248.
Domenjoz, R. (1971). *In* "Rheumatoid Arthritis: Pathogenetic Mechanisms and Consequences in Therapeutics" (W. Müller, H.-G. Harwerth, and K. Fehr, eds.), pp. 513–550. Academic Press, New York.
Dreser, H. (1899). *Pfluegers Arch. Gesamte Physiol. Menschen Tiere* **76,** 306–318.
Duncan, M. W., Person, D. A., Rich, R. R., and Sharp, J. T. (1977). *Arthritis Rheum.* **20,** 1174–1178.
Eckenfels, A., and Vane, J. R. (1972). *Br. J. Pharmacol.* **45,** 451–462.
Egan, R. W., Paxton, J., and Kuehl, F. A. (1976). *J. Biol. Chem.* **251,** 7329–7335.
Eisen, V., Walker, D. I., Binysh, S. G., and Tedder, R. S. (1977). *Agents Actions, Suppl. AAS* **2,** 99–108.
Ezer, E., Palosi, E., Hajos, Gy., and Szporny, L. (1976). *J. Pharm. Pharmacol.* **28,** 655–656.
Famaey, J.-P., and Whitehouse, M. W. (1973). *Biochem. Pharmacol.* **22,** 2707–2717.
Famaey, J.-P., and Whitehouse, M. W. (1976). *Arch. Int. Physiol. Biochim.* **84,** 719–734.
Farmer, J. B., Farrar, D. G., and Wilson, J. (1974). *Br. J. Pharmacol.* **52,** 559–565.
Feldberg, W. (1974). *In* "Prostaglandin Synthetase Inhibitors" (H. J. Robinson and J. R. Vane, eds.), pp. 197–203. Raven, New York.
Feldberg, W., and Gupta, K. P. (1972). *J. Physiol. (London)* **222,** 126P–129P.
Feldberg, W., and Gupta, K. P. (1973). *J. Physiol. (London)* **228,** 41–53.
Feldberg, W., and Saxena, P. N. (1971a). *J. Physiol. (London)* **217,** 547–556.
Feldberg, W., and Saxena, P. N. (1971b). *J. Physiol. (London)* **219,** 739–745.
Feldberg, W., and Saxena, P. N. (1975). *J. Physiol. (London)* **249,** 601–615.
Feldberg, W., Gupta, K. P., Milton, A. S., and Wendlandt, S. (1973). *J. Physiol. (London)* **234,** 279–303.
Ferreira, S. H. (1972). *Nature (London) New Biol.* **240,** 200–203.
Ferreira, S. H., and Nakamura, M. (1979). *In* "Advances in Inflammation Research" (G. Weissmann, B. Samuelsson, and R. Paoletti, eds.), Vol. I, pp. 317–329. Raven, New York.
Ferreira, S. H., Moncada, S., and Vane, J. R. (1971). *Nature (London) New Biol.* **231,** 237–239.
Ferreira, S. H., Moncada, S., and Vane, J. R. (1973). *Br. J. Pharmacol.* **49,** 86–97.
Ferreira, S. H., Flower, R. J., Parsons, M. F., and Vane, J. R. (1974). *Prostaglandins* **8,** 433–437.
Ferreira, S. H., Nakamura, M., and Castro, M. S. A. (1978). *Prostaglandins* **16,** 31–37.
Filshie, G. (1971). *Ann. N. Y. Acad. Sci.* **180,** 553.
Floersheim, G. L. (1965). *In* "Non-Steroidal Anti-Inflammatory Drugs" (S. Garattini and M. N. G. Dukes, eds.), pp. 232–235. Excerpta Medica Foundation, Amsterdam.
Flower, R. J., and Vane, J. R. (1972). *Nature (London)* **240,** 410–411.
Flower, R. J., and Vane, J. R. (1974a). *Biochem. Pharmacol.* **23,** 1439–1450.
Flower, R. J., and Vane, J. R. (1974b). *In* "Prostaglandin Synthetase Inhibitors" (H. J. Robinson and J. R. Vane, eds.), pp. 9–31. Raven, New York.
Flower, R. J., Gryglewski, R., Herbaczynska-Cedro, K., and Vane, J. R. (1972). *Nature (London) New Biol.* **238,** 104–106.
Flower, R. J., Cheung, H. S., and Cushman, D. W. (1973). *Prostaglandins* **4,** 325–341.
Forbes, I. J., and Smith, J. L. (1967). *Lancet* **2,** 334–337.
Ford-Hutchinson, A. W., Walker, J. R., Davidson, E. M., and Smith, M. J. H. (1978). *Prostaglandins* **16,** 253–258.
Frederickson, R. C. A. (1977). *Life Sci.* **21,** 23–41.
Frens, J., van Miert, A. S. J. P. A. M., and van Duin, C. Th. M. (1978). *Br. J. Pharmacol.* **64,** 439P.
Garcia Leme, J., Bechara, G. H., and Sudo, L. S. (1977). *Br. J. Exp. Pathol.* **58,** 703–711.

Gardiner, P. J., and Collier, H. O. J. (1980a). *Prostaglandins* **19,** 819–841.
Gardiner, P. J., and Collier, H. O. J. (1980b). *In* "Advances in Prostaglandin and Thromboxane Research" (B. Samuelsson and R. Paoletti, eds.), Vol. VII, pp. 1003–1008. Raven, New York.
Gilfoil, T. M., Klavins, I., and Grumbach, L. (1963). *J. Pharmacol. Exp. Ther.* **142,** 1–5.
Gillespie, A. (1972). *Br. Med. J.* **1,** 150–152.
Glenn, E. M., and Rohloff, N. (1972). *Proc. Soc. Exp. Biol. Med.* **139,** 290–294.
Goetzl, E. J., and Gorman, R. R. (1978). *J. Immunol.* **120,** 526–531.
Goldlust, M. B., and Schreiber, W. F. (1975). *Agents Actions* **5,** 39–47.
Goldstein, A. (1976). *Science* **193,** 1081–1086.
Goldstein, S., DeMeo, R., Shemano, I., and Beiler, J. M. (1966). *Proc. Soc. Exp. Biol. Med.* **123,** 712–715.
Gordon, D., Bray, M. A., and Morley, J. (1976). *Nature (London)* **262,** 401–402.
Graf, P., Glatt, M., and Brune, K. (1975). *Experientia* **31,** 951–953.
Greaves, M. W., Sondergaard, J., and McDonald-Gibson, W. (1971). *Br. Med. J.* **2,** 258–260.
Gryglewski, R. J., Bunting, S., Moncada, S., Flower, R. J., and Vane, J. R. (1976). *Prostaglandins* **12,** 685–713.
Hales, J. R. S., Bennett, J. W., Baird, J. A., and Fawcett, A. A. (1973). *Pfluegers Arch. Gesamte Physiol. Menschen Tiere* **339,** 125–133.
Ham, E. A., Cirillo, V. J., Zanetti, M., Shen, T. Y., and Kuehl, F. A. (1972). *In* "Prostaglandins in Cellular Biology" (P. W. Ramwell and B. B. Pharriss, eds.), pp. 345–352. Plenum, New York.
Hamberg, M. (1972). *Biochem. Biophys. Res. Commun.* **49,** 720–726.
Hamberg, M., and Samuelsson, B. (1974). *Proc. Natl. Acad. Sci. U.S.A.* **71,** 3400–3404.
Hamberg, M., Svensson, J., and Samuelsson, B. (1974a). *Proc. Natl. Acad. Sci. U.S.A.* **71,** 3824–3828.
Hamberg, M., Svensson, J., Wakabayashi, T., and Samuelsson, B. (1974b). *Proc. Natl. Acad. Sci. U.S.A.* **71,** 345–349.
Hamberg, M., Hedqvist, P., Strandberg, K., Svensson, J., and Samuelsson, B. (1975a). *Life Sci.* **16,** 451–461.
Hamberg, M., Svensson, J., and Samuelsson, B. (1975b). *Proc. Natl. Acad. Sci. U.S.A.* **72,** 2994–2998.
Harter, H. R., Burch, J. W., Majerus, P. W., Stanford, N., Delmez, J. A., Anderson, C. B., and Weerts, C. A. (1979). *New Engl. J. Med.* **301,** 577–579.
Hawkins, M., and Lipton, J. M. (1977). *Prostaglandins* **13,** 209–218.
Helfer, H., and Jaques, R. (1968). *Helv. Physiol. Pharmacol. Acta* **26,** 137–144.
Herman, A. G., and Vane, J. R. (1975). *Arch. Int. Pharmacodyn. Ther.* **213,** 328–329.
Hichens, M. (1974). *In* "Anti-Inflammatory Agents: Chemistry and Pharmacology" (R. A. Scherrer and M. W. Whitehouse, eds.), Vol. II, pp. 263–302. Academic Press, New York.
Higgs, G. A., and Salmon, J. A. (1979). *Prostaglandins* **17,** 737–746.
Higgs, G. A., and Youlten, L. J. F. (1972). *Br. J. Pharmacol.* **44,** 330P.
Higgs, G. A., Vane, J. R., Hart, F. D., and Wojtulewski, J. A. (1974). *In* "Prostaglandin Synthetase Inhibitors" (H. J. Robinson and J. R. Vane, eds.), pp. 165–173. Raven, New York.
Higgs, G. A., McCall, E., and Youlten, L. J. F. (1975). *Br. J. Pharmacol.* **53,** 539–546.
Higgs, G. A., Harvey, E. A., Ferreira, S. H., and Vane, J. R. (1976). *In* "Advances in Prostaglandin and Thromboxane Research" (B. Samuelsson and R. Paoletti, eds.), Vol. I, pp. 105–110. Raven, New York.
Higgs, E. A., Moncada, S., and Vane, J. R. (1978). *Prostaglandins* **16,** 153–162.
Hitchens, J. T., Goldstein, S., Shemano, I., and Beiler, J. M. (1967). *Arch. Int. Pharmacodyn. Ther.* **169,** 384–393.

Holmes, S. W., and Horton, E. W. (1968). *J. Physiol. (London)* **195,** 731–741.
Horodniak, J. W., Julius, M., Zarembo, J. E., and Bender, A. D. (1974). *Biochem. Biophys. Res. Commun.* **57,** 539–545.
Horton, E. W. (1963). *Nature (London)* **200,** 892–893.
Horton, E. W., Main, I. H. M., Thompson, C. J., and Wright, P. M. (1968). *Gut* **9,** 655–658.
Ignarro, L. J. (1971). *Biochem. Pharmacol.* **20,** 2847–2860.
Jaques, R. (1965). *Helv. Physiol. Pharmacol. Acta* **23,** 156–162.
Jaques, R. (1969). *Experientia* **25,** 1059–1060.
Johnson, R. A., Morton, D. R., Kinner, J. H., Gorman, R. R., McGuire, J. C., Sun, F. F., Whittaker, N., Bunting, S., Salmon, J. A., Moncada, S., and Vane, J. R. (1976). *Prostaglandins* **12,** 915–928.
Johnston, M. G., Hay, J. B., and Movat, H. Z. (1976). *Agents Actions* **6,** 705–711.
Jori, A., and Bernardi, D. (1966). *Med. Pharmacol. Exp.* **14,** 500–506.
Juan, H., and Lembeck, F. (1974). *Naunyn-Schmiedebergs Arch. Exp. Pathol. Pharmakol.* **283,** 151–164.
Juan, H., and Lembeck, F. (1977). *Br. J. Pharmacol.* **59,** 385–391.
Juhlin, L., and Michaelsson, G. (1969). *Acta Derm. Venereol.* **49,** 251–261.
Kalbhen, D. A., Domenjoz, R., and Ehlers, K. (1967). *Life Sci.* **6,** 1883–1886.
Kaley, G., and Weiner, R. (1968). *In* "Prostaglandin Symposium of the Worcester Foundation for Experimental Biology" (P. W. Ramwell and J. E. Shaw, eds.), pp. 321–328. Wiley (Interscience), New York.
Kaley, G., and Weiner, R. (1971). *Ann. N.Y. Acad. Sci.* **180,** 338–350.
Karim, S. M. M. (1971). *Ann. N.Y. Acad. Sci.* **180,** 483–498.
Kitchen, E. A., Boot, J. R., and Dawson, W. (1978). *Prostaglandins* **16,** 239–244.
Klee, W. A. (1977). *In* "Peptides in Neurobiology" (H. Gainer, ed.), pp. 375–396. Plenum, New York.
Kloeze, J. (1967). *In* "Prostaglandins" (S. Bergström and B. Samuelsson, eds.), pp. 241–252. Almqvist & Wiksell, Stockholm.
Kloeze, J. (1969). *Biochim. Biophys. Acta* **187,** 285–292.
Kocsis, J. J., Hernandovich, J., Silver, M. J., Smith, J. B., and Ingerman, C. (1973). *Prostaglandins* **3,** 141–153.
Komoriya, K., Ohmori, H., Azuma, A., Kurozumi, S., Hashimoto, Y., Nicolaou, K. C., Barnette, W. E., and Magolda, R. L. (1978). *Prostaglandins* **15,** 557–564.
Ku, E. C., and Wasvary, J. M. (1973). *Fed. Proc. Fed. Am. Soc. Exp. Biol.* **32,** 803 (Abstr.).
Kuehl, F. A., Egan, R. W., Humes, J. L., Beveridge, G. C., and Van Arman, C. G. (1977a). *In* "Biochemical Aspects of Prostaglandins and Thromboxanes" (N. Kharasch and J. Fried, eds.), pp. 55–74. Academic Press, New York.
Kuehl, F. A., Humes, J. L., Egan, R. W., Ham, E. A., Beveridge, G. C., and Van Arman, C. G. (1977b). *Nature (London)* **265,** 170–173.
Laburn, H., Woolf, C. J., Willies, G. H., and Rosendorff, C. (1975). *Neuropharmacology* **14,** 405–411.
Laburn, H., Mitchell, D., and Rosendorff, C. (1977). *J. Physiol. (London)* **267,** 559–570.
Lands, W. E. M., Le Tellier, P. R., Rome, L. H., and Vanderhoek, J. Y. (1973). *Adv. Biosci.* **9,** 15–28.
Leduc, L. E., and Needleman, P. (1979). *J. Pharmacol. Exp. Ther.* **211,** 181–188.
Lehmeyer, J. E., and Johnston, R. B. (1978). *Clin. Immunol. Immunopathol.* **9,** 482–490.
Lembeck, F., and Juan, H. (1974). *Naunyn-Schmiedebergs Arch. Exp. Pathol. Pharmakol.* **285,** 301–313.
Lembeck, F., Popper, H., and Juan, H. (1976). *Naunyn-Schmiedebergs Arch. Exp. Pathol. Pharmakol.* **294,** 69–73.
Lester, D., Lolli, G., and Greenberg, L. A. (1946). *J. Pharmacol.* **87,** 329–342.
Lewis, A. J. (1978). *Agents Actions* **8,** 244–250.

Lewis, A. J., Nelson, D. J., and Sugrue, M. F. (1974). *Br. J. Pharmacol.* **50,** 468P–469P.
Lewis, D. A. (1977). *Biochem. Pharmacol.* **26,** 693–698.
Lichtenstein, L. M., and DeBernardo, R. (1971). *J. Immunol.* **107,** 1131–1136.
Lieb, J. (1978). *Lancet* **2,** 157.
Lim, R. K. S. (1966). *In* "The Salicylates: A Critical Bibliographic Review" (M. J. H. Smith and P. K. Smith, eds.), pp. 155–202. Wiley (Interscience), New York.
Lim, R. K. S., Guzman, F., Rodgers, D. W., Goto, K., Braun, C., Dickerson, G. D., and Engle, R. J. (1964). *Arch. Int. Pharmacodyn. Ther.* **152,** 25–58.
Lim, R. K. S., Leung, P. M., and Guy, J. L. (1967). *Fed. Proc. Fed. Am. Soc. Exp. Biol.* **26,** 619.
Luderer, J. R., Demers, L. M., Bonnem, E. M., Saleem, A., and Jeffries, G. H. (1976). *New Engl. J. Med.* **295,** 1179.
McArthur, J. N., and Dawkins, P. D. (1969). *J. Pharm. Pharmacol.* **21,** 744–750.
McArthur, J. N., Dawkins, P. D., and Smith, M. J. H. (1971a). *J. Pharm. Pharmacol.* **23,** 393–398.
McArthur, J. N., Dawkins, P. D., Smith, M. J. H., and Hamilton, E. B. D. (1971b). *Br. Med. J.* **2,** 677–679.
McArthur, J. N., Smith, M. J. H., and Freeman, P. C. (1972). *J. Pharm. Pharmacol.* **24,** 669–671.
McCall, E., and Youlten, L. J. F. (1973). *J. Physiol. (London)* **234,** 98P–100P.
McCall, E., and Youlten, L. J. F. (1974). *Br. J. Pharmacol.* **52,** 452P.
McCord, J. M. (1974). *Science* **185,** 529–531.
McDonald-Gibson, W. J., and Collier, H. O. J. (1979). *Eur. J. Pharmacol.* **58,** 497–500.
Maguire, E. D., and Wallis, R. B. (1977). *Br. J. Pharmacol.* **59,** 261–268.
Majerus, P. W. (1976). *Circulation* **54,** 357–359.
Malmsten, C., Hamberg, M., Svensson, J., and Samuelsson, B. (1975). *Proc. Natl. Acad. Sci. U.S.A.* **72,** 1446–1450.
Marks, V., Smith, M. J. H., and Cunliffe, A. C. (1961). *J. Pharm. Pharmacol.* **13,** 218–223.
Masotti, G., Galanti, G., Poggesi, L., Abbate, R., and Neri Serneri, G. G. (1979). *Lancet* **2,** 1213–1216.
Matuchansky, C., and Bernier, J.-J. (1973). *Gastroenterology* **64,** 1111–1118.
Matuchansky, C., Mary, J.-Y., and Bernier, J.-J. (1976). *Gastroenterology* **71,** 274–281.
Menguy, R., and Masters, Y. F. (1965). *Surg. Gynecol. Obstet.* **120,** 92–98.
Mennie, A. T., Dalley, V. M., Dinneen, L. C., and Collier, H. O. J. (1975). *Lancet* **2,** 942–943.
Mielke, C. H., Kaneshiro, M. M., Maher, I. A., Weiner, J. M., and Rapaport, S. I. (1969). *Blood* **34,** 204–215.
Miller, W. S., and Smith, J. G. (1966). *Proc. Soc. Exp. Biol. Med.* **122,** 634–636.
Mills, D. G., Hirst, M., and Philp, R. B. (1974). *Life Sci.* **14,** 673–684.
Milton, A. S., and Wendlandt, S. (1970). *J. Physiol. (London)* **207,** 76P–77P.
Milton, A. S., and Wendlandt, S. (1971). *J. Physiol. (London)* **218,** 325–336.
Misiewicz, J. J., Waller, S. L., Kiley, N., and Horton, E. W. (1969). *Lancet* **1,** 648–651.
Misra, H. P., and Fridovich, I. (1972). *J. Biol. Chem.* **247,** 188–192.
Mizushima, Y. (1964). *Arch. Int. Pharmacodyn. Ther.* **149,** 1–7.
Mizushima, Y., and Suzuki, H. (1965). *Arch. Int. Pharmacodyn. Ther.* **157,** 115–124.
Moncada, S., Ferreira, S. H., and Vane, J. R. (1973). *Nature (London)* **246,** 217–219.
Moncada, S., Ferreira, S. H., and Vane, J. R. (1975). *Eur. J. Pharmacol.* **31,** 250–260.
Moncada, S., Gryglewski, R., Bunting, S., and Vane, J. R. (1976). *Nature (London)* **263,** 663–665.
Moncada, S., Higgs, E. A., and Vane, J. R. (1977). *Lancet* **1,** 18–21.

Morley, J. (1974). *Prostaglandins* **8,** 315–326.
Morley, J. (1975). *In* "Proceedings of the Aspirin Symposium" (T. L. C. Dale, ed.), pp. 19–22. Aspirin Foundation, London.
Morley, J. (1976). *Nurs. Mirror* **143,** 57–59.
Murota, S., Morita, I., Tsurufuji, S., Sato, H., and Sugio, K. (1978). *Prostaglandins* **15,** 297–301.
Murota, S., Chang, W.-C., Tsurufuji, S., and Morita, I. (1979). *In* "Advances in Inflammation Research" (G. Weissmann, B. Samuelsson, and R. Paoletti, eds.), Vol. I, pp. 439–455. Raven, New York.
Murphy, R. C., Hammarström, S., and Samuelsson, B. (1979). *Proc. Natl. Acad. Sci. U.S.A.* **76,** 4275–4279.
Myers, R. D. (1976). Cited in *Nature (London)* **264,** 213–214.
Myers, R. D., Rudy, T. A., and Yaksh, T. L. (1974). *J. Physiol. (London)* **243,** 167–193.
Nijkamp, F. P., Flower, R. J., Moncada, S., and Vane, J. R. (1976). *Nature (London)* **263,** 479–482.
Northover, B. J. (1964). *J. Pathol. Bacteriol.* **88,** 332–335.
Nugteren, D. H. (1975). *Biochim. Biophys. Acta* **380,** 299–307.
O'Brien, J. R. (1968). *Lancet* **1,** 779–783.
Opelz, G., Terasaki, P. I., and Hirata, A. A. (1973). *Lancet* **2,** 478–480.
Orange, R. P., Austen, W. G., and Austen, K. F. (1971). *J. Exp. Med.* **134,** 136s–148s.
Oyanagui, Y. (1976a). *Biochem. Pharmacol.* **25,** 1465–1472.
Oyanagui, Y. (1976b). *Biochem. Pharmacol.* **25,** 1473–1480.
Oyanagui, Y. (1978). *Biochem. Pharmacol.* **27,** 777–782.
Pace-Asciak, C. R. (1973). *Adv. Biosci.* **9,** 29–33.
Pace-Asciak, C., and Wolfe, L. S. (1971). *Biochemistry* **10,** 3657–3664.
Packham, M. A., and Mustard, J. F. (1977). *Blood* **50,** 555–573.
Palmer, M. A., Piper, P. J., and Vane, J. R. (1970a). *Br. J. Pharmacol.* **40,** 547P–548P.
Palmer, M. A., Piper, P. J., and Vane, J. R. (1970b). *Br. J. Pharmacol.* **40,** 581P–582P.
Panganamala, R. V., Brownlee, N. R., Sprecher, H., and Cornwell, D. G. (1974a). *Prostaglandins* **7,** 21–28.
Panganamala, R. V., Sharma, H. M., Sprecher, H., Geer, J. C., and Cornwell, D. G. (1974b). *Prostaglandins* **8,** 3–11.
Peskar, B. M. (1977). *Biochim. Biophys. Acta* **487,** 307–314.
Pinckard, R. N., Hawkins, D., and Farr, R. S. (1968). *Nature (London)* **219,** 68–69.
Piper, P. J., and Vane, J. R. (1969). *Nature (London)* **223,** 29–37.
Piper, P. J., and Vane, J. R. (1971). *Ann. N.Y. Acad. Sci.* **180,** 363–383.
Potts, W. J., and East, P. F. (1972). *Arch. Int. Pharmacodyn, Ther.* **197,** 31–36.
Puig-Parellada, P., and Planus, J. M. (1978). *Biochem. Pharmacol.* **27,** 535–537.
Rainsford, K. D., and Whitehouse, M. W. (1976). *J. Pharm. Pharmacol.* **28,** 83–86.
Ramwell, P. W., and Shaw, J. E. (1968). *J. Physiol. (London)* **195,** 34P–36P.
Randall, L. O., and Selitto, J. J. (1957). *Arch. Int. Pharmacodyn. Ther.* **111,** 409–419.
Rask-Madsen, J. (1980). *In* "Prostaglandin Synthetase Inhibitors in Clinical Medicine" (P. W. Ramwell, ed.), pp. 375–396. Liss, New York.
Rask-Madsen, J., and Bukhave, K. (1978). *Gut* **19,** A448–A449.
Rawlins, M. D., Luff, R. H., and Cranston, W. I. (1973). *Biochem. Pharmacol.* **22,** 2639–2642.
Ribeiro dos Santos, R., Garcia Leme, J., Ferreira, S. H., Bechara, G. H., and Sudo, L. (1976). *Agents Actions* **6,** 690–693.
Robak, J., Wieckowski, A., and Gryglewski, R. (1978). *Biochem. Pharmacol.* **27,** 393–396.
Robert, A., and Asano, T. (1977). *Gastroenterology* **72,** A97/1120.

Robinson, D. R., and Levine, L. (1974). *J. Clin. Invest.* **53,** 65a–66a.

Rooney, P. J., Lee, P., Brookes, P., and Dick, W. C. (1973). *Curr. Med. Res. Opin.* **1,** 501–516.

Rosenthale, M. E., and Nagra, C. L. (1967). *Proc. Soc. Exp. Biol. Med.* **125,** 149–153.

Roth, G. J., and Majerus, P. W. (1975). *J. Clin. Invest.* **56,** 624–632.

Roth, G. J., Stanford, N., and Majerus, P. W. (1975). *Proc. Natl. Acad. Sci. U.S.A.* **72,** 3073–3076.

Roth, G. J., Stanford, N., Jacobs, J. W., and Majerus, P. W. (1977). *Biochemistry* **16,** 4244–4248.

Saeed, S. A., McDonald-Gibson, W. J., Cuthbert, J., Copas, J. L., Schneider, C., Gardiner, P. J., Butt, N. M., and Collier, H. O. J. (1977). *Nature (London)* **270,** 32–36.

Schoener, E. P., and Wang, S. C. (1974). *Experientia* **30,** 383–384.

Shanahan, R. W. (1968). *Arch. Int. Pharmacodyn. Ther.* **175,** 186–192.

Shio, H., and Ramwell, P. (1972). *Nature (London) New Biol.* **236,** 45–46.

Sicuteri, F. (1970). *In* "Bradykinin, Kallidin and Kallikrein" (E. G. Erdös, ed.), pp. 482–515. Springer Verlag, Berlin and New York.

Siegel, M. I., McConnell, R. T., and Cuatrecasas, P. (1979). *Proc. Natl. Acad. Sci. U.S.A.* **76,** 3774–3778.

Silver, M. J., Smith, J. B., Ingerman, C., and Kocsis, J. J. (1973). *Prostaglandins* **4,** 863–875.

Simchowitz, L., Mehta, J., and Spilberg, I. (1979). *Arthritis Rheum.* **22,** 755–763.

Smith, J. B., and Willis, A. L. (1971). *Nature (London) New Biol.* **231,** 235–237.

Smith, J. L., and Forbes, I. J. (1967). *Nature (London)* **215,** 538–539.

Smith, M. J. H. (1963). *In* "Salicylates: An International Symposium" (A. St. J. Dixon, B. K. Martin, M. J. H. Smith, and P. H. N. Wood, eds.), pp. 47–54. Little, Brown, Boston, Massachusetts.

Smith, M. J. H., and Dawkins, P. D. (1971). *J. Pharm. Pharmacol.* **23,** 729–744.

Smith, M. J. H., and Ford-Hutchinson, A. W. (1975). *Agents Actions* **5,** 318–321.

Smith, M. J. H., and Smith, P. K., eds. (1966). "The Salicylates: A Critical Bibliographic Review." Wiley (Interscience), New York.

Smith, M. J. H., Dawkins, P. D., and McArthur, J. N. (1971). *J. Pharm. Pharmacol.* **23,** 451.

Smith, M. J. H., Ford-Hutchinson, A. W., and Elliott, P. N. C. (1975). *J. Pharm. Pharmacol.* **27,** 473–478.

Smith, M. J. H., Walker, J. R., Ford-Hutchinson, A. W., and Penington, D. G. (1976). *Agents Actions* **6,** 701–704.

Smythies, J. R., and Russell, R. O. (1974). *Lancet* **2,** 963.

Solomon, L. M., Juhlin, L., and Kirschenbaum, M. B. (1968). *J. Invest. Dermatol.* **51,** 280–282.

Sondergaard, J., and Wolf-Jurgensen, P. (1972). *Acta Derm. Venereol.* **52,** 361–364.

Sorenson, J. R. J. (1974a). *Nat. Meet. Am. Chem. Soc. Med. Chem. Div., 167th.* Abstr. No. 73.

Sorenson, J. R. J. (1974b). *In* "Trace Substances in Environmental Health-VIII" (D. D. Hemphill, ed.), pp. 305–311. Univ. of Missouri Press, Columbia.

Sorenson, J. R. J. (1976a). *J. Med. Chem.* **19,** 135–148.

Sorenson, J. R. J. (1976b). *Inflammation* **1,** 317–331.

Stecher, V. J., and Chinea, G. L. (1978). *Agents Actions* **8,** 258–262.

Stitt, J. T. (1973). *J. Physiol. (London)* **232,** 163–179.

Sweatman, W. J. F., and Collier, H. O. J. (1968). *Nature (London)* **217,** 69.

Sykes, J. A. C., and Maddox, I. S. (1972). *Nature (London) New Biol.* **237,** 59–61.

Takeguchi, C., and Sih, C. J. (1972). *Prostaglandins* **2,** 169–184.

Tauber, A. I., Kaliner, M., Stechschulte, D. J., and Austen, K. F. (1973). *J. Immunol.* **111,** 27–32.
Thomas, G., and West, G. B. (1973). *J. Pharm. Pharmacol.* **25,** 747–748.
Tomlinson, R. V., Ringold, H. J., Qureshi, M. C., and Forchielli, E. (1972). *Biochem. Biophys. Res. Commun.* **46,** 552–559.
Turker, K., and Kiran, B. K. (1964). *Arzneim. Forsch.* **14,** 1318–1319.
Turner, S. R., Tainer, J. A., and Lynn, W. S. (1975). *Nature (London)* **257,** 680–681.
Twomey, J. J., Mena, H., and Lazar, S. (1974). *Lancet* **1,** 684–685.
Vane, J. R. (1971). *Nature (London) New Biol.* **231,** 232–235.
Vane, J. R. (1972). *Hosp. Pract.* **7**(3), 61–71.
Vane, J. R. (1974). *In* "Prostaglandin Synthetase Inhibitors" (H. J. Robinson and J. R. Vane, eds.), p. 70. Raven, New York.
Vane, J. R., and Ferreira, S. H. (1976). *In* "Chemistry and Biology of the Kallikrein-Kinin System in Health and Disease, Fogarty International Center Proceedings No. 27" (J. J. Pisano and K. F. Austen, eds.), pp. 255–266. U.S. Gov. Printing Office, Washington, D.C.
Vargaftig, B. B. (1966). *Experientia* **22,** 182–183.
Vargaftig, B. B., and Dao, N. (1971). *Pharmacology* **6,** 99–108.
Vargaftig, B. B., and Zirinis, P. (1973). *Nature (London) New Biol.* **244,** 114–116.
Vaughan, J. H., and Chihara, T. (1975). *Arch. Intern. Med.* **135,** 1324–1328.
Veale, W. L., and Cooper, K. E. (1974). *J. Appl. Physiol.* **37,** 942–945.
Velo, G. P., Dunn, C. J., Giroud, J.-P., Timsit, J., and Willoughby, D. A. (1973). *J. Pathol.* **111,** 149–158.
Verstraete, M. (1976). *Am. J. Med.* **61,** 897–914.
Villa, S., Livio, M., and de Gaetano, G. (1979). *Br. J. Haematol.* **42,** 425–431.
Vincent, J. E., Zijlstra, F. J., and Bonta, I. L. (1975). *Prostaglandins* **10,** 899–911.
Vincent, J. E., Bonta, I. L., and Zijlstra, F. J. (1978). *Agents Actions* **8,** 291–295.
Vinegar, R., Truax, J. F., and Selph, J. L. (1973). *Proc. Soc. Exp. Biol. Med.* **143,** 711–714.
Vinegar, R., Truax, J. F., and Selph, J. L. (1976). *Fed. Proc. Fed. Am. Soc. Exp. Biol.* **35,** 2447–2454.
Walker, D. I., and Eisen, V. (1979). *Int. J. Radiat. Biol.* **36,** 399–407.
Walker, J. R. (1979). *Int. Arch. Allergy Appl. Immunol.* **60,** 44–49.
Walker, J. R., Smith, M. J. H., and Ford-Hutchinson, A. W. (1976). *Agents Actions* **6,** 602–606.
Warne, P. J., and West, G. B. (1978). *J. Pharm. Pharmacol.* **30,** 783–785.
Wasserman, M. A. (1976). *Eur. J. Pharmacol.* **36,** 103–114.
Weiss, H. J. (1976). *Am. Heart J.* **92,** 86–102.
Weiss, H. J., Aledort, L. M., and Kochwa, S. (1968). *J. Clin. Invest.* **47,** 2169–2180.
Weissmann, G. (1972). *New Engl. J. Med.* **286,** 141–147.
Weissmann, G., Zurier, R. B., Spieler, P. J., and Goldstein, I. M. (1971). *J. Exp. Med.* **134,** 149s–165s.
Weksler, B. B. (1974). *In* "Platelets: Production, Function, Transfusion and Storage" (M. G. Baldini and S. Ebbe, eds.), pp. 277–285. Grune & Stratton, New York.
Whelan, C. J. (1974). *J. Pharm. Pharmacol.* **26,** 355–356.
Whitehouse, M. W. (1965). *Fortschr. Arzneimittelforsch.* **8,** 321–429.
Whitehouse, M. W. (1971). *In* "Rheumatoid Arthritis: Pathogenetic Mechanisms and Consequences in Therapeutics" (W. Müller, H.-G. Harwerth, and K. Fehr, eds.), pp. 197–208. Academic Press, New York.
Williams, D. A., Waltz, D. T., and Foye, W. O. (1976). *J. Pharm. Sci.* **65,** 126–128.
Williams, T. J. (1976). *Br. J. Pharmacol.* **56,** 341P–342P.
Williams, T. J. (1979). *Br. J. Pharmacol.* **65,** 517–524.

Williams, T. J., and Morley, J. (1973). *Nature (London)* **246,** 215–217.
Willis, A. L. (1969). *In* "In Prostaglandins, Peptides and Amines" (P. Mantegazza and E. W. Horton, eds.), pp. 31–38. Academic Press, New York.
Willis, A. L., Davison, P., Ramwell, P. W., Brocklehurst, W. E., and Smith, B. (1972). *In* "Prostaglandins in Cellular Biology" (P. W. Ramwell and B. B. Pharriss, eds.), pp. 227–259. Plenum, New York.
Willis, A. L., Vane, F. M., Kuhn, D. C., Scott, C. G., and Petrin, M. (1974). *Prostaglandins* **8,** 453–507.
Willoughby, D. A. (1968). *J. Pathol. Bacteriol.* **96,** 381–387.
Winder, C. V. (1959). *Nature (London)* **184,** 494–497.
Winter, C. A. (1965). *In* "Non-Steroidal Anti-Inflammatory Drugs" (S. Garattini and M. N. G. Dukes, eds.), pp. 190–202. Excerpta Medica Foundation, Amsterdam.
Winter, C. A., and Flataker, L. (1965). *J. Pharmacol. Exp. Ther.* **148,** 373–379.
Woolf, C. J., Willies, G. H., Laburn, H., and Rosendorff, C. (1975). *Neuropharmacology* **14,** 397–403.
Zucker, M. B., and Peterson, J. (1968). *Proc. Soc. Exp. Biol. Med.* **127,** 547–551.
Zurier, R. B. (1974). *In* "Mediators of Inflammation" (G. Weissmann, ed.), pp. 163–180. Plenum, New York.
Zurier, R. B., and Sayadoff, D. M. (1975). *Inflammation* **1,** 93–101.
Zurier, R. B., Hoffstein, S., and Weissmann, G. (1973). *Arthritis Rheum.* **16,** 606–618.
Zurier, R. B., Doty, J., and Goldenberg, A. (1977). *Prostaglandins* **13,** 25–31.

ADVANCES IN PHARMACOLOGY AND CHEMOTHERAPY, VOL. 17

Physiological and Pharmacological Determinants of Sensitivity and Resistance to 5-Fluorouracil in Lower Animals and Man

BACH ARDALAN

Laboratory of Toxicology, Developmental Therapeutics Program
Division of Cancer Treatment, National Cancer Institute
Bethesda, Maryland
and
Department of Medical Oncology
City of Hope National Medical Center
Duarte, California

DAVID COONEY

Laboratory of Medicinal Chemistry and Biology, Developmental Therapeutics Program
Division of Cancer Treatment, National Cancer Institute
Bethesda, Maryland

JOHN S. MACDONALD

Cancer Therapy Evaluation Program, Division of Cancer Treatment
National Cancer Institute
Bethesda, Maryland

I. Introduction

The biological activation of 5-fluorouracil (5-FU)[1] is dependent on the operation of several enzymes; these can be aggregated into three principal

[1] Abbreviations: 5-FU, 5-fluorouracil; 5-FUR, 5-fluorouridine; 5-FUdR, 5-fluorodeoxyuridine; 5-FUMP, 5-fluorouridine 5′-monophosphate; 5-FUDP, 5-fluorouridine, 5′-diphos-

ISBN 0-12-032917-4

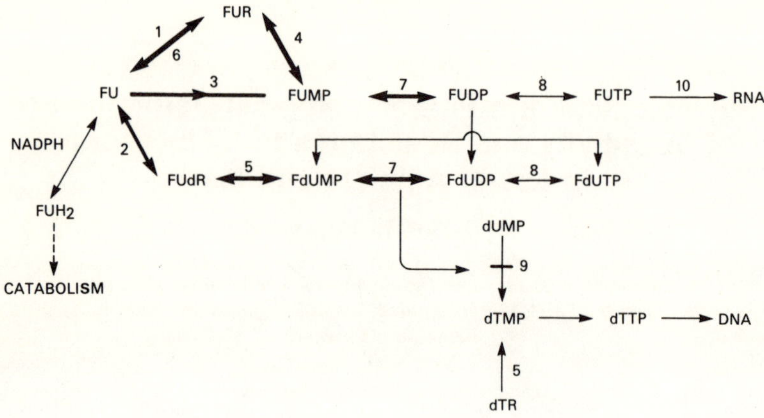

FIG. 1. Interrelationship of metabolism of 5-FU and pharmacological actions. 1, Uridine phosphorylase; 2, thymidine phosphorylase; 3, phosphoribosyltransferase; 4, uridine kinase; 5, thymidine kinase; 6, ribonucleotide reductase; 7, pyrimidine monophosphate kinase; 8, pyrimidine diphosphate kinase; 9, thymidylate synthetase; 10, RNA–polymerase.

groups: those which anabolize the drug; those which catabolize it, or its anabolites; and "target" enzymes whose function is finally interrupted following treatment. These families of enzymes are susceptible, in turn, to two general types of regulation: physiologic control, which is used here to encompass genetic or biochemical modulation, and pharmacologic control, which is used to designate the synergistic or antagonistic actions of one drug on the activity of the other. As 5-FU continues to be used in the palliation of breast and gastrointestinal malignancies, more information is being gathered on these classes of enzymes, as well as on the manner in which they are regulated. It is the purpose of this article to discuss selected aspects of such regulation, with emphasis both on published and original findings in the field. Whenever possible, absolute specific activities of the enzymes involved will be presented in order that reasonable

---

phate; 5-FUTP, 5-fluorouridine, 5′-triphosphate; 5-FdUMP, 5-fluorodeoxyuridine, 5′-monophosphate; 5-FdUDP, 5-fluorodeoxyuridine, 5′-diphosphate; 5-dUTP, 5-fluorodeoxyuridine, 5′-triphosphate; PRPP, 5-phosphoribosyl-1-pyrophosphate; 5-BrUdR, 5-bromodeoxyuridine; 5-ClUdR, 5-chlorodeoxyuridine; ATP, adenosine 5′-triphosphate; dATP, deoxyadenosine 5′-triphosphate; 5-FdCTP, 5-fluorodeoxycytidine 5′-triphosphate; dUMP, deoxyuridine, 5′-monophosphate; RNA, ribonucleic acid; DNA, deoxyribonucleic acid; NADPH, nicotinamide-adenine dinucleotide phosphate, reduced form; dTR, deoxythymidine; dTMP, deoxythymidine, 5′-monophosphate; dTTP, deoxythymidine, 5′-triphosphate; R-1-P, ribose 1-phosphate; dR-1-P, deoxyribose 1-phosphate; OPRTase; orotate phosphoribosyltransferase.

TABLE I

SPECIFIC ACTIVITIES OF NUCLEOSIDE KINASE AND PHOSPHORYLASE IN A PANEL OF MURINE TUMORS

Tumor	Nucleoside kinase activity (nmoles/mg protein/hour)		Nucleoside phosphorylase activity (nmoles/mg protein/hour)	
	Uridine	Thymidine	Uridine	Thymidine
L 1210	8.3 ± 3.5	—	17.21 ± 1.5	5.6 ± 7.3
L5178Y/AR	22.8 ± 0.6	—	41.2 ± 8.9	8.5 ± 4.9
B.16	5.2 ± 3.8	—	12.59 ± 0.7	1.2
Lewis lung	35.1 ± 7.9	6.6 ± 1.2	—	—
Mouse ovarian teratocarcinoma	58.6 ± 8.3	2.4 ± 0.8	—	—
Ehrlich ascites sarcoma	49.3 ± 4.3	3.57 ± 0.30	—	—
P388/0	23.2 ± 4.1	0.91 ± 0.11	—	—
P388/5-FU	32.7 ± 6.7	1.36 ± 0.17		

TABLE II

SPECIFIC ACTIVITY OF NUCLEOSIDE PHOSPHORYLASE IN HUMAN BREAST TUMORS

Human breast tumor	Nucleoside phosphorylase activity (nmoles/mg protein/hour)	
	Uridine	Thymidine
1	21.84	94.6
2	157.4	397.5
3	17.44	38.57
4	178.2	563.8
5	21.5	71.75
6	25.9	107.31
7	16.11	4.56
8	153.9	486.4
9	79.2	203.83
10	287.8	307.5
11	1489.4	1240.80
12	1.92	255.8
13	1817.3	604.5
14	752.5	1377.5
15	224.8	539.8

intercomparisons can be made of their relative contributions to the metabolism of 5-FU.

Figure 1 is a diagram of the routes known to be involved in the anabolism and catabolism of 5-FU. Indicated in the bold arrows on this figure are enzymic steps whose modulation is associated with resistance to the drug under physiologic circumstances. The specific activities of some of these enzymes, in a panel of widely used mouse tumors, are presented in Table I: comparable values for a group of human breast carcinomas are shown in Table II. These values were generated *in vitro* under conditions of substrate saturation. At this junction, each of these enzymic steps will be examined in turn.

II. Preclinical Studies

A. Anabolic Enzymes

1. *Uridine Phosphorylase*

Uridine phosphorylase catalyzes the following reaction:

$$\text{U or 5-FU} + \text{Ribose 1-Phosphate} \leftrightharpoons \text{UR or 5-FUR} + \text{Phosphate}$$

Uridine phosphorylase occupies a central role in the degradation of pyrimidine nucleotides as well as in the "salvage" pathway for nucleic acid synthesis. The enzyme is essentially cytoplasmic and has been reported to be widely distributed in many rat organs, with the highest activity demonstrable in the small intestine: 16.5 nmoles of uracil are formed per minute per milligram protein (Kraut *et al.*, unpublished data).

The specific activity of this enzyme in murine tumors ranges from 12.5 ± 0.7 to 41.2 ± 8.9 nmoles/mg protein/hour in the B 16 melanoma and L5178Y/AR, respectively (Table I). In studies reported by Reichard *et al.* (1959, 1962), resistance to 5-FU in cells of the Ehrlich ascites tumor and L1210 leukemia was accompanied by a decrease in the activities both of uridine phosphorylase and uridine kinase.

In a series of human breast tumors, the specific activity of uridine phosphorylase was, on the average, substantially higher than the comparable value for rodents with rates ranging from 1.92 to 1489.4 nmoles/mg protein/hour (Table II). Moreover, in a retrospective analysis of 11 patients treated with 5-FU, the responders were generally those demonstrating high specific activation of uridine phosphorylase (Table III). This suggests that the enzyme is likely to play a quantitatively important role in the inauguration of the metabolism of 5-FU and that any depression of its activity might have negative therapeutic effects.

TABLE III

SYNTHESIS OF FUdR, FUR, AND FUMP FROM 5-FU AND CYTOSOLS FROM HUMAN BREAST CANCER *in Vitro*[a]

Precursor	Product	Responders	Nonresponders
		(nmoles of product formed/mg protein/hour)	
dR-1-P	5-FUdR	307.0[b] ±121.2	275.2 ±125.1
R-1-P	5-FUR	272.3 ± 98.2	81.5 ± 29.2
PRPP	5-FUMP	1.43 ± 0.59	1.67 ± 0.72

[a] Cytosol fraction of human breast cancer incubated with [2-^{14}C]5-FU, and buffer mix containing either dR-1-P or R-1-P or PRPP.

[b] Mean ± SD.

2. *Thymidine Phosphorylase*

Through the action of thymidine phosphorylase, a deoxyribose moiety is coupled with U or 5-FU:

$$\text{U or 5-FU + Deoxyribose 1-phosphate} \rightleftharpoons \text{UdR or 5-FUdR + Phosphate}$$

This enzyme can also accept deoxyuridine as an alternate substrate and is present in many human tissues, most notably liver (86 nmoles/mg/hour), and spleen (80 nmoles/mg/hour) (Zimmerman *et al.*, 1964). It also has been measured in the plasma of normal mice and human beings at a calculated specific activity of approximately 0.2 nmoles/mg protein/hour (Pauly *et al.*, 1977). (Since these studies were carried out at a thymidine concentration of 12 μM, they probably do not reflect the velocity at saturation.) Interestingly, the activity of plasmatic thymidine phosphorylase increases up to 10-fold in the course of uncontrolled neoplastic growth (Pauly *et al.*, 1978). Relevant to the present vogue in the chemotherapeutic use of thymidine together with 5-FU is the recent observation of Salser *et al.* (1979) that thymidine phosphorylase activity was also induced promptly and markedly (3–20×) by parenteral doses of thymidine, and that the enzyme, so induced, persisted at elevated levels even after the inducing stimulus, i.e., thymidine, had disappeared from the circulation. Since this enzyme can shunt 5-FU in the direction of 5-FdUMP via 5-FUdR, and since 5-FUdR has cytotoxic and therapeutic properties different than 5-FU, e.g., it is 1000 times more cytotoxic *in vitro,* this persistent effect could have profound therapeutic and toxicologic consequences (B. Ardalan, unpublished data).

In murine tumors, the specific activity of thymidine phosphorylase is, in general, lower than that of uridine phosphorylase (Table I); however, the rate at which extracts of human breast carcinomas catalyzed the conjugation of deoxyribose 1-phosphate to 5-FU was somewhat higher than the corresponding rate with ribose 1-phosphate (Table III). In one other study, human neoplasms originating in the kidney and stomach exhibited specific activities in the neighborhood of 125 μmoles/gm/hour. In certain rapidly growing rodent hepatomas, the enzyme is present at a level approximately three times lower than in normal liver. Moreover, depression of the specific activity of thymidine phosphorylase has been shown to have therapeutic consequences in at least one experimental setting. Ohnuma *et al.* (1978) have shown that B lymphocytes are 1000 times more sensitive to killing by 5-FU than are T cells. Subsequently, Fox *et al.* (1979) determined that thymidine phosphorylase levels in T cells are either absent or many fold more feeble than those of B cells; this difference, therefore, assumes causal importance to the state of resistance to 5-FU.

3. *Phosphoribosyl Transferase*

5-FU can acquire a ribose moiety phosphorylated in the 5′ position through the operation of one, or possibly several phosphoribosyltransferases:

$$\text{U or 5-FU + PRPP} \xrightleftharpoons{Mg^{2+}} \text{UMP or 5-FUMP + Ribose 5-Phosphate}$$

Orotic acid phosphoribosyltransferase is generally acknowledged to be the enzyme principally responsible for this step. Greenberg *et al.* (1956) was the first worker to demonstrate that an ultracentrifugally homogeneous preparation of the phosphoribosyltransferase from calf thymus could accept 5-FU as a substrate. Subsequently, Kessel *et al.* (1965) isolated the enzyme from P388 leukemic blasts and characterized its substrate specificity: orotic acid, 5-fluoroorotic acid, 5-fluorouracil, and uracil were all utilized, with K_is of 400, 600, 300, and 70 μmoles/mg protein/minute, respectively.[2] Thus, at least as far as velocity at saturation is concerned, 5-FU is the preferred substrate.

All of the phosphoribosyltransferases examined to date have exhibited an absolute requirement for magnesium or manganese ions, with an opti-

[2] These maximal velocities are perplexingly high especially in view of the fact that the specific activity of the best preparation of enzyme purified by these workers was approximately 3 nmoles/mg protein/hour. Reyes and Gugani (1975) purified orotate phosphoribosyltransferase from other murine leukemia, P15345; these workers did not provide V_{max} values, but the specific activities of their enzyme toward 5-FU, orotic acid, and uracil (at pH 10) were 120, 96, and 47 nmoles/mg protein/hour.

mal concentration of approximately 2 m*M*. The K_m for PRPP ranges from 25 to 100 μM depending on the source, but is independent of the cosubstrate, at least within the family of pyrimidines mentioned earlier. The pH optima of the two well-characterized tumoral phosphotransferases were alkaline, but rather markedly dependent on substrate; thus, in glycine buffer, maximal activity with oratic acid and fluorouracil was observed at or near pH 9.0, while the corresponding value with uracil fell between pH 10 and 11.

Orotic phosphoribosyltransferase, as an essential participating enzyme in the *de novo* pathway of pyrimidine biosynthesis, is widely distributed in normal tissues, especially those with contingents of rapidly dividing cells. Thus, mouse liver and brain exhibited specific activities of this enzyme at birth which approach 120 and 50 nmoles/mg protein/hour, respectively; these activities decreased by 20% of their neonatal values in the adult of this species. Tissues with a presumably lower rate of DNA synthesis also exhibited notable levels of activities; these included erythrocytes of humans and cows. Orotic acid phosphoribosyltransferase purified from each of the above mentioned sources invariably exhibits the ability to decarboxylate OMP; this feature has warranted the conclusion that both of the aforementioned activities are catalyzed by a single enzyme or multienzyme complex, *in vivo*. The ability of red cells to activate 5-FU could serve as a means of trapping the drug in these cells (Fig. 2). As a consequence of their impermeability to nucleotides, erythrocytes could then function as a reservoir from which drug might be slowly released as the cells senesce.

From the standpoint of predictive enzymology, it is noteworthy that the specific activities of orotate phosphoribosyltransferase in a panel of mouse neoplasms correlated in an imperfect but, nevertheless, significant way with sensitivity to the oncolytic activity of 5-FU. Thus, the P388 and P1534 J leukemias both exhibited a high specific activity of approximately 8 nmoles/mg protein/hour, as well as notable increases in survival ranging from 125 to 200% when 5-FU was given intraperitoneally at the maximally effective doses (5–20 mg/kg) on days 1–10 after the implantation of 10^6 cells. Conversely, the Mecca lymphosarcoma contained orotate phosphoribosyltransferase at a specific activity of only approximately 1 nmole/mg/hour and responded to optimal doses of 5-FU with a negligible (25%) increase in survival. More dramatic, still, were the correlations observed in a variant of L1210 rendered resistant to 5-FU where the drug was wholly inactive, and orotate phosphoribosyltransferase was wholly absent. The fact that an enzyme essential for pyrimidine biosynthesis was lacking in these rapidly dividing cells is perplexing and raises several possibilities; (1) that the *de novo* pathway was, in fact, defunct in such mu-

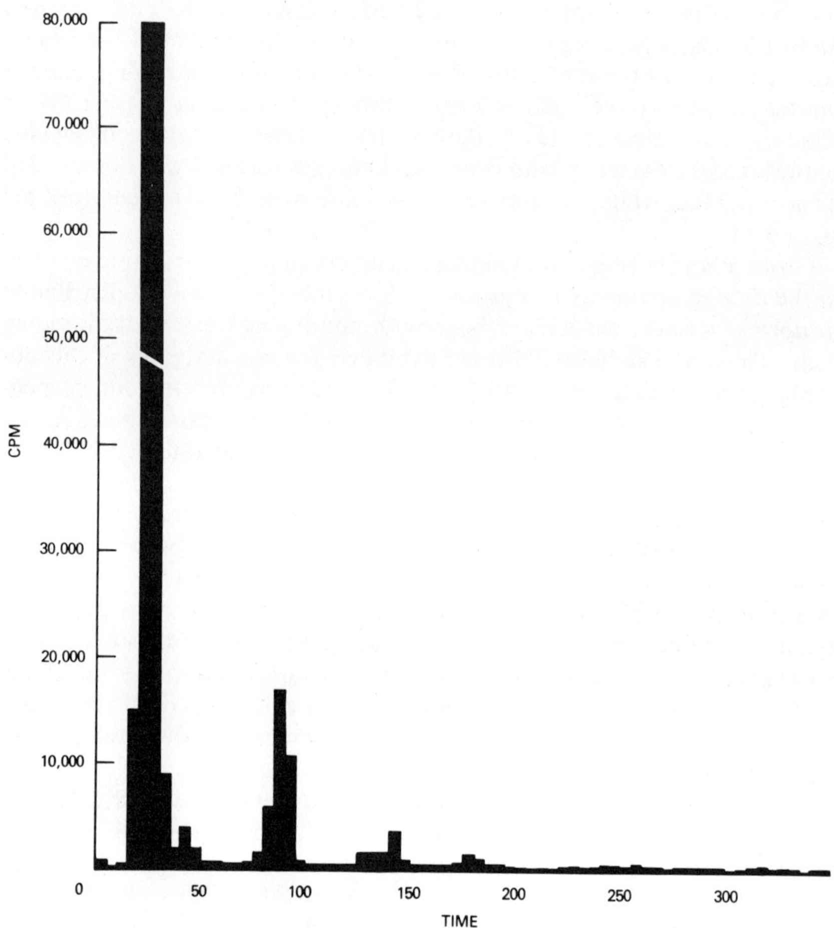

FIG. 2. Formation of fluorinated nucleotides from [2-^{14}C]5-FU by human red cells. Human red cell preparation was incubated with [2-^{14}C]5-FU, 30 μCi, specific activity 13.1 mCi/mmole for 2 hours; thereafter red cells were washed twice with physiological saline, lysed, and protein percipitated with 5% percholic acid; 12,000 *g* supernatant was loaded on an automatic chromatography analyzer (Ardalan *et al.*, 1980). Approximately 3% of the total radioactivity appeared in the fluorinated monophosphate elution time of 90 minutes, with minimal formation of either diphosphate or triphosphate.

tants or (2) that the catalytic properties of orotate phosphoribosyltransferase had changed in L1210/FU, so that 5-FU was no longer accepted as a substrate.

Although the correlations between sensitivity to 5-FU and phosphoribosyltransferase activity were significant, salient exceptions were documented. Thus, leukemia 5178Y contained the title enzyme at the highest specific activity of any murine neoplasm examined, yet 5-FU produces only a modest increase of survival *versus* this tumor. When this exception was removed from the computations, the correlation coefficient between sensitivity or resistance to 5-FU and specific activity of orotate phosphoribosyltransferase in the remaining 11 neoplasms improved to 0.82. This correlative study, although not comprehensive in scope, remains the most definitive in the literature on the predictive enzymology of mouse tumors to 5-FU. It raised, not unexpectedly, the expectation that measurements of orotic acid phosphoribosyltransferase might be of value in determining which patients might undergo remission on exposure to 5-FU. Since the customary response rate in breast and bowel cancers is approximately 20%, and since 5-FU can produce pronounced side-effects at therapeutic doses, this knowledge is of more than biochemical interest; it would permit 80% of the potential recipients of a toxic antimetabolite to be spared such exposure. However, contrary to expectations, it was very soon apparent that the specific activity of orotic acid phosphoribosyltransferase in human neoplasms was markedly lower than the comparable activity in the rodent series (Ardalan *et al.*, 1979). Indeed, the feebleness of this activity makes accurate measurement of the enzyme difficult and renders questionable any prediction made on such measurements. These features are underscored in Table III, where it can be seen that OPRTasc is present in human breast tumors at mean levels of 1.5 nmole/mg protein/hour which is 5-fold lower than those reported for most mouse neoplasms irrespective of their responsiveness to 5-FU. In addition, no correlation was found between the 10 specimens in the series with the highest activity and response to 5-FU. These results notwithstanding, it is only fair to stress that with superior analytical methodology, and in the setting of a prospective therapeutic trial, measurements of orotic acid phosphoribosyltransferase, *inter alia,* might assume predictive importance.

4. *Uridine Kinase*

Once the ribosyl group is acquired by 5-FU, further anabolism requires phosphorylation of the 5′ position; this step is accomplished by uridine kinase:

$$\text{UR, CY, or 5-FUR} + \text{ATP-Mg}^{2+} \rightleftharpoons \text{UMP, CMP, or 5-FUMP} + \text{ADP-Mg}^{2+}$$

Because it is present at exceptionally high specific activities in a broad variety of tumors and tissues, uridine kinase is likely to be one of the principal determinants of the ultimate anabolic fates of 5-FU; in other words, this enzyme may serve to shunt the drug in the direction of ribonucleotides; these, in turn, can be used for RNA synthesis. Since this fate (i.e., incorporation of 5-FU into RNA) has been considered by Martin and others (1978) to govern the oncolytic actions of 5-FU, it is likely to be of pivotal therapeutic importance. Indeed, depressions of its activity are thought to be associated with impaired anabolism of 5-FU and resistance to the drug. Thus, using sublines of Ehrlich ascites tumor cells and in L1210 leukemia, Reichard *et al.* (1959, 1962) were able to correlate successful therapy with 5-FU and near normal levels of uridine kinase; conversely, mutants lacking normal complements of this kinase proved to be refractory to chemotherapy. It is significant in this regard that, in cells of the Ehrlich ascites carcinoma, 95% of the nucleotides incorporated into RNA originate from the so-called salvage pathway.

As a prominent participant in this pathway, uridine kinase can exert profound control over such critical cellular processes as transcription and protein synthesis. Conversely, it is, in turn, subject to feedback control by its ultimate products: thus UTP and CTP inhibit uridine kinase profoundly with K_is of 60 and 50 μM, respectively (Lee, 1976). ATP is the preferred energy donor; however, ITP and GTP can, under certain conditions, replace it. Similarly, magnesium is the preferred metal ion cofactor, but manganese and iron are utilized by the enzyme, although at diminished velocities. In general, uridine is phosphorylated at a rate roughly twice that seen with cytidine; thymidine is not utilized by the purest preparation of the enzyme from murine tumors.

From a chemotherapeutic standpoint, the importance of uridine kinase derives from its ability to phosphorylate 5′-fluorouridine (5-FUdR). Indeed, the enzyme from Ehrlich ascites tumor cells exhibits a greater affinity for this fluorinated pyrimidine (K_m = 23 μM) than for either uridine (K_m = 48 μM) or cytidine (K_m = 90 μM) (Sköld *et al.*, 1962). However, FUR produces substrate inhibition at concentrations above $5 \times 10^{-4}\ M$, whereas uridine is noninhibitory at concentrations four times this; it follows that doses of 5-FUdR capable of achieving the former concentration *in vivo* might retard the anabolism of the drug.

5. *Thymidine Kinase*

Thymidine kinase catalyzes the phosphorylation of deoxythymidine and a number of congeneric molecules, among them the whole family of halogenated pyrimidines, to form the corresponding deoxyribonucleotides:

$$\begin{matrix} \text{TdR} & & \text{TMP} & \\ \text{or} & + \text{ATP-Mg}^{2+} \rightarrow & \text{or} & + \text{ADP-Mg}^{2+} \\ \text{5-FUdR} & & \text{5-FdUMP.} & \end{matrix}$$

In mammals, thymidine kinase is found both in the cytoplasm and in the mitochondria (Okazaki *et al.*, 1964).

With thymidine as substrate, the enzyme plays an important and obvious role in pyrimidine nucleoside salvage; with FUdR as substrate, it directly generates 5-FdUMP, a metabolite that is of profound chemotherapeutic importance by virtue of its efficacious inhibition of thymidylate synthetase.

Thymidine kinase activity is closely correlated with the proliferative capacity of the normal and neoplastic cells; for example, it has been observed that marked elevations in its activity accompany hepatic regeneration (Bresnick, 1971), neoplastic tissues (Sneider, 1969; Bresnick, 1965; Bukovsyk, 1965; Hashimoto, 1972), virally infected cells entering the S-phase of the cell cycle (Brent, 1971), tissues undergoing dietary and diurnal variation (Sheinin, 1966), and the embryonic liver (Klemperer *et al.*, 1968; Taylor *et al.*, 1972).

This kind of correlation has laid the foundation for the expectation that 5-FU or 5-FUdR might be maximally metabolized and, therefore, maximally therapeutic in aggressive malignancies; however, this expectation has not always been met in man (Heidelberger, 1973).

The substrate specificity of the mammalian thymidine kinase extends to the halogenated pyrimidines; however, whereas 5-BrUdR, 5-ClUdR, and 5-IUdR are equal to thymidine as substrates, 5-FUdR is phosphorylated at only 60% of the rate measured with thymidine; uridine is not a substrate for the enzyme from regenerating rate liver.

In general, ATP or dATP is the preferred source of energy for the phosphorylation of thymidine and, presumably, FUdR; magnesium ions are the preferred metal cofactor (K_m = 0.8 mM). The pyrimidine deoxyribonucleosides UdR and 5-FUdR, in their capacity as alternate substrates, are competitive inhibitors of thymidine kinase from liver with K_is of 110 and 20 μM, respectively. In addition, certain pyrimidine nucleoside triphosphates are powerful inhibitors of mitochondrial thymidine kinase; for example, the K_is of dTTP and dCTP are 10 and 2 μM, respectively. Now, 5-FU is known to be metabolized to 5-FdUTP and 5-FdCTP at a slow but finite rate. By analogy to the natural pyrimidine nucleotides mentioned above, it is likely that these fraudulent pyrimidines might be capable of inhibiting thymidine kinase, and that the onset of such inhibition might be delayed as a consequence of the slow rate of their generation. In point of fact, Sawyer *et al.* (1979) and their collaborators have shown that treatment with 5-FUdR is accompanied by an apparently delayed loss of thymidine kinase activity to levels 10% of those seen in untreated tumors. This fall in enzyme activity was accompanied by a parallel fall in the rate of DNA synthesis.

Although thymidine kinase is present in fetal organs at comparatively high specific activities (ranging from 120 nmoles/mg protein/hour in the embryonic rat liver to 58 nmoles/mg protein/hour in the liver of aborted

TABLE IV

Specific Activity of Thymidine Kinase in a Spectrum of Murine Target Tissues

Number	Thymidine kinase	
	10 Weeks old (nmoles/mg protein/hour)	4 Weeks old (nmoles/mg protein/hour)
1. Brain	0.081 ± 0.03	0.911 ± 0.05
2. Heart	0.214 ± 0.10	0.101 ± 0.05
3. Lung	0.152 ± 0.10	0.226 ± 0.05
4. Stomach	0.48 ± 0.22	0.291 ± 0.12
5. Large intestine	0.703 ± 0.20	0.488 ± 0.22
6. Small intestine	4.07 ± 0.36	10.80 ± 0.01
7. Pancreas	0.311 ± 0.05	0.598 ± 0.30
8. Spleen	2.138 ± 1.25	18.85 ± 3.60
9. Liver	3.160 ± 0.45	0.472 ± 0.08
10. Kidney	0.181 ± 0.14	0.158 ± 0.07

human fetuses), the abundance of this enzyme falls dramatically at and following birth to levels less than 1% of those measurable in tissues taken antepartum. Calf thymus, in fact, is one of the few normal organs from which thymidine kinase has been purified so far, and even in this case, its starting specific activity is low (12 nmoles/mg protein/hour). In the interest of completeness, we have determined the distribution of thymidine kinase in a rather thorough survey of the organs of 4- and 12-week-old BDF_1 mice.

Table IV presents the results of our studies of the enzyme. The specific activity of thymidine kinase in most organs is already low in the 4-week-old mouse, but falls to even lower levels with maturation. The sole adult organ with levels of the kinase approximating those of the fetus is small intestine, followed in order by spleen. Since the former organ is well known as being a target for the toxic actions of 5-FU, it is likely that the comparative abundance of thymidine kinase contributes to the adverse effects of the drug. More relevant to the therapeutic use of 5-fluorouracil are levels of thymidine kinase in tumors. However, measurements of such levels are relevant only when a significant fraction of the injected drug is metabolized to 5-fluorouridine, either because of an abundance of thymidine phosphorylase and/or by virtue of the conjoint administration of donors of the deoxyribose moiety, such as thymidine.

Sarcoma 180 in the ascitic form contained the enzyme at the highest native specific activity so far reported: 222 nmoles/mg protein/hour (Lih-Syng Lee *et al.*, 1976), while blasts from patients with acute myeloblastic leukemia exhibited activities around 4.5 nmoles/mg protein/hour (Lih-Syng Lee, 1976), as did most of the Morris hepatomas studied by Sneider *et al.* (1969). In connection with this last study, it is worthwhile stressing that tumoral thymidine kinase was the only enzyme whose activity was invariably elevated over the levels seen in host liver; if this feature is true for human hepatomas, it ought to confer on 5-FU (or, more properly, on 5-FUdR) selective therapeutic advantage in the treatment of hepatic tumors without undue hepatic toxicity. Indeed, intravascular infusions of 5-FU through the hepatic artery are reportedly of palliative value in the treatment of hepatocellular carcinoma.

6. *Ribonucleotide Reductase*

$$\begin{matrix}\text{UMP}\\ \text{or}\\ \text{FUMP}\end{matrix} + \text{ATP-Mg}^{2+} \rightleftharpoons \begin{matrix}\text{dUMP}\\ \text{or}\\ \text{FdUMP}\end{matrix} + \text{ADP-Mg}^{2+}$$

This enzyme catalyzes the conversion of deoxyribonucleotides from ribonucleotides at the level of nucleoside diphosphates. It thus plays an active, if indirect, role in the conversion of FUMP to FdUMP, and serves to direct the anabolism of 5-FU away from its subsequent incorporation into RNA. Hydroxyurea is a powerful inhibitor of ribonucleotide reductase; thus, in theory at least, it should serve to shunt the fluorinated necleotides in the direction of ribonucleotides and hence promote their incorporation into RNA. The preliminary data on the combination studies of 5-FU and hydroxyurea in murine tumor bearing animal models (Lerner *et al.*, 1974) are suggestive of increased antitumor activity from the combination as contrasted with its constituents used singly.

7. *Pyrimidine Monophosphate Kinase*

This phosphorylating enzyme, the first of the so-called "higher kinases," is responsible for the conversion of 5-FUMP to FUDP. At a variably diminished rate, depending on its source, it may accept 5-FdUMP as substrate:

$$\begin{matrix}\text{UMP}\\ \text{or}\\ \text{FUMP}\end{matrix} \xrightleftharpoons{\text{ATP-Mg}^{2+}} \begin{matrix}\text{UDP}\\ \text{or}\\ \text{FUDP}\end{matrix}$$

$$\text{or} \qquad\qquad \text{or}$$

$$\text{FdUMP} \longleftrightarrow \text{FdUMP}$$

Although the specific activity of this kinase is high in many tumors and tissues, such abundance is not universally observed; thus, we have recently shown that the conversion of 5-FUMP to 5-FUDP is dramatically impaired in a subline of the P388 murine leukemic rendered resistant to

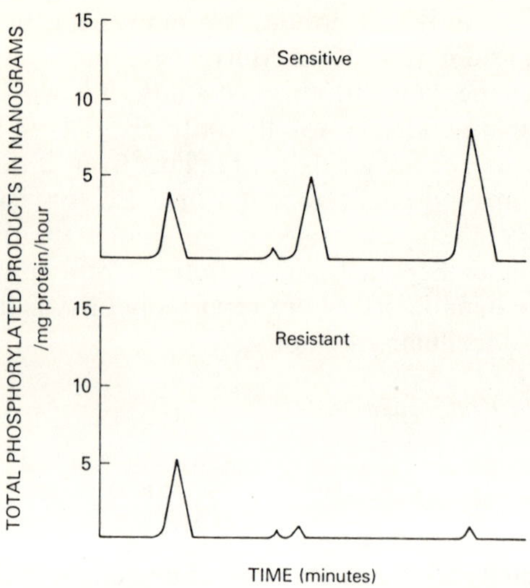

FIG. 3. Formation of nucleoside mono-, di-, and triphosphates from [2-^{14}C]5-FU P388/0 and P388/FU cells *in vitro*. Cell-free extracts from P388/0 and P388/FU were incubated with [2-^{14}C]5-FU and buffer mix, and nucleotides of 5-FU were separated by high-resolution ion-exchange chromatography (Ardalan *et al.*, 1980).

5-FU by repeated subcurative injections of the drug. In this instance, resistance was specifically attributed to the low capacity of the subline to phosphorylate FUMP. This defect is illustrated in Fig. 3, which is a chromatogram of a perchloric acid extract of P388 cells (sensitive and resistant to 5-FU) incubated with radioactive drug for 30 minutes. It can be appreciated that both lines generate equivalent amounts of monophosphate, but that only the sensitive line phosphorylated this nucleotide further.

8. *Pyrimidine Nucleoside Diphosphate Kinase*

This kinase is responsible for the generation of the nucleoside triphosphates of 5-FU; these, in turn, are utilized as substrates by ribonucleotide reductase and RNA polymerases. Despite this dual importance, no subline has so far been shown to be resistant to 5-FU on the basis of absence or depression of pyrimidine nucleoside diphosphate kinase.

$$\begin{array}{ccc} \text{UDP} & & \text{UTP} \\ \text{or} & \xrightarrow[\text{ATP-Mg}^{2+}]{} & \text{or} \\ \text{FUDP} & & \text{FUTP} \\ \text{or} & & \text{or} \\ \text{FdUDP} & \longrightarrow & \text{FdUTP} \end{array}$$

B. Target Enzymes

Two other enzymes, not directly involved either in the anabolism or catabolism of 5-FU, are nevertheless important to its mechanism of action. These are the target enzymes thymidylate synthetase and the RNA polymerases. As was mentioned, the phosphorylated anabolites of 5-FU are substrates for inhibitors of these enzymes. If, through mutation or selection, altered enzyme molecules are synthesized, and if these molecules do not accept the fluorinated pyrimidine nucleotides with the same affinity as the native enzymes did, diminished activity at the molecular level would ensue. In fact, Heidelberger (1973) has shown that a variant of P388 resistant to 5-FU synthesizes a thymidylate synthetase so altered that its affinity for FdUMP is 5-fold lower than that of the parental strain. The effects of 5-FU on DNA synthesis via inhibition of thymidylate synthetase (Danneberg *et al.*, 1958; Bosch *et al.*, 1958; Hartman and Heidelberger, 1961) and its incorporation into RNA (Chaudhuri *et al.*, 1958; Bosch *et al.*, 1958) probably both play a role in the chemotherapeutic activity of the antimetabolite.

Early studies of the effect of 5-FU on total RNA in Ehrlich ascites tumor cells indicated that 5-FU replaced uracil in RNA (Danneberg *et al.*, 1958; Harbers *et al.*, 1959), but did not affect the incorporation of ^{32}P into RNA (Bosch *et al.*, 1958). These results suggested that transcription per se was not inhibited by 5-FU, even though extensive incorporation of the drug occurred. The amount of incorporation of 5-FU into RNA also correlated inversely with the degree of resistance of the Ehrlich ascites tumor to the drug (Heidelberger *et al.*, 1960b). Similar results were observed by Kessel *et al.* (1966) in a wide spectrum of transplanted tumors, by Goldberg *et al.* (1966) in sensitive and resistant variants of L1210 leukemia, and by Wilkinson and Crumley (1977) with wild type and thymidine kinase-deficient Novikoff hepatoma cells. The general correlation between drug sensitivity and incorporation of 5-FU into RNA is predominantly a function of the ability of the tumor cell to anabolize 5-FU to 5-FUTP (Laskin *et al.*, 1979); however, the latter parameter is not necessarily a determinant of tumor responsiveness. As shown by Kessel *et al.* (1969), two variants of P388 leukemia which responded similarly to 5-FU differed 5-fold in their capacity to incorporate 5-FU. Although not yet demonstrated, it is conceivable that an analogous situation could affect one or more of the RNA polymerases which ordinarily accept 5-FUTP as substrate.

C. Catabolic Enzymology

The catabolyzing enzymes fall into two classes: those destroying 5-FU and those destroying its anabolites. The importance of both classes of enzyme resides in their ability to preclude the oncolytic action of the drug by degrading the therapeutic species or its precursors.

1. *The Uracil-Degradative Pathway*

The uracil-degradative pathway consists of a series of enzymes which first reduce the pyrimidine ring, open it, and dismantle the resultant α-fluoro-β-ureidopropionic acid. These operations are carried out at a vigorous rate in the liver and may serve there as a means of preventing the toxicity of 5-FU, especially when the drug has been given orally. However, in most tumors examined, 5-FU is catabolized at a very much slower rate than in the liver. For example, P388 cells generated $[^{14}C]O_2$ from $[5\text{-}^{14}C]$FU at a rate of only 250 fmoles/10^6 cells/hour, irrespective of their sensitivity or resistance to the drug. Such sluggish catabolism would suggest that the uracil degradative route is not the primary mechanism used by tumors to control the intracellular concentration of 5-FU.

2. *Phosphatases*

A simple review of the anabolic steps presented earlier will reconfirm the number of phosphorylated intermediates involved in the metabolism of 5-FU. Each of these phosphorylated intermediates is susceptible to destruction by one or another of the plentiful cytoplasmic acid or alkaline phosphatases, as well as by the more specific 5′ nucleotidases. So plentiful are these phosphohydrolyses, and so broad is their substrate specificity, that attempts to determine which enzyme is principally responsible *in vivo* for the dephosphorylation of FdUMP, as opposed to FUTP, have not met with success. Nevertheless, the conjoint action of this whole family of phosphatases appears to be of cardinal importance to the expression of the antitumor activity by 5-FU. For example, it is not unreasonable to suggest that phosphatases, by controlling the intracellular molarity of FdUMP, determine the extent of inhibition of thymidylate synthetase produced by parenteral doses of the drug. It will be recalled that, although FdUMP binds very tightly to this enzymic target, it dissociates at a finite rate. If phosphatases attack the free species, they will drive the reaction to completion and ultimately free the cytoplasm of FdUMP (Ardalan *et al.*, 1978). In fact, this appears to be the case. Thus, despite *in vitro* kinetic data which would suggest the likelihood of very long lasting inhibition by FdUMP, *in vivo* the duration of this effect is relatively brief. Phosphatases doubtless play a role in this clearance.

Phosphatases have also been invoked to explain the susceptibility of certain tumors (versus their tissues of origin) to 5-FU. Thus, it has recently been demonstrated that extracts of human colonic tumors dephosphorylate FdUMP at a significantly slower rate than extracts of adjacent, normal mucosa. This finding was considered to explain the favorable therapeutic index of 5-FU in the treatment of tumors of the large intestine.

D. Pharmacologic Modulators of the Activity of 5-FU

As complicated as are the physiologic determinants of responsiveness to 5-FU, the pharmacologic determinants are more complicated still. This is so because of the numerous antimetabolites available to the present day chemotherapist. Although this complexity can be bewildering to medical oncologists, it can also contribute substantive therapeutic gains under properly controlled circumstances. For this reason, the area will be treated here in some detail.

Organizationally, these pharmacologic determinants can be grouped into three main categories: (1) those second drugs that interrupt uptake of 5-FU or its metabolites; (2) those agents that alter the anabolisms of 5-FU; and (3) those agents that influence the catabolism of the drug. These three main areas will be considered in turn.

1. *Agents That Impede Uptake of 5-FU and Nucleosides*

Paterson *et al.* (1977, 1979) have reported a number of studies in which nitrobenzylthioinosine has been used to impede the uptake of nucleoside drugs, including ribosides, deoxyribosides, and arabinosides of therapeutically important purines and pyrimidines. While this agent should be without affect on the diffusion-mediated transport of 5-FU itself, it would impede the interiolocation of FUR and FUdR, and might also disturb the rate of efflux of these nucleotides.

2. *Agents Modulating the Anabolism of 5-FU*

a. Agents That Alter the Acquisition of Sugars by 5-FU. In the category of agents that modulate the anabolism of 5-FU by altering the rate at which this fluorinated base acquires a pentose or deoxypentose moiety can be included a number of "natural" and unnatural ribosides: thymidine, uridine, deoxyuridine, and inosine fall into the former category; pyrazofurin into the latter. Of these nucleosides, thymidine has been the principal agent to be used in conjunction with 5-FU (Martin *et al.*, 1977, 1978). Although the actions of thymidine are complex, at least one of its roles is to donate a deoxyribose functionality to 5-FU. Although this donation could be accomplished by a direct transglycosylation:

$$\text{Thymidine} + \text{5-FU} \rightarrow \text{Thymine} + \text{5-FUdR}$$

It is likely that a two step process is operative in most tumors:

(1) Thymidine + Phosphate → Thymine + Deoxyribose 1-Phosphate
(2) Deoxyribose 1-Phosphate + 5-FU → 5-FUdR + Phosphate

Lee *et al.* (1979) have quantitated the generation of these reactions *in vivo* by demonstrating that uridine (5 mg/kg) given 5 minutes before 5-FU (100 mg/kg) increased the concentration of 5-FUR in plasma by 80-fold (from 0.4 to 35 μM); thymidine (2.5 gm/kg) given in like manner increased the concentration of 5-FUdR in plasma by 50-fold (from 0.9 to 33 μM). Such measurements leave little doubt that is is possible to augment the early anabolism of 5-FU to an important degree by the coadministration of sugar donors.

Pharmacologic manipulations can also depress the degree to which 5-FU is glycosylated. Thus, studies in our laboratory have demonstrated that pyrazofurin, an antineoplastic nucleoside in its own right, inhibits the rate at which 5-FU acquires a ribosyl moiety in short-term explant cultures of Leukemia P388. This effect is illustrated in Fig. 4 where it can be seen that prior exposure of these cells to pyrazofurin results in a time-dependent depression in the rate at which 5-FU (added subsequent to pyrazofurin) is converted to 5-FUR. Such dependence on time suggests that pyrazofurin must be metabolized before the effect observed can be produced, or else that some intermediary metabolite must accumulate before inhibition can be expected. This agent will be further discussed later.

b. Agents That Alter the Utilization of PRPP. The second class of pharmacologic agents capable of modulating the anabolism of 5-FU encompasses those drugs that alter the rate and the extent of utilization of phosphoribosylpyriphosphate (PRPP). These agents fall into two classes: those augmenting the concentration of PRPP, of which methotrexate is the example, and those diminishing the availability of PRPP, of which hypoxanthine may be an example. These classes of agents will be considered in turn.

Cadman *et al.* (1979) have demonstrated that pretreatment of L1210 cells with methotrexate results in enhanced intracellular accumulation of 5-FU nucleotides, and that this sequence is synergistic in killing cells as measured by the soft-agar cloning assay. Such pretreatment was also found to augment the pool size of PRPP by factors of up to six, depending on the concentration of antifol used, and it was to such augmentation that these workers attributed the enhanced anabolism of 5-FU. In parallel studies, it was observed that hypoxanthine was capable of blocking the enhanced glycosylation of 5-FU engendered by prior exposure to MTX, and also of diminishing PRPP pools. This effect is almost certainly achieved by the operation of guanine–hypoxanthine phosphoribosyltransferase. Relevant in this connection was the observation of Leyva *et al.* (1979) that MTX decreases the pool size of PRPP in L1210 cells.

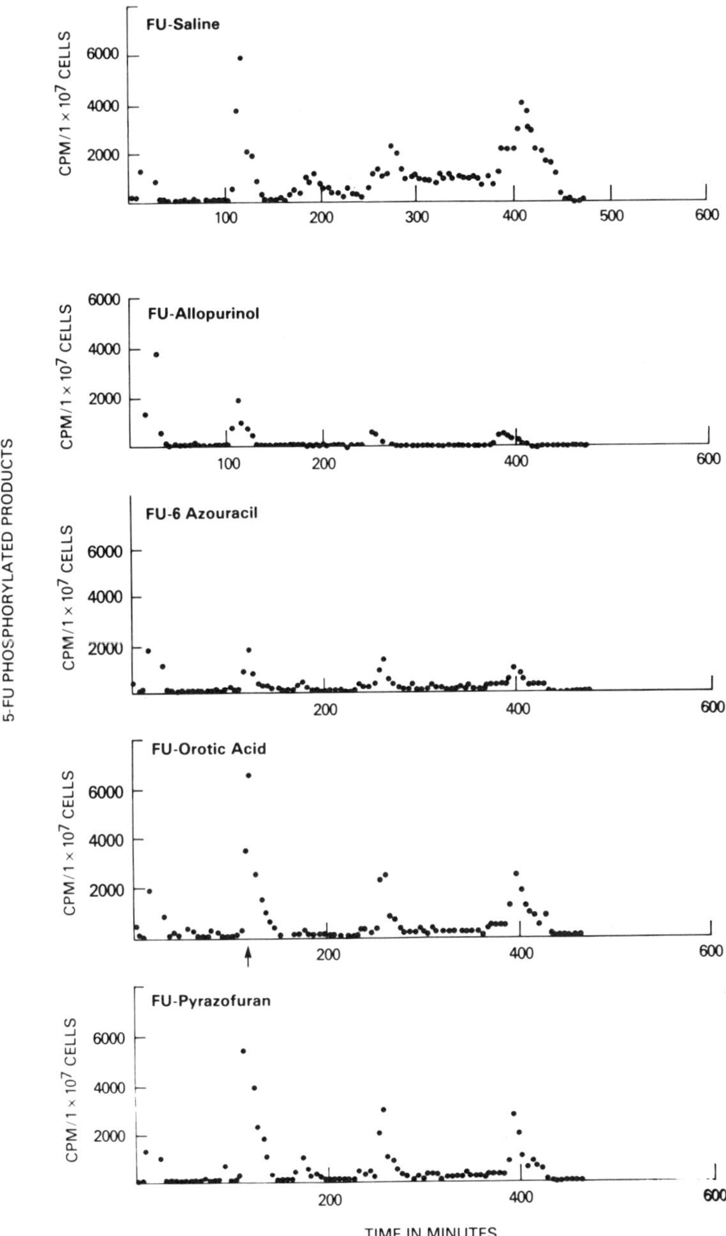

FIG. 4. P388/0 cells were incubated with [2-^{14}C]5-FU for 15 minutes; acid-soluble extract was then loaded on analyzer as before.

c. Inhibitors of Orotidylic Decarboxylase. Three clinically important chemotherapeutic agents are known to be strong inhibitors of orotidylic decarboxylase: they are pyrazofurin, 6-azauracil, and allopurinol. All three of these drugs provoke an accumulation of orotic acid *in vivo;* all three also markedly impair the anabolism of 5-FU. This effect is illustrated in Fig. 4 which demonstrates that 1 hour after exposure to any of the three drugs, phosphorylation of 5-FU is reduced by 80%. It can also be seen that orotic acid and hypoxanthine produce an analogous effect. With briefer exposures, differences in potency emerge: 6-azauracil still curtails the anabolism of 5-FU, whereas pyrazofurin and allopurinol do not. This sensitivity to timing is taken to indicate that the latter two drugs require time-consuming anabolism before they can interact with their target enzyme. Indeed, it is as the 5′-monophosphates that pyrazofurin and allopurinol are thought to interact with OMP-decarboxylase (Schwartz *et al.*, 1979).

Since it is either known or likely that all three of these agents provoke an increase in the intratumoral concentration of orotic acid, it might be supposed that they are acting by lowering the PRPP pools via the reaction:

$$\text{Orotic acid} + \text{PRPP} \rightarrow \text{OMP} + \text{Pyrophosphate.}$$

However, Schwartz and Handschumacher (1979) have demonstrated that this is not so, at least in the case of pyrazofurin and allopurinol; (as was shown earlier, augmentation of hypoxanthine pools can depress PRPP levels; however, the hypoxanthine accumulating after inhibition of xanthine oxidase by allopurinol must not reach the requisite concentration to exert this effect under the conditions used by these workers). Such failure to depress PRPP levels makes it likely that orotic acid is acting at some other site, perhaps at the level of uridine phosphorylase.

d. Agents Promoting the Binding of Fluoropyrimidine Nucleotides to Their Target Enzymes. Only a limited number of studies are available in this area; however, Evans and Hakela (1979) did demonstrate that citrovorum factor at concentration of 300 μM could increase the growth inhibitory potency of 5-FU versus murine and human cells in culture by 400%. This augmented cytotoxicity was correlated with increased inhibition of thymidylate synthetase, and is very likely moderated by a greater saturation of the FH_4 site on the enzyme; this, in turn, probably serves to promote more efficient or tenacious binding of any FdUMP finding its way into the catalytic center.

In this context it is relevant to speculate that at least a part of the synergistic action of methotrexate and 5-FU (given in the proper temporal relationship) may derive from an analogous promotion: namely, promotion of the binding of FdUMP to the active site of its target enzyme.

e. Inhibitors of Ribonucleotide Reductase. As was mentioned earlier, there are two routes by which 5-FU can acquire a deoxyribose moiety via thymidine phosphorylase and via ribonucleotide reductase. By using inhibitors of this latter enzyme, it should be possible to discriminate which of these routes is mainly operative in a given case. In fact, in addition to the *in vivo* schedules cited earlier, Fox *et al.* (1979) and co-workers have utilized hydroxyurea toward this end in their study of 5-FU metabolism by human lymphocytes *in vitro*. In these experiments, hydroxyurea was without substantial influence in the cytotoxicity of 5-FU toward B cells, a finding which was taken to mean that thymidine phosphorylase was largely responsible for the conveyance to the base of a deoxyribose moiety in these cells.

Thymidine, in the form of TTP, is also capable of inhibiting ribonucleotide reductase, thereby restricting intracellular pools of deoxyribonucleotides (Morris *et al.*, 1963; Mathias *et al.*, 1962; Morse *et al.*, 1965; Izutsu *et al.*, 1966; Lee *et al.*, 1977). However, the extent to which thymidine and 5-FU interact at this level has yet to be assessed.

3. *Agents Modulating the Catabolism of 5-FU*

Thymidine, after its phosphorylytic conversion to thymine, is also capable of impeding the catabolism of 5-FU; such inhibition is most likely exerted at the level of the uracil degrative pathway, for which both pyrimidines compete. Chaudhuri *et al.* (1958a) have quantitated the extent of this competition *in vivo* by measuring the rate of appearance of dihydro-5-FU in the plasma of mice given 5-FU along and in conjunction with thymidine. The rate of appearance of reduced pyrimidine was markedly depressed by thymidine in these studies. The clinical trials of combination of 5-FU and thymidine will be discussed later.

III. Clinical Studies

The fluorinated pyrimidines are important drugs in the clinical management of cancer. 5-Fluorouracil, the oldest of these agents, has been shown to be capable of producing palliative effects in 30 to 50% of patients with advanced gastrointestinal, breast, and ovarian adenocarcinomas (Heidelberger, 1974). Since approximately 250,000 cases of breast and gastrointestinal cancer occur in the United States each year (Silverberg, 1977), discussion of useful drugs in these diseases is of obvious importance.

This section will first discuss the appropriate clinical use of the commercially available, single-agent fluorinated pyrimidines; subsequently, initial findings in a series of studies aimed at exploiting biochemical and pharmacologic interactions between fluorinated pyrimidines and other agents in the treatment of cancer will be described.

There are two preparations of fluorinated pyrimidine antineoplastic currently available in the United States. These are 5-fluorouracil (5-FU) and its deoxynucleoside, 5-fluoro-2′-deoxyuridine (FUdR).[3] By far, the largest clinical experience is available with 5-FU. Since it was first used clinically in the late 1950s, there has been substantial debate over the most appropriate way to administer 5-FU. The originally described method of administration was an intravenous (iv) loading dose entailing injection of 15 mg/kg/day for 5 days followed by four half doses every other day (Moertel *et al.*, 1969). However, this schedule was associated with very significant toxicity. Bone marrow depression resulting in clinically apparent thrombocytopenia and leukopenia was observed in more than 70% of patients, and gastrointestinal toxicity including nausea, vomiting, and stomatitis was seen in 50–60% of patients (Moertel *et al.*, 1969; Moertel, 1975).

Other approaches to the administration of 5-FU have included the oral route (Khung *et al.*, 1966; Lahiri *et al.*, 1971; Leone, 1974), the use of lesser doses in iv loading schedules (Moertel, 1975; Carter, 1976), continuous intravenous infusions (Seiffert *et al.*, 1975), and weekly iv infusion (Jacobs *et al.*, 1971).

Oral 5-FU was initially of considerable interest for patients with liver metastases. The assumption was that the drug would be delivered by the portal circulation directly to liver metastases. In early uncontrolled trials of oral 5-FU, dramatic response rates, especially of hepatic metastases, were reported (Khung *et al.*, 1966; Lahiri *et al.*, 1971; Leone, 1974). However, in three controlled trials comparing oral and intravenous 5-FU, a superiority of intravenous administration was shown both in response rate

[3] The second fluorinated pyrimidine available for clinical use in the United States is FUdR. This drug is a deoxynucleoside of 5-FU and was designed with an understanding of the previously described steps in the *in vivo* activation of 5-FU. It was reasoned that the nucleoside form would be easily activated *in vivo* to the active antimetabolite, FdUMP (5-fluorodeoxyuridylate). However, it has been demonstrated that FUdR is rapidly converted to FU *in vivo* (Heidelberger, 1973) thus obviating at least a fraction of theoretical advantage of this nucleoside. FUdR is approved only for intraarterial infusion; since it is significantly more expensive than 5-FU, it would be necessary to demonstrate increased antitumor activity to justify its use in preference to 5-FU. In some animal tumors, FUdR was shown to be superior to 5-FU; however, in human tumors, FUdR has not been demonstrated to have any advantages over 5-FU (Heidelberger, 1973). It is worth noting, however, that FUdR has been used via hepatic artery infusion to treat patients who were exhibiting progressive liver metastases while receiving systemic 5-FU. Buroker *et al.* (1976) reported on 21 such patients. Eight of 21 (38%) showed objective response of liver metastases to intraarterial FUdR therapy. These results would suggest that the question of cross-resistance between 5-FU and FUdR should be further investigated.

and in response duration (Bateman *et al.*, 1975; Hahn *et al.*, 1975; Ansfield *et al.*, 1977). Oral 5-FU was also not superior for the treatment of liver metastases in these trials. This is not a surprising finding since liver metastases have been demonstrated to be dependent upon blood supply via the hepatic artery and not the portal vein (Ackerman *et al.*, 1969; Bierman *et al.*, 1951, 1952). It should also be emphasized that the absorption of 5-fluorouracil from the gastrointestinal tract is inconsistent (Hahn *et al.*, 1975).

The use of prolonged intravenous infusion of 5-FU has been of interest since this method of administration may modify the clinical toxicity of the drug. Lemon (1960) and Moertel *et al.* (1972) presented data demonstrating that prolonged intravenous infusion (usually over 120 hours) of 5-FU allows larger total doses of drug to be given and changes the dose-limiting toxicity from bone marrow suppression to mucositis. Moertel *et al.* (1972) state that infusion of 5-FU, as opposed to iv bolus, increases the total tolerable dose 6-fold. However, the ability to administer larger total doses would have clinical importance only if increased response rates resulted from intravenous infusion of 5-FU. Seifert *et al.* (1975) performed a randomized trial comparing a 5 day "loading course" of 12 mg/kg/day 5-FU with a 96 hour continous infusion of 30 mg/kg/day. The infusion produced more stomatitis but much reduced marrow suppression and, in this study, 44% of patients treated by infusion responded to chemotherapy. The response rate in patients receiving iv bolus therapy was 19%. Seifert *et al.* (1975) state that the difference in response rates was explainable by unequal distribution of patients with different prognostic characteristics between the two treatment groups. Other studies confirmed the advantage of infusion in terms of bone marrow suppression but have failed to support the suggestion of therapeutic advantage (Moertel *et al.*, 1969, 1972).

Although prolonged iv administration of 5-FU is more expensive than iv bolus therapy and offers no clinical benefit when the drug is used as a single agent, it may be useful in combination chemotherapy. The decreased myelosuppression with intravenous infusions of 5-FU permits the drug to be used in combination with potentially bone marrow suppressive drugs. Such studies are now underway.

In an attempt to define the optimal method of administration of 5-FU, the Central Oncology Group (Ansfield *et al.*, 1977) performed a study comparing four commonly used dose schedules. Four hundred and sixty-two patients with advanced, measurable colorectal or breast cancer were randomly allocated to the following 5-FU treatment schedules. Treatment *one* consisted of five intravenous doses of 12 mg/kg/day followed by half doses every other day to toxicity or a total of 11 half doses. Then weekly doses of 15 mg/kg were given. Treatment *two* consisted of weekly intravenous 5-Fu doses of 15 mg/kg. Treatment *three* consisted of 5-FU at 500 mg/day intravenously for 4 days followed by 500 mg weekly. This schedule had previously gained some popularity because of its lack of toxicity. Treatment *four* was orally administered, 5-FU 15 mg/kg/day for 6 days and then 15 mg/kg once weekly. A preliminary analysis showed a statistically superior response rate of 33% in colorectal patients receiving the "loading course" (treatment one) but at the expense of increased toxicity including leukopenia classed as severe or life-threatening in 18%. Survival was also prolonged in patients receiving treatment *one* (projected incremental survival 4–6 months as compared with the other treatment arms), however, this prolongation was marginally significant ($p < 0.09$). The "loading course" response rate of 33% was impressive not only in comparison with the other treatment arms but also in comparison with the accumulated 5-FU experience of other workers. Although this study suggests that the loading dose schedule is superior to other schedules, one must question the advantage of this mode of administration in view of the incidence of severe toxicity, the marginal survival benefit and the inconvenience of the schedule.

Because of the frequency of liver metastases in many adenocarcinomas, there has been much interest in regional chemotherapy of the liver with fluorinated pyrimidines (Ansfield *et al.*, 1971, 1975; Buroker *et al.*, 1976). It was felt that the delivery of high concentrations of drug to hepatic tumors by hepatic arterial infusion would result in superior antitumor response when compared to the intravenous administration of the same drug. 5-Fluourouracil administered by hepatic artery infusion has been extensively studied in Phase II trials (Ansfield *et al.*, 1971, 1975). Ansfield's group has reported response rates of 50–60% with this approach. Burrow (1967) reported slight survival benefit to patients evidencing antitumor response to hepatic infusion. However, it should be emphasized that the percutaneous or surgical placement of hepatic artery catheter may be difficult and patients frequently require hospitalization for 15 to 30 days while the infusion is being carried out. Also, significant complications including hepatic artery thrombosis, hemorrhage, and infection have been reported with this technique (Ansfield *et al.*, (1975). A controlled randomized trial of intravenous versus hepatic arterial administration of 5-FU has been initiated by the Central Oncology Group. The results of this study have not yet been published but will be very helpful in defining the role of 5-FU via hepatic artery perfusion in the clinical management of patients with liver metastases.

As described previously, an understanding of the biochemical pharmacology of the fluorinated pyrimidines has allowed for the design of combinations of these drugs with other agents to produce pharmacologic syner-

TABLE V

SYNERGISTIC DRUG COMBINATIONS OF POTENTIAL CLINICAL IMPORTANCE

Drugs	Reference
5-FU + spironolactone	Waddell (1973)
5-FU + hydroxyurea	Engstrom *et al.* (1978)
5-FU + thymidine	Martin *et al.* (1977, 1978)
5-FU + methotrexate	Cadman *et al.* (1978)
5-FU + PALA	Nayak *et al.* (1978)

gism or antagonism in lower animals. The development of clinical trials combining fluorinated pyrimidines with a number of oncolytic and nononcolytic drug combinations manifesting pharmacologic interactions is at an early stage. However, as illustrated in Table V, there are several combinations that merit clinical trials. The remainder of this article will examine the results of these trials.

One of the earliest attempts to exploit potential pharmacologic synergism in 5-FU-containing regimens was reported by Waddell (1973). This worker reported a series of pancreatic cancer patients treated with weekly iv 5-FU and daily oral testolactone and/or spironolactone. The rationale for this combination was evidence that testolactone inhibited pyrimidine biosynthesis. Van Rymenant *et al.* (1971) demonstrated that testolactone inhibited the activity of L-aspartate transcarbamylase, an enzyme essential for the synthesis of nucleic acid basis. The drug may, therefore, significantly inhibit DNA and RNA synthesis. Since one important mechanism of action of 5-FU is to decrease thymidine synthesis, it was felt that concomitant inhibition of nucleic acid synthesis by testolactone might result in synergistic antitumor activity.

Waddell (1973) reported a total of 13 patients with pancreatic cancer treated with 5-FU + lactones. The survival of these patients was compared to that of matched historical control patients treated with an identical 5-FU regimen without lactones. The median survival in the control group was 5 months, whereas the median survival of the 5-FU + lactones-treated group had not been reached after 21 months of follow-up. This difference was highly significant ($p < 0.001$). Because of this provocative result, the 5-FU + lactone regimen was taken into a prospectively randomized controlled trial by the Eastern Cooperative Oncology Group (ECOG) (Moertel *et al.*, 1977). In this trial, 160 patients with advanced pancreatic cancer were randomized to receive 5-FU alone or 5-FU + spironolactone. Patients in both arms were also randomly allocated to either receive or not receive spironolactone, 50 mg three times per day. The results indicated no benefit from the use of lactones. The median survival of all pancreatic patients was 15 weeks, whether or not lactones had been administered. The results of the ECOG study emphasize the need to test a new chemotherapy regimen rigorously in carefully controlled prospectively randomized trials before conclusions about efficacy are drawn.

A well-designed randomized trial has been completed to test the efficacy of the combination of 5-FU + hydroxyurea. As described previously, hydroxyurea is an inhibitor of the enzyme ribonucleotide reductase. This combination of drugs was reported to have synergistic antitumor activity in an Ehrlich ascites tumor model (Lerner, 1974). The mechanism of this observation has been discussed earlier.

The ECOG has tested the efficacy of 5-FU + hydroxyurea in patients with advanced colon cancer (Engstrom *et al.*, 1978). In an earlier study, patients were randomly allocated to treatment with either 5-FU + hydroxyurea, 5-FU + methyl-CCNU, 5-FU + methyl-CCNU + vincristine, 5-FU + methyl-CCNU + dacarbazine, or 5-FU + methyl-CCNU + dacarbazine + vincristine. Results of this trial revealed 5-FU + hydroxyurea to be the superior treatment. Twenty-one percent of patients treated with this regimen developed an objective partial regression. The response rates of the methyl-CCNU-containing regimens varied from 10 to 15%. Although the superiority of 5-FU + hydroxyurea was not statistically significant, the regimen was well tolerated and had acceptable toxicity. This treatment program is now undergoing further evaluation in a Phase III study by the Veterans Administration Surgical Oncology Group (VASOG). In their study, 5-FU + hydroxyurea will be compared to 5-FU alone in a surgical adjuvant chemotherapy study of patients with resected colon cancer. This protocol has just been activated and disease-free survival data are not yet available.

The use of thymidine and 5-FU in combination chemotherapy has recently stirred considerable interest. Martin *et al.* (1977, 1978) reported augmentation of *in vivo* anticancer activity when 5-FU was given in conjunction with thymidine to tumor-bearing animals. The mechanism of this apparent synergism is not entirely clear but may be related to two major factors. Pharmacokinetic studies (Kirkwood *et al.*, 1978) have demonstrated that 5-FU clearance from plasma is markedly impaired when the drug is given with thymidine. This prolongation of 5-FU plasma levels may be due to competition for pyrimidine degradation enzymes between 5-FU and thymidine (Chaudhuri *et al.*, 1958b). It may also be important that in the presence of thymidine, the qualitative nature of 5-FU-induced cytotoxicity is being changed. Data (Nayak *et al.*, 1978) show that excess thymidine in the form of deoxythymidine triphosphate results in feedback inhibition of the ribonucleotide reductase and pyrimidine kinase enzymes.

This results in a decrease in the conversion of 5-FU to deoxy derivatives and therefore makes it more likely that 5-FU would be anabolized to ribose derivatives and hence be incorporated into RNA. Animal data (Nayak *et al.*, 1978) confirm that 5-FU + thymidine treatment results in increased incorporation of the fluorinated pyrimidine into RNA.

Because of the striking increases in 5-FU efficacy seen in animal systems (Martin *et al.*, 1977, 1978) when the drug is administered with thymidine, clinical trials have been initiated (Kirkwood *et al.*, 1978; Woodcock *et al.*, 1978; Vogel *et al.*, 1979). All of these trials have been Phase I clinical studies to define the toxicity of thymidine + 5-FU combinations in man. In two studies the 5-FU and thymidine were given by continuous infusion (Kirkwood *et al.*, 1978; Vogel *et al.*, 1979). In one study (Woodcock *et al.*, 1978), the thymidine was administered by 30 minute infusion followed by iv bolus 5-FU. The results in all studies were similar. The combination of 5-FU and thymidine markedly increased the myelosuppressive toxicity of 5-FU. Severe toxicity was seen at 5-FU doses of 7.5 mg/kg. Under normal conditions, a single bolus dose of 15 mg/kg 5-FU is tolerated with minimal toxicity. Drug-related deaths secondary to myelosuppression were seen in 1/4 (Kirkwood *et al.*, 1978) and 2/8 patients (Vogel *et al.*, 1978). 5-Fluorouracil plasma levels were studied in two of the Phase I trials. Kirkwood *et al.* (1978) noted that thymidine + 5-FU prolonged the $t_{1/2}$ of 5-FU to 150–400% of the baseline $t_{1/2}$ measured when 5-FU was administered alone. Woodcock *et al.* (1978) demonstrated analogous results. These workers showed that the second phase $t_{1/2}$ of 5-FU was 340 minutes in patients given thymidine in contrast to less than 10 minutes if the same dose of 5-FU was given alone.

The clinical studies described clearly demonstrate that the addition of thymidine to 5-FU changes the pharmacokinetic characteristics of the fluorinated pyrimidine. However, the prolonged plasma drug levels appear to increase toxicity significantly with no clear indication that therapeutic efficacy is also increased. Cautiously performed Phase II trials to assess response will be necessary before the question of the efficacy of this combination can be answered.

As was mentioned earlier, the combination of 5-FU and methotrexate has been investigated in animal systems (Bertino *et al.*, 1977; Cadman *et al.*, 1978). Recently, clinical studies have been proposed and initiated (Freedman *et al.*, 1978, 1979; Tisman and Wu, 1979). The clinical interest in the combination of 5-FU and methotrexate developed from animal and *in vitro* work performed by the group at Yale University (Bertino *et al.*, 1977; Cadman *et al.*, 1978). These workers showed that if 5-FU is given 1 to 2 hours following methotrexate to L1210 mouse leukemia cells (Cadman *et al.*, 1978) or to animals bearing the mouse sarcoma 180 (Bertino *et al.*, 1977), there was an increased cytotoxic effect of the 5-FU. The mechanism of this finding is not entirely clear although there are several possible events that may produce pharmacologic synergism. Cadman *et al.* (1978) have demonstrated that pretreatment with methotrexate markedly increases the intracellular levels of subsequently administered 5-FU in the L1210 system. Cadman and colleagues (1979) also demonstrated that the combination of methotrexate followed by 5-FU resulted in a 6-fold increase in the intracellular concentration of phosphoribosylpyrophosphate (PRPP), a sugar utilized, in part, for the activation of 5-FU to its active cytotoxic nucleotide forms. These workers demonstrated that the increased concentration of PRPP results in markedly elevated levels of 5-FU nucleosides and nucleotides in cells treated with methotrexate followed by 5-FU.

Clinical trials of methotrexate followed by 5-FU have only recently been initiated. This treatment program has been referred to as "methotrexate directed 5-FU." Tisman and Wu (1979) have reported the results of a pilot study in patients with advanced colorectal cancer. These authors used high dose methotrexate (1500 mg/m^2 iv) followed in 1 hour by 5-FU 1500 mg/m^2. Twenty-four hours after the completion of the methotrexate infusion, oral calcium leukovorin "rescue" was initiated. The preliminary report by Tisman and Wu (1979) was quite promising. Of four patients with advanced metastatic colorectal cancer, three objective responses were recorded. A somewhat different schedule of "methotrexate directed 5-FU" has been reported by Friedman *et al.* (1979). These workers treated 12 patients with advanced cancer (11 colon cancer and 1 adrenal cortical carcinoma patients). Although only two partial responses to therapy were observed, all of the responding patients had previously failed to respond to 5-FU therapy.

As is readily apparent, the clinical studies with the combination of methotrexate followed by 5-FU are at an early stage. There are several important questions that must be answered by further trials: (1) is this regimen indeed effective in 5-FU resistant patients? (2) will there be a therapeutic advantage to this program in the more chemotherapeutically sensitive tumors such as breast and ovarian cancer? and finally (3) what is the optimal clinical schedule for these drugs? For example, will relatively low-dose methotrexate also be effective in producing a synergistic effect with 5-FU? The answers to these questions will be awaited with interest.

Another approach to the use of biochemical interaction of 5-FU and other drugs in clinical chemotherapy would be to search for ways in which such interaction could selectively decrease the host toxicity caused by 5-FU but not affect the drug's antitumor activity. Utilizing this approach would allow for escalation of 5-FU dose without increasing patient toxicity. The potential for such an interaction exists between 5-FU and allopurinol. Schwartz and Handschumacher (1979) have demonstrated in cell culture experiments that allopurinol inhibits the cytotoxicity of 5-FU in certain tumor cell lines. These workers demonstrated that this inhibition resulted from decreased production of the active nucleotide 5-fluorodeoxyuridine 5′-phosphate (F-dUMP). Allopurinol was shown to inhibit orotidylate decarboxylase resulting in accumulation of intracellular orotate which competes with 5-FU for conversion to nucleotide forms. The net result is a decrease in intracellular nucleotides of 5-FU and thus decreased cytotoxicity. Schwartz and Handschumacher (1979) observed antagonism between 5-FU and allopurinol in the L5178Y tumor line but not in the Walker 256 sarcoma or HeLa cell lines. It is presumed that the latter two tumors do not have high levels of orotic acid phosphoribosyltransferase decarboxylase but rather activate 5-FU via a uridine phosphorylase–uridine kinase enzyme system not inhibited by allopurinol.

These findings present intriguing possibilities for clinical trials. If orotic acid phosphoribosyltransferase is an enzyme of central importance to the activation of 5-FU in normal tissues, it should be possible to decrease the drug's toxicity by treating patients with allopurinol. It also should be possible to evaluate human tumor samples *in vitro* for 5-FU–allopurinol antagonism. Thus, one could select patients with tumors analogous to the Walker 256 sarcoma and HeLA lines which are not sensitive to 5-FU–allopurinal pharmacologic antagonism. Patients with such tumors could be treated with allopurinol and escalating doses of 5-FU in an attempt to increase the therapeutic index of this drug while decreasing patient toxicity. Such Phase I–II trials are under consideration at present.

A recently developed drug, *N*-(phosphonacetyl)-L-aspartate (PALA), (Johnson *et al.*, 1977, 1978) would appear to be another excellent candidate for combination with the fluorinated pyrimidines. This drug is an inhibitor of L-aspartic acid transcarbamylase (ATCase), the second enzyme in the *de novo* pyrimidine synthesic pathway. 5-FU blocks DNA synthesis through inhibition of thymidylate synthetase, and its combinations with PALA could result in synergistic cytotoxicity since the synthesis of pyrimidine bases would be inhibited at two points. It should be noted that PALA interacts with the same enzyme, ATCase, that lactones do. This interaction was the basis of the clinical trials of lactones + 5-FU reported by Waddell (1973) and Moertel *et al.* (1977).

PALA has undergone Phase I trials (Ehrlichman *et al.*, 1979; Ervin *et al.*, 1979) and early Phase II trials (Gralla *et al.*, 1979). The Phase I trials showed similar results. The dose-limiting toxicity of PALA is gastrointestinal with diarrhea being most marked. Mucositis and dermatitis also occur in up to 50% of patients. Of particular relevance to planning the use of PALA in a combination chemotherapy program is the finding that the drug did not produce myelosuppression. The results of large Phase II trials with PALA are not yet available; however, in one preliminary report (Gralla *et al.,* 1979), minor responses were seen in 3/21 patients with non-oat cell lung cancer and 2/20 patients with bladder carcinoma.

No clinical trials of PALA + 5-FU have been completed. However, there are animal data to suggest that the combination of these two drugs does alter the mechanism of antitumor activity of 5-FU (Nayak *et al.*, 1978). These workers showed that, in the mouse mammary cancer model, the addition of PALA to 5-FU results in markedly increased incorporation of the fluorinated pyrimidine into nuclear RNA. This correlated with significantly increased antitumor effect. These animal data are encouraging, and the results of clinical trials of 5-FU + PALA are awaited with interest.

IV. Summary and Prospects

It can be appreciated from the preceding discourse that physiological, i.e., biochemical, resistance to 5-FU can occur by mutations at any one of a plenitude of loci: those catalyzing acquisition of a sugar, of a sugar phosphate, or of one or more phosphate esters, as well as the level of the target enzyme(s), and one or more of the catabolic enzymes. This complexity is exemplified by thymidine which acts to promote the cytotoxicity of FU by donating a deoxyribose moiety impeding catabolism, but also impeding the anabolism of 5-FU by inhibiting ribonucleotide reductase (as TTP) and depressing the available pools of PRPP (via hypoxanthine). Such antagonistic actions can promote or depress the cytotoxicity of 5-FU depending on the basic enzymologic equipment of the tumor under study. One unifying system appears to emerge: any agent that provokes a marked rise in the pool-size of orotic acid is apt to impair the activity of 5-FU. As the practice of polypharmacy continues, it is likely that further such generalizations will be appreciated.

References

Ackerman, N. B., Lien, W. M., Kondi, E. S., and Silverman, N. A. (1969). *Surgery* **66,** 1067–1072.

Ansfield, F. J., Ramirez, G., Skibba, J. L., Bryan, G. T., Davis, H. L., and Wirtanen, G. W. (1971). *Cancer* **28,** 1147–1151.

Ansfield, F. J., Ramirez, G., Davis, H. L., Wirtanen, G. W., Johnson, R. O., Bryan, G. T., Manalo, F. B., Borden, E. C., Davis, T. G., and Esmaili, M. (1975). *Cancer* **36,** 2413–2417.

Ansfield, R., Klotz, J., Nealon, T., Ramirez, G., Minton, J., Hill, G., Wilson, W., Davis, H., and Cornell, G. (1977). *Cancer* **39,** 34–40.

Ardalan, B., Buscaglia, M. D., and Schein, P. S. (1977). *Biochem. Pharmacol.* **27,** 2009–2013.

Ardalan, B., Cooney, D. A., Lippman, M., Macdonald, J. S., and Schein, P. S. (1978). *Bull. Cancer (Paris)* (in press).

Ardalan, B., Cooney, D. A., Jayaram, N. H., Carrico, C. K., Glazer, R. I., Macdonald, J., and Schein, P. S. (1980). *Cancer Res.* **40,** 1431–1437.

Bateman, J., Irwin, L., Pugh, R., *et al.* (1975). *Proc. Am. Assoc. Cancer Res.* **16,** 242.

Bertino, J. R., Sawicki, W. L., Lindquist, C. A., and Gupta, V. A. (1977). *Cancer Res.* **37,** 327–334.

Bierman, H. R., Byron, R. L., Kelley, K. H., and Grady, A. (1951–1952). *J. Natl. Cancer Inst.* **12,** 107.

Bosch, L., Harbers, E., and Heidelberger, C. (1958). *Cancer Res.* **18,** 335–343.

Brent, T. P. (1977). *Cell Tissue Kinet.* **4,** 297.

Bresnick, E. (1971). *Methods Cancer Res.* **6,** 347.

Bresnick, E., and Thompson, V. B. (1965). *J. Biol. Chem.* **240,** 3967.

Bresnick, E., and Mainigi, K. D., Buccino, R., and Burleson, S. S. (1970). *Cancer Res.* **30,** 2506.

Bukovsky, J., and Roth, J. S. (1965). *Cancer Res.* **25,** 358.

Buroker, T., Samson, M., Correa, J., Fraile, R., and Vaitkevicius, V. K. (1976). *Cancer Treat. Rep.* **60,** 1277–1279.

Burrow, J. H., Talley, R. W., and Drake, E. H. (1967). *Cancer* **20,** 1886–1892.

Cadman, E., Davis, L., and Heimer, R. (1978). *Proc. Am. Assoc. Cancer Res. Am. Soc. Clin. Oncol.* **19,** 211.

Cadman, E., Benz, C., and Heiner, R. (1979). *Proc. Am. Assoc. Cancer Res.* **20,** 258.

Carter, S. K. (1976). *J. Natl. Cancer Inst.* **56,** 3–10.

Chaudhuri, N. K., Montag, B. J., and Heidelberger, C. (1958a). *Cancer Res.* **18,** 318–328.

Chaudhuri, N. K., Mukherjee, K. L., and Heidelberger, C. (1958b). *Biochem. Pharmacol.* **1,** 328–341.

Danneberg, P. B., Montag, B. J., and Heidelberger, C. (1958). *Cancer Res.* **18,** 329–334.

Ehrlichman, C., Strong, J., Wiernik, P., Edwards, L., Cohen, M., Levine, A., Hubbard, S., and Chabner, B. (1979). *Proc. Am. Assoc. Cancer Res. Am. Soc. Clin. Oncol.* **20,** 314.

Engstrom, P., MacIntyre, J., Douglass, H., and Carbone, P. (1978). *Proc. Am. Assoc. Cancer Res. Am. Soc. Clin. Oncol.* **19,** 384.

Ervin, T. J., Blum, R. H., and Canellos, G. P. (1979). *Proc. Am. Assoc. Cancer Res. Am. Soc. Clin. Oncol.* **20,** 200.

Evans, R. M., and Hakela, M. T. (1979). *Proc. Am. Assoc. Cancer Res.* **623.**

Fox, R. M., Piddington, S. K., and Pioer, A. A. (1979). *Proc. Am. Assoc Cancer Res.* **20,** 262.

Friedman, M. A., and Sadel, W. (1978). *Cancer Chemother. Pharmacol.* **1,** 77–82.

Friedman, M. A., Ignoffo, R. J., Resser, K. J., and Carter, S. K. (1979). *Proc. Am. Assoc. Cancer Res. Am. Soc. Clin. Oncol.* **20,** 24.

Goldberg, A. R., Macheldt, J. H., Jr., and Pardee, A. B. (1966). *Cancer Res.* **26,** 1611–1615.

Greenberg, G. R. (1956). *J. Biol. Chem.* **219,** 423.

Gralla, R. J., Casper, E. S., Golbey, R. B., and Young, C. W. (1979). *Proc. Am. Assoc. Cancer Res. Am. Soc. Clin. Oncol.* **20,** 115.

Hahn, R. G., Moertel, C. G., Schutt, A. J., and Bruckner, H. W. (1975). *Cancer* **35,** 1031–1035.

Harbers, E., Chaudhuri, N. K., and Heidelberger, C. (1959). *J. Biol. Chem.* **234,** 1255–1262.

Hartman, K. V., and Heidelberger, C. (1961). *J. Biol. Chem.* **236,** 3006–3013.

Hashimoto, T., Arima, T., Okuda, H., and Fujii, S. (1972). *Cancer Res.* **32,** 67.

Heidelberger, C. (1973). *In* "Cancer Medicine" (J. F. Holland and E. Frei, III, eds.), pp. 768–791. Lea & Febiger, Philadelphia.

Heidelberger, C. (1974). *In* "Antineoplastic and Immunosuppressive Agents. Handbook of Experimental Pharmacology" (A. C. Sartorelli and D. G. Johns, eds.), Vol. 38, pp. 193–231. Springer-Verlag, Berlin and New York.

Heidelberger, C., Ghobar, A., Baker, R. K., and Mukherjee, K. L. (1960a). *Cancer Res.* **20,** 897–902.

Heidelberger, C., Kaldor, G., Murkherjee, K. L., and Danneberg, P. B. (1960b). *Cancer Res.* **20,** 903–909.

Izutsu, K., and Bieselle, J. J. (1966). *Cancer Res.* **26,** 910–928.

Jacobs, E. M., Reeves, W. J., Wood, D. A., Pugh, R., Braunwald, J., and Bateman, J. R. (1971). *Cancer* **27,** 1302–1305.

Johnson, R. K. (1977). *Biochem. Pharmacol.* **26,** 81–84.

Johnson, R. K., Swyryd, E. A., and Stark, G. R. (1978). *Cancer Res.* **38,** 371–378.

Kara, J., and Weil, R. (1967). *Proc. Natl. Acad. Sci. U.S.A.* **57,** 63.

Kessel, D., Hall, T. C., and Reyes, P. (1965). *Mol. Pharmacol.* **5,** 481–486.

Kessel, D., Hall, T. C., and Wodinsky, I. (1966). *Science* **154,** 911–913.

Khung, C. L., Hall, T. C., Piro, A. J., and Dederick, M. M. (1966). *Clin. Pharmacol. Ther.* **7,** 527–533.

Kirkwood, J. M., and Frei, E., III. (1978). *Proc. Am. Assoc. Cancer Res. Am. Soc. Clin. Oncol.* **19,** 159.

Kit, S., Dubbs, D. R., and Frearson, P. M. (1966). *Cancer Res.* **26,** 638.

Klemperer, H. G., and Haynes, G. R. (1968). *Biochem. J.* **108,** 541.

Kraut, A., Rose, R., and Yamada, E. W. Unpublished data.

Lahiri, S. R., Boileau, G., and Hall, T. C. (1971). *Cancer* **28,** 902–906.

Lee, L.-S., and Cheng, Y.-C. (1976). *J. Biol. Chem.* **251,** 2600.

Lee, S. S., Giovanella, B. C., and Stehlin, J. S. (1977). *J. Cell Physiol.* **92,** 401–405.

Lemon, H. M. (1960). *Cancer Chemother. Rep.* **8,** 97–101.

Leone, L. A. (1974). *Cancer* **34,** 972–976.

Lerner, H. J. (1974). *Proc. Am. Assoc. Cancer Res. Am. Soc. Clin. Oncol.* **15,** 258.

Leyva, A., Weiss, R., Schornagel, J. H., and Pinedo, H. M. (1979). *Proc. Am. Assoc. Cancer Res.* **20,** 250.

McAuslan, B. R. (1963). *Virology* **20,** 162.

Martin, D., and Stolfi, R. L. (1977). *Proc. Am. Assoc. Cancer Res. Am. Soc. Clin. Oncol.* **18,** 126.

Martin, D., Stolfi, R. L., and Spiegelman, S. (1978). *Proc. Am. Assoc. Cancer Res. Am. Soc. Clin. Oncol.* **18,** 221.

Mathias, A. P., and Fischer, G. A. (1962). *Biochem. Pharmacol.* **11,** 57–58.

Moertel, C. G. (1975). *Cancer* **36,** 675–682.

Moertel, C. G., and Lavin, P. T. (1977). *Proc. Am. Assoc. Cancer Res. Am. Soc. Clin. Oncol.* **18,** 344.

Moertel, C. G., Reitemeier, R. J., and Hahn, R. G. (1969). *In* "Advanced Gastrointestinal Cancer" C. G. Moertel and R. J. Reitemeier, eds.), pp. 86–107. Koeber, New York.

Moertel, C. G., Schutt, A. J., Reitemeier, R. J., and Hahn, R. G. (1972). *Cancer Res.* **32,** 2717–2719.

Morris, N. R., Reichard, P., and Fischer, G. A. (1963). *Biochem. Biophys Acta* **68,** 93–99.

Morse, P. A., and Potter, V. R. (1965). *Cancer Res.* **25,** 499–507.

Nayak, R., Martin, D., Stolfi, R., Furth, J., and Spiegelman, S. (1978). *Proc. Am. Assoc. Cancer Res. Am. Soc. Clin. Oncol.* **19,** 63.

Ohnuma, T., Arkin, H., Minowada, J., and Holland J. F. (1978). *J. Natl. Cancer Inst.* **60,** 749.

Okazaki, R., and Kornberg, A. (1964). *J. Biol. Chem.* **239,** 275.

Paterson, A. R. P., Babb, L. R., Paran, J. H., and Cass, C. E. (1977). *Mol. Pharmacol.* **13,** 1147.
Paterson, A. R. P., Paran, J. H., Yang, S., and Lynch, T. P. (1979). *Cancer Res.* **39,** 3607.
Pauly, J. L., Schuller, M. G., Zelcer, A. A., Kirss, T. A., Gore, S. S., and Germain, M. J. (1977). *J. Natl. Cancer Inst.* **58,** 1587–1590.
Pauly, J., Paolini, N. S., Ebrab, R. L., and Germain, M. J. (1978). *Proc. Soc. Exp. Biol. Med.* **157,** 262.
Reichard, P., Sköld, O., and Klein, G. (1959). *Nature (London)* **183,** 939.
Reichard, P., Sköld, O., Klein, G., and Revesz, L. (1962). *Cancer Res.* **22,** 235.
Reyes, P., and Guganik, M. E. (1975). *J. Biol. Chem.* **250,** 5097.
Salser, J. S., and Balis, M. E. (1979). *Prom. Am. Assoc. Cancer Res.* **20,** 127.
Sawyer, R., Nayak, R., Spiegelman, S., and Martini, D. (1979). *Proc. Am. Assoc. Cancer Res.* **20,** 263.
Schwartz, P. M., and Handschumacher, R. E. (1979). *Cancer Res.* **39,** 3095–3101.
Seifert, P., Baker, L. H., Reed, M. L., and Vaitkevicius, V. K. (1975). *Cancer* **36,** 123–128.
Sheinin, R. (1966). *Virology* **28,** 47.
Silverberg, E. (1977). *Cancer* **27,** 26–41.
Sköld, O., Magnusson, P. H., and Revesz, L. (1962). *Cancer Res.* **22,** 407.
Sneider, T. W., Potter, V. R., and Morris, H. P. (1969). *Cancer Res.* **29,** 40.
Taylor, A. T., Stafford, M. A., and Jones, O. W. (1972). *J. Biol. Chem.* **247,** 1930.
Tisman, G., and Wu, S. J. G. (1979). *Clin. Res.* **27,** 54A.
Van Rymenant, M., Keymolen, P., Procheret, J., DeSchutter, A., and Kram, R. (1971). *Acta Endocrinol. (Copenhagen)* **66,** 498–507.
Vogel, S. J., Presant, E. A., Ratkin, G. A., and Klahr, C. (1979). *Cancer Treat. Rep.* **63,** 1–5.
Waddell, W. R. (1973). *Surgery* **74,** 420–429.
Wilkinson, D. S., and Crumley, J. (1977). *J. Biol. Chem.* **252,** 1051–1056.
Woodcock, T. M., Martin, D. S., Kemeng, N., and Young, C. (1978). *Proc. Am. Assoc. Cancer Res. Am. Soc. Clin. Oncol.* **19,** 351.
Zimmerman, M., and Seidenberg, J. (1964). *J. Biol. Chem.* **239,** 2618.

Index

D

E

F

G

H

R

S

T

V

X